Ego Mechanisms of Defense:
A Guide for Clinicians
and Researchers

Ego Mechanisms of Defense: A Guide for Clinicians and Researchers

By

George E. Vaillant, M.D.

Raymond Sobel Professor of Psychiatry
Dartmouth Medical School
Hanover, New Hampshire;
Director, Study of Adult Development
Harvard University Health Services
Cambridge, Massachusetts

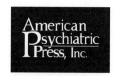

Washington, DC
London, England

Copyright © 1992 American Psychiatric Press, Inc.
ALL RIGHTS RESERVED
Manufactured in the United States of America on acid-free paper.
94 93 92 91 4 3 2 1
First Edition

American Psychiatric Press, Inc.
1400 K Street, N.W., Washington, DC 20005

Library of Congress Cataloging-in-Publication Data
Vaillant, George E., 1934–
  Ego mechanisms of defense : a guide for clinicians and researchers / by George E. Vaillant. — 1st ed.
    p. cm.
  Outgrowth from the 1985 Annual Meeting of the American Psychiatric Association held in Dallas.
  Includes bibliographical references and index.
  ISBN 0-88048-404-7 (alk. paper)
  1. Defense mechanisms (Psychology)—Congresses. I. American Psychiatric Association. Meeting (138th : 1985 : Dallas, Tex.) II. Title.
  [DNLM: 1. Defense Mechanisms—congresses. 2. Psychotherapy—congresses. WM 193 V131e 1985]
RC455.4.D43V35 1992
616.89—dc20
DNLM/DLC   91-33137
for Library of Congress   CIP

British Library Cataloguing in Publication Data
A CIP record is available from the British Library.

This book is dedicated to Caroline Officer Vaillant, whose companionship at home and at work for 20 years has made its creation possible.

Contents

Appendixes: Seven Assessment Schemes
for Defense Mechanisms

Contributors

William Beardslee, M.D.
Associate Professor of Psychiatry
Harvard Medical School and Children's Hospital
Boston, Massachusetts

Michael Bond, M.D.
Associate Professor of Psychiatry, McGill University;
Director of Education and Residency Training
Sir Mortimer B. Davis Jewish General Hospital
Montreal, Canada

Steven Cooper, Ph.D.
Assisant Professor of Psychology in Psychiatry
Beth Israel Hospital
Boston, Massachusetts

Elizabeth Gelfand, Ed.D.
Research Associate in Psychiatry
Massachusetts Mental Health Center
Harvard Medical School
Boston, Massachusetts

Stuart T. Hauser, M.D., Ph.D.
Professor of Psychiatry
Massachusetts Mental Health Center
Harvard Medical School
Boston, Massachusetts

Alan M. Jacobson, M.D.
Director, Mental Health Unit
Joslin Diabetes Center;
Associate Professor of Psychiatry
Harvard Medical School
Boston, Massachusetts

Kimberly A. Lee, A.B.
Research Assistant
Dartmouth Medical School
Hanover, New Hampshire

Leigh McCullough, Ph.D.
Assistant Professor of Psychology in Psychiatry
University of Pennsylvania Medical School
Philadelphia, Pennsylvania

Gil G. Noam, Dipl.Psych.
Assistant Professor of Psychology
Harvard Medical School;
Director, Hall-Mercer Laboratory of Developmental Psychology
   and Developmental Psychopathology
McLean Hospital
Belmont, Massachusetts

J. Christopher Perry, M.D., M.P.H.
Associate Professor of Psychiatry
Cambridge Hospital
Harvard Medical School
Cambridge, Massachusetts

Sally I. Powers, Ed.D.
Associate Professor of Psychology
University of Massachusetts
Amherst, Massachusetts;
Instructor in Psychiatry
Harvard Medical School
Cambridge, Massachusetts

Diane Roston, M.D.
Lecturer
Dartmouth Medical School
Hanover, New Hampshire

Caroline O. Vaillant, M.S.S.W.
Research Associate
Dartmouth Medical School
Hanover, New Hampshire

George E. Vaillant, M.D.
Raymond Sobel Professor of Psychiatry
Dartmouth Medical School
Hanover, New Hampshire;
Director, Study of Adult Development
Harvard University Health Services
Cambridge, Massachusetts

Preface

This book began as a symposium at the American Psychiatric Association (APA) annual meeting in Dallas in 1985. At that time, Stuart T. Hauser, J. Christopher Perry, Leigh McCullough, Michael Bond, and I each presented a paper on the empirical assessment of defenses. In 1986, these five papers were published by the American Psychiatric Press, Inc. (APPI) as a Clinical Insights monograph that was edited by me. Their general context can be found in Chapters 7 to 11 of this book. In 1989, Timothy Clancy of APPI asked me if I would be willing to expand the monograph into a full-length book on the subject of ego defenses. This I have done, but the result has been to create a hybrid; this book is half a single-authored book and half an edited volume. I acknowledge my debt to the *International Review of Psychoanalysis,* to the *Journal of Psychotherapy Practice and Research,* and to the *Archives of General Psychiatry* for permission to publish Chapters 1, 4, and 11, respectively.

The book has three main goals. First, it tries to remind clinical psychiatry that full appreciation of defense mechanisms is integral to diagnosis, case formulation, and treatment. Paying attention to defense mechanisms will bring psychiatry closer to, not further from, the rest of modern medicine. The second intent of the book is to help psychiatry move toward the common language for defenses; this process was begun in DSM-III-R. Third, the book tries to lay a foundation for and offer an impetus to future empirical research in defense mechanisms.

The book's multiple authorship extends beyond the acknowledged coauthors. As should be clear from Chapters 1 and 2, the ideas and theoretical basis for this book owe much to Sigmund Freud and Anna Freud, and to Elvin Semrad. The empirical underpinnings for this book would not have been possible without the selfless patience of the members of the Harvard Grant Study of Adult Development, the Gluecks' study of inner city youth, and the Terman study of gifted women. The book also owes much to the many dedicated individuals—especially Clark Heath, Sheldon and Eleanor Glueck, and Lewis Terman—who created these studies and maintained them for a lifetime. Albert Hastorf and Eleanor Walker at the Terman study at Stanford deserve special thanks for making the Terman archives available to myself and Caroline Vaillant. There have also been many recent co-workers in my own continuation of the Study of Adult Development. Some of them are included as authors of Chapters 6, 9, and 12. Other co-workers to whom I owe much are Sylvia Singh, Phyllis Remalador, Eva Milofsky, Sara Koury, Tara Mitchell, and Sally Allen. These research associates have allowed my own work on the defenses to bear fruit. Throughout the preparation of this book, Mardi Horowitz and Bram Fridhandler and their colleagues at the Program on Conscious and Unconscious Mental Processes of the John D. and Catherine T. MacArthur Foundation have been a sustaining source of intellectual stimulation.

As the editor of this book I have opted not to strive for consensus. Each of the authors of the empirical chapters (7 through 12) introduces defenses in a slightly different manner. Similarly, each of the seven appendixes defines defenses a little differently. My hope is that these differences in points of view will facilitate fresh thought and synthesis in the next generation of empirical research on the defenses. If there were clear answers regarding the study of defenses, this book would not be necessary.

As the editor of this book I must also acknowledge two final debts. First, Tara Mitchell patiently and flawlessly typed and retyped the entire manuscript. Second, the National Institutes of Mental Health and Aging have supported the preparation of this book and much of its underlying research through Grants K05-MH0364 and MH42248, respectively.

Section I: Clinical Applications

Chapter 1

The Historical Origins of Sigmund Freud's Concept of the Mechanisms of Defense

George E. Vaillant, M.D.

erhaps Freud's most original contribution to human psychology was his inductive postulation that unconscious "defense mechanisms" protect the individual from painful emotions, ideas, and drives. In delineating the nature of ego mechanisms of defense, Freud not only established that upsetting affects, as well as ideas, underlie psychopathology, but he also established that much of what is perceived as psychopathology reflects a potentially healing process. Today, no mental status or clinical formulation should be considered complete without an effort to identify the patient's dominant defense mechanism.

During Freud's lifetime, his readers became increasingly impressed with his discoveries of dream interpretation, of childhood sexuality, of the psychoanalytic method, and of the profound effect of unconscious conflict and "phantasy." In contrast, both Freud and his readers, with the exception of his daughter, tended to ignore the importance of his elucidation of defense mechanisms. Even after Freud's death, both Fenichel (1945) and Jones (1953–1957) paid relatively scant attention to the importance of Freud's discovery of a spectrum of defense mechanisms. Indeed, psychoanalysts from Freud on have had an ambivalent attitude toward the defenses. On the one hand, there seem to be discrete defense mechanisms, and these mechanisms can be understood both as building blocks of psychopathology and as potential stepping-stones of ego development. On the other hand, defenses are elusive: the more closely you look at them, the harder they

This chapter is reprinted with permission from Vaillant GE: "The Historical Origins and Future Potential of Sigmund Freud's Concept of the Mechanism of Defence." *International Review of Psycho-analysis,* Vol. 19, Part 1, 1992. Copyright © 1992, Institute of Psycho-Analysis.

become to study and to verify. Thus, over the years many writers, including Wallerstein (1983), Van der Leeuw (1971), and especially Brenner (1976, 1981), have pointed out difficulties with the concept of defense mechanisms. But clear conceptualization of a variety of relatively discrete defense mechanisms is critical if we are to appreciate the hierarchical development of the ego and its function. Also, only as we differentiate defensive processes in a disciplined fashion can we gain full understanding of our patients' symptoms.

Because I believe that psychiatry has more to gain than to lose from retaining the concept of differentiated defense mechanisms, this introductory chapter will chart Freud's discovery of 17 distinct defenses and his tentative effort to arrange them in a developmental hierarchy. My hope is that such review of the past will make future progress possible. But besides documenting Freud's discovery of a variety of defense mechanisms, my purpose in this chapter is to direct attention in two fresh directions. First, previous writers have not sufficiently stressed the importance of differentiating individual defenses from one another. Yet it is no coincidence that Freud's decision in 1926 to redifferentiate ego mechanisms of defense from nonspecific terms like "repression" (circa 1915) and "countercathexis" occurred simultaneously with the birth of ego psychology. Second, sometimes psychiatry has been reluctant to view defenses as adaptive as well as pathological. This difficulty has slowed our understanding of the maturation of ego mechanisms of defense.

Freud's Discovery of the Concept of Defense

That emotions were significant to man had been known since ancient times, but our understanding of unconscious mechanisms of defense originated with Freud. Neither Aristotle nor Hippocrates, neither Schopenhauer nor Shakespeare, neither Montaigne nor Janet had anticipated Freud in recognizing even such simple psychological mechanisms as those of isolation and projection. Over a period of 40 years, Freud discovered most of the defense mechanisms that we speak of today and identified five of their important properties:

1. Defenses are a major means of managing instinct and affect.
2. They are unconscious.
3. They are discrete (from one another).
4. Although often the hallmarks of major psychiatric syndromes, defenses are dynamic and reversible.
5. They can be adaptive as well as pathological.

These properties of defenses continue to be rediscovered by every new student of psychiatry.

It was difficult to develop a concept of defense, however, until psychology could imagine that cortical ideas gain color, temperature, and importance from limbic affect. For example, in their influential textbooks the two greatest psychologists of the 19th century, Wilhelm Wundt (1894) and William James (1890), persisted in discussing a psychology that consisted of only cognition, not emotion. Psychology needed to replace neutral terms like intellect, will, moral sentiment, higher feelings, and cognition for terms suffused with affect (e.g., sadness, lust, rage, and guilty fantasy). From the beginning, Freud's work effected this change. In 1894 Freud observed that not only could affect be "dislocated or transposed" from ideas (by the mechanisms that Freud would later call *dissociation, repression,* and *isolation*), but it could be "reattached" to other ideas (i.e., by displacement). He wrote that

> between the patient's effort of will, which succeeds in repressing the unacceptable sexual idea, and the emergence of the obsessional idea, which, though having little intensity in itself, is now supplied with an incomprehensibly strong affect, yawns the gap which the theory here developed seeks to fill. The separation of the sexual idea from its affect and the attachment of the latter to another, suitable but not incompatible idea—these are processes which occur without consciousness. (Freud 1894, p. 53)

Freud's contribution, then, went far beyond merely probing the unconscious. He drew the attention of psychology to "incomprehensibly strong affect" without the understanding of which there can be no understanding of psychopathology. But perhaps precisely because defenses manage such affectively charged processes, the "regulatory" mechanisms discovered by Freud were often, and still are often, lost to view (i.e., repressed or disavowed). For example, Sherrington and Pavlov had also observed and defined "unconscious" psychological mechanisms. From the very beginning, their students had given their full attention to these postulated unconscious mechanisms—for they did not deal with feelings, only reflexes. In contrast, Freud and those after him repeatedly "forgot" differentiated defense mechanisms.

Indeed, Freud even encountered difficulty himself believing that defenses were wholly unconscious. For example, *vergessen wollen* (to wish to forget) was implicit in his early formulation of repression. It was difficult for any 19th-century man to conceive how someone could perform maneuvers as ingenious, and as convenient, as the deployment of ego defenses without assistance from consciousness.

Although Strachey disagrees, I interpret Freud's first use of the term "repressed" (*verdrängt*) as implying conscious process: Freud wrote that "it was a question of things which the patient wished to forget, and therefore intentionally repressed [*absichtlicht verdrängt*] from his conscious thought and inhibited and suppressed" (Breuer and Freud 1893, p. 10). Three years later, however, Freud (1896b) wrote that the symptoms of a variety of neuroses "arose through the psychical mechanism of (unconscious) *defence*—that is, in an attempt to repress an incompatible idea which had come into distressing opposition to the patient's ego" (p. 162).

Early in his career, Freud (1896a) suggested that "there is a normal trend towards defence—that is, an aversion to directing psychical energy in such a way that unpleasure results" (p. 221). Nevertheless, Freud could not always believe that the distortions created by defenses could serve healthy adaptation. For example, he wrote that "defensive processes are the psychical correlative of the flight reflex and perform the task of preventing the generation of unpleasure from internal sources. In fulfilling this task they serve mental events as an automatic regulation, which in the end, incidentally, turns out to be detrimental . . . " (Freud 1905b, p. 233). Freud, however, was focusing his scientific attention toward the etiology of symptoms rather than toward normal character, and thus he concentrated his attention upon pathology.

As early as 1901, however, Freud conceived of a special class of defense mechanisms that were to transmute libido, not into a source of pathology, but into culture and virtue. "The sexual life of each one of us," wrote Freud,

> extends to a slight degree—now in this direction, now in that—beyond the narrow lines imposed as the standard of normality. The perversions are neither bestial nor degenerate in the emotional sense of the word. They are a development of germs all of which are contained in the undifferentiated sexual disposition of the child, and which, by being suppressed or by being diverted to higher, asexual aims—by being "sublimated"—are destined to provide the energy for a great number of our cultural achievements. (Freud 1905a, p. 50)

Yet even today the glossary of defenses of DSM-III-R (American Psychiatric Association 1987) excludes sublimation because the defense is considered "healthy."

During the first decade after he postulated their existence, Freud definitely conceptualized defense mechanisms as being distinct from one another. Thus, by 1905 in the single work *Jokes and Their Relation to the Unconscious*, Freud (1905b) described seven different mechanisms of defense: humor, distortion, displacement, repression, suppression, phantasy, and isolation. After 1905, however, the term defense (*abwehr*) no longer figured prominently in Freud's work and was replaced by "'repression' (as I now began to say instead of 'defence')" (Freud 1906, p. 276). For 20 years, the distinction between ego mechanisms remained blurred.

In his *Introductory Lectures on Psycho-Analysis,* Freud (1916–1917) made little formal mention of the defenses and shrouded the concept behind general terms like "repression," "anticathexis," "censorship," and "resistance." He stated that the mechanism of cure in psychoanalysis is "the revival of the pathogenic conflict and the overcoming of the resistance due to repression . . ." (p. 447). Elsewhere, Freud (1914) suggested that "the theory of repression is the corner-stone on which the whole structure of psycho-analysis rests" (p. 16). The ego's defenses, thus, were all condensed under the single term "repression." In his *Introductory Lectures,* Freud does not mention isolation, dissociation, denial, reaction formation, and turning against the self.

For the next 10 years the elegance and power of one of Freud's most brilliant discoveries remained in eclipse. Freud offered only occasional hints of what had been initially so clear to him, namely that "no experience could have a pathogenic effect unless it appeared intolerable to the patient's ego and gave rise to efforts at defence" (Freud 1906, p. 276). During these later years he could ask, "In particular we want to know whether there is a single mechanism only, or more than one, and whether perhaps each of the psychoneuroses is distinguished by a mechanism of repression peculiar to it" (Freud 1917, p. 154). However, in contrast to his earliest papers in 1894 and 1896, Freud failed to elaborate on how one "mechanism of repression" or "mechanisms of forming substitutes" differed from another. Freud suggested that the subunits of behavior that he was calling "neuroses" might bear the same relation to the actual clinical states as the chemical elements bear to compound minerals. But he did not, as he had in his earlier papers, assign consistent labels to these defensive subunits.

In 1926, Freud did an abrupt about-face. In *Inhibitions, Symptoms and Anxiety,* he formally suggested that the concept of defense be reintroduced as the term under which specifically defined individual ego mechanisms such as "repression" and "isolation" were to be subsumed. Freud pointed out that these two mechanisms represented very different ways of handling the same disturbing affects: "I have revived a concept," Freud wrote,

> . . . of which I made exclusive use thirty years ago when I first began to study the subject [of anxiety] but which I later abandoned. I refer to the term "defensive process." I afterwards replaced it by the word "repression," but the relation between the two remained uncertain. It will be an undoubted advantage, I think, to revert to the old concept of "defence," provided we employ it explicitly as a general designation for all the techniques which the ego makes use of in conflicts which may lead to a neurosis. . . .

These observations provide good enough grounds for re-introducing the old concept of *defence,* which can cover all these processes that have the same purpose—namely, the protection of the ego against instinctual demands—and for subsuming repression under it [defence] as a special case. (Freud 1926, pp. 163–164)

Despite Freud's decision to reemphasize the differences between the defense mechanisms, other workers for decades continued to wish, consciously or not, to subsume all defenses under the term "repression." For example, in the first English edition of *Inhibitions, Symptoms and Anxiety,* Henry Bunker's translation of Freud's about-face read as follows: "I now think that it confers a *distinct disadvantage* to re-adopt the old concept of defense if in doing so it is laid down that this shall be the general designation for all the techniques of which the ego makes use in the conflicts which potentially lead to neurosis . . ." (Freud 1936b, p. 144; emphasis added). Compare Bunker's phrasing with the Strachey translation—"an undoubted advantage"—quoted previously. Thirty years later, in a panel on defenses sponsored by the American Psychoanalytic Association, more than one contemporary writer continued to insist that repression is the major defense and that all the others are somehow secondary (Wallerstein 1967). More recently still, Charles Brenner (1981) has suggested that we abandon the whole concept of defense.

Freud's Discovery of Individual Defenses

In trying to date Freud's discovery of individual defenses, inevitable semantic problems arise. These problems arise both from ambiguities inherent in translation from German to English and from the fact that the psychiatric argot used to describe defensive maneuvers changes over time. To circumvent these difficulties I will employ three rather arbitrary strategies. First, no special effort will be made to emphasize when Freud first used a given term but rather when he first described a given process. The terms used will reflect my own semantic bias. Rather than dispute my choice of words, readers are asked to substitute terms that are suitable to them. Second, for this discussion, the processes of introjection, identification, and regression are considered to be so intimately bound up with the normal maturational process that they will not be grouped with the mechanisms of defense. Third, because Freud, unlike Wallerstein (1983), does not distinguish the forever invisible defense mechanism or process from the sometimes visible defense contents or defensive behaviors, I, too, have chosen to ignore the distinction. Similarly, the difference between momentary projection during an analytic session and chronic projection by a paranoid character will be viewed as quantitative, not qualitative. My argument is that it is the discernible compromise formations and symptoms that allow clinicians to infer the underlying mental mechanisms. We can see fire; from that we infer combustion.

By 1915, Sigmund Freud had, if only in passing, identified almost all the mechanisms of defense that Anna Freud was to catalogue 20 years later. I shall describe these defenses not in order of discovery but in order of their possible maturity. I shall begin with the least mature—and most often pathological—defenses first and end with the most mature—and the least pathological—defenses. For although Freud rarely bothered to differentiate defenses unambiguously or to bring a list of defenses together in a single paper, he had hinted that defense mechanisms bore a hierarchical relationship to each other.

In 1926, Freud had raised an issue that remains one of the most important unanswered problems in ego psychology: the ontogeny of the ego mechanisms of defense. "It may well be," Freud noted, "that before its sharp cleavage into an ego and an id, and before the formation of a super-ego, the mental apparatus makes use of different methods of defence from those which it employs after it has reached these stages of organization" (Freud 1926, p. 164). As will be documented below, for Freud, the defenses of denial, distortion, and projection were the defenses of psychosis. At the opposite end of the continuum, sublimation, altruism, humor, and suppression were the defenses of maturity. Between these two groups of defense mechanisms were splitting, hypochondriasis, turning against the self, phantasy, dissociation, repression, isolation, undoing, displacement, and reaction formation—defenses that Freud believed to be the hallmarks of neurosis.

Denial (Verleugnung)

In 1894, Freud gave an excellent example of how psychotic denial is used defensively and how recognition of this defense renders some psychotic episodes intelligible. Freud did not use the term "denial"; nevertheless, he described the role of the process of denial in hallucinations. He wrote of the case of a young girl in love with a man who does not return the sentiment:

> Finally, in a state of great tension, she awaited his arrival. . . . When all the trains by which he could arrive had come and gone, she passed into a state of hallucinatory confusion: he had arrived, she heard his voice in the garden, she hurried down in her nightdress to receive him. From that time on she lived for two months in a happy dream, whose content was that he was there, always at her side . . . (Freud 1894, pp. 58–59)

He sharply differentiated this defense against external reality from the mechanisms of displacement, repression, and isolation.

In 1915, Freud used Theodor Meynert's old term "amentia" synonymously with his own term "wish psychosis" to describe a state synonymous with the remitting (reactive) psychoses. "Amentia," Freud wrote,

> is the reaction to a loss which reality affirms, but which the ego has to deny, since it finds it insupportable. Thereupon the ego breaks off its relation to reality; . . . the wishful phantasies are able to press forward into the system, and they are there regarded as a better reality. Such a withdrawal may be put on a par with the processes of repression. (Freud 1915d, p. 233)

In 1924, Freud introduced the formal term "denial of external reality" (*verleugnung*), or "disavowal" as James Strachey chose to translate it in order to distinguish it from *verneinen* (or negation). Freud pointed out that a woman in love with her dead sister's husband could master her guilt in two ways. The neurotic solution of the conflict was "by repressing the instinctual demand which had emerged—that is, her love for her brother-in-law. The psychotic reaction would have been a disavowal of the fact of her sister's death" (Freud 1924, p. 184).

Thus, Freud first seriously introduced into psychopathology the idea of a psychopathological hierarchy of defenses and expanded the point that he had made regarding amentia as a defensive process qualitatively different from repression. In contrast to neurotic defenses, psychotic defenses were those that distorted external reality. This distinction is important in separation. Later, Freud (1927) developed this distinction further by pointing out that *verdrängung* (repression) was used to control affects, while *verleugnung* (denial) was used to control the idea or the perception of a disturbing external reality (e.g., that girls lacked penises). This precise definition of denial contrasts with the nonspecific and often careless use of the term in which denial is almost synonymous with "defense." For example, reaction formation, projection, dissociation, and undoing all involve "denial" as the term is defined in a general dictionary. Anna Freud made the distinction between repression and denial still more explicit: "Repression gets rid of instinctual derivatives, just as external stimuli are abolished by denial" (A. Freud 1937, p. 90).

Two years later, Freud himself affirmed Anna Freud's distinction. "The childish ego," Freud wrote,

> under the domination of the real world, gets rid of undesirable instinctual demands by what are called repressions . . . during the same period of life, the ego often enough finds itself in the position of fending off some

demand from the external world which it feels distressing and that this is effected by means of a *disavowal* of the perceptions which bring to knowledge this demand from reality. (Freud 1938, pp. 203–204)

Because in modern psychoanalytic discussions confusion regarding the difference between the semantic terms "denial" and "repression" still persists, Freud's distinction among these processes remains timely.

Distortion

Although his chief concern with distortion was with its role in the dream work, Freud early recognized that the mechanism was operative in the waking life of a psychotic individual. For example, he had observed that "hysteria is in the habit of repeating its mnemic symbols without modification, whereas mnemic hallucinations in paranoia undergo a distortion similar to that in obsessional neurosis: an analogous modern image takes the place of the repressed one" (Freud 1896b, p. 184).

Projection

In his correspondence with Fliess, Freud first defined the process of projection as follows: "The purpose of paranoia is thus to fend off an idea that is incompatible with the ego, by projecting its substance into the external world" (Freud 1895, p. 209). Later in the same draft, however, he underscored that it was "affect" more than "ideas" that he was discussing. The next year Freud wrote: "In paranoia, the self-reproach is repressed in a manner which may be described as *projection*. It is repressed by erecting the defensive symptom of *distrust of other people*. In this way the subject withdraws his acknowledgement of the self-reproach . . ." (Freud 1896b, p. 184).

The concept of *projection* is so marvelously simple and so easily verified. Today, projection is recognized by many well-educated high school students. Yet Freud can take virtually full credit for its discovery. Shakespeare, in his portrayal of the central character in *Richard III*, and the German Hegelian philosopher Ludwig Feuerbach (1841), in his suggestion that man's conception of God was an outward reflection of his own inner nature, had both only hinted at the nature of projection.

Splitting (Ichspaltung)

Splitting of the ego is a defensive process that Freud recognized only at the end of his life. He saw the process as less pathological than the total denial of reality in psychosis but as more primitive than the neurotic defenses described below. As was his usual custom, Freud illustrated the splitting of the ego in relation to conflict between instinct and reality rather than in relation to conflicting object and self representations as is more common today. Thus, Freud's use of the term may seem a little outmoded to those grown accustomed to the advances in the understanding of object relations that occurred after his death.

Freud described the process of splitting as follows:

> Thus, there is a conflict between the demand by the instinct and the prohibition by reality. But in fact the child takes neither course, or rather he takes both simultaneously. . . . He replies to the conflict with two contrary reactions, both of which are valid and effective. . . . the instinct is allowed to retain its satisfaction and proper respect is shown to reality. (Freud 1940, p. 275)

Freud suggested that such use of splitting might lead to chronic impairment and to "a rift in the ego which never heals but increases as times goes on" (Freud 1940, p. 276). However, he also appreciated that splitting could be used in the sphere of object relations and described splitting in a case of pathological jealousy in which "[t]wo psychical attitudes . . . one . . . which takes account of reality, and another which under the influence of the instincts detached the ego from reality" (Freud 1938, p. 202).

Hypochondriasis

In his correspondence with Fliess, Freud had first conceived of hypochondriasis as a symptom and not as a defense. But later he wrote, "The affect of the self-reproach may be transformed by various psychical processes [ego mechanisms] into other affects, which then enter consciousness more clearly than the affect itself: for instance, into . . . *hypochondria* . . ." (Freud 1896a, p. 224). This statement demonstrates also what was so very original about the concept of defense. It was not painful *ideas* or thoughts that were transformed, but, rather, it was painful *affects* that were transformed. In addition, Freud offered medicine a lesson that continues to be rediscovered even today. Namely, hypochondriasis has far more to do with covert reproach than with secondary gain.

Turning Against the Self (Passive Aggression)

From the beginning, Freud saw turning against the self as a defense against aggression. In 1905, Freud wrote: "[I]t may be doubted at first whether it [masochism] can ever occur as a primary phenomenon or whether, on the contrary, it may not invariably arise from a transformation of sadism . . . turned round upon the subject's own self, which thus, to begin with, takes the place of the sexual object" (Freud 1905c, p. 158). A decade later, Freud outlined four possible "vicissitudes" of an instinct. Besides being controlled by repression, sublimation, and reaction formation, an instinct could undergo a process of "[t]urning round upon the subject's own self": ". . . we may also regard these vicissitudes as modes of defence against the instincts" (Freud 1915a, pp. 126–127). Thus, Freud points out that masochism is actually hostility turned round upon the subject. In the same paper, Freud anticipates the concept of covert hostility implicit in the term *passive-aggressive*: "The earlier active direction of the instinct persists to some degree side by side with its later passive direction, even when the process of its transformation has been very extensive" (Freud 1915a, p. 130).

Phantasy

Freud, in his correspondence with Fliess, suggested that "phantasies" referred only to the content of what was repressed or defended against. Except in dreams, phantasies did not themselves seem to represent a restitutive or defensive ego mechanism. However, by 1901 Freud offered a tentative example of a man with a waking fantasy of marriage to his physician's daughter; in reality, this man had no further relations with women and "took a dislike to marriage and lasting love-relationships" (Freud 1901, p. 172). In other words, Freud conceived that the defense of phantasy could allow an imagined—an autistic—object to substitute fully for a real relationship.

Later, Freud (1908) examined the autistic implications of daydreaming in greater detail. In contrast to the child, "who likes to link his imagined objects . . . to the tangible and visible things of the real world," the creative writer "creates a world of phantasy which he takes very seriously—that is, which he invests with large amounts of emotion—while separating it sharply from reality" (Freud 1908, p. 144). Three years later he sharpened the concept of autistic fantasy as a means of remaking a conflictual relationship in one's own mind: "*phantasying, which begins already in children's play, and later, continued as day-dreaming,* abandons dependence on real objects" (Freud 1911, p. 222). In the same paper he captures the process more clearly in a footnoted analogy: "A neat example of a psychical system shut off from the stimuli of the external world, and able to satisfy even its nutritional requirements autistically (to use Bleuler's term), is afforded by a bird's egg . . ." (Freud 1911, p. 220, n. 4).

Dissociation

For Benjamin Rush (1835), the process of dissociation had implied a pathological entity analogous to a DSM-III Axis I disorder. Pierre Janet also perceived dissociation as a diagnostic entity resulting from genetic defect. But as early as 1888, Freud had perceived that dissociation could function as a dynamic defense against affects. Freud later wrote:

> . . . in every case of hysterical paralysis, we find that *the paralysed organ* [arm] *or the lost function is involved in a subconscious association which is provided with a large quota of affect and it can be shown that the arm is liberated as soon as this quota is wiped out.* (Freud 1893, p. 171)

In other words, a conversion symptom could free the user of responsibility or awareness of a quota of affect (*valeur affective* or *affektbetrag*) that was not repressed so much as it was dissociated from its original attachment yet remaining in consciousness.

At the same time, Josef Breuer further developed the concept of dissociation—"splitting of the mind" or "double conscience" as it was variously called:

> Janet regards a particular form of congenital mental weakness as the disposition to hysteria . . . [but] . . . it is not the case that the splitting of consciousness occurs because the patients are weak-minded; they appear to be weak-minded because their mental activity is divided. (Breuer and Freud 1893, p. 231)

Defense, according to Breuer, was a dynamic function of the ego, not evidence of being weak-minded. Only an intact, thoroughly alert possum can play dead. And so, dissociation, the first ego mechanism to be recognized, was to set the stage for all the rest.

Repression (Verdrängung)

Unlike most of the defense mechanisms, the concept of repression was not original to Freud. J. F. Herbart had written extensively on the *verdrängung* (Freud's term for repression, also) of ideas. Herbart's *Psychology as a Science* (1824) may have influenced Freud indirectly through Freud's psychiatric mentor, Theodor Meynert. Schopenhauer had also perceived that defensive forgetting had something to do with psychopathology; but he, too, wrote of forgetting ideas and circumstances, not feelings. In 1818, Schopenhauer noted: "How unwillingly we think of things which powerfully injure our interests, wound our pride or interfere with our wishes. . . . In that resistance of the will to allowing what is contrary to it to come under the examination of our intellect lies the place at which madness can break in upon the mind" (Whyte 1960, p. 140).

It was Freud, however, who first pointed out that repression was used against *ideas* in order to manage *affects*:

> The affect from which the ego has suffered remains as it was before, unaltered and undiminished, the only difference being that the incompatible idea is kept down and shut out from recollection. The repressed ideas . . . form the nucleus of a second psychical group, which, I believe, is accessible even without the help of hypnosis. (Freud 1894, pp. 54–55)

At the same time, Freud wrote that

> in the course of our therapeutic work, we have been led to the view that hysteria originates through the repression of an incompatible idea from a motive of defence. On this view, the repressed idea would persist as a memory trace that is weak (has little intensity), while the affect that is torn from it would be used for a somatic innervation. (That is, the excitation is "converted.") . . . A hysteria exhibiting this psychical mechanism may be given the name of "defence hysteria." (Breuer and Freud 1893, p. 285)

Isolation

In 1894, with astonishing clarity Freud identified the mechanism of isolation as the obverse of repression. The concept of isolation, Freud believed, was necessary to distinguish the defensive operations present in obsessional states from those present in conversion hysteria. If the ego could not simply eradicate a distressing idea, it could achieve approximate success by removing from it all affective charge, or, as Freud wrote, "if the ego succeeds in *turning this powerful idea into a weak one,* in robbing it of the affect—the sum of excitation—with which it is loaded" (Freud 1894, p. 48). In the same paper he continued, "If someone with a disposition [to neurosis] lacks the aptitude for conversion, but if, nevertheless, in order to fend off an incompatible idea, he sets about separating it from its affect, then *that affect is obliged to remain in the psychical sphere.* The idea, now weakened, is still left in consciousness, separated from all association" (pp. 51–52). Repression banished the idea from consciousness while preserving the affect; isolation spared the idea but banished the affect. Dissociation kept both affect and idea in consciousness, but the significance of such association was obscured (e.g., fugues and conversions).

Later, in keeping with his decision to abandon the term *defence* for *repression,* Freud described isolation in new words but the same melody:

"Repression makes use of another, and in reality a simpler, mechanism. The trauma, instead of being forgotten, is deprived of its affective cathexis; so that what remains in consciousness is nothing but its ideational content, which is perfectly colourless and is judged to be unimportant" (Freud 1909, p. 196). In the same paper he first gave the process its modern name: "And similarly other patients will endeavor to '*isolate*' all such protective acts from other things" (p. 243). By "things," of course, Freud meant affects.

Almost 20 years later, Freud again elucidated this identical concept of isolation, but he wrote as if he was discovering what he had never known before: "The second of these techniques *which we are setting out to describe for the first time,* that of isolation, is peculiar to obsessional neurosis" (Freud 1926, p. 120; emphasis added).

Undoing (Ungeschenmachen)

This defense bears close kinship to isolation, both in Freud's writing and in its clinical occurrence. Undoing provides a means of reversing hostile wishes, or as Freud (1909, p. 192) put it: "Compulsive acts like this, in two successive stages, of which the second neutralizes the first, are a typical occurrence in obsessional neuroses." Later in the same case history Freud used the term *undoing* for the first time; he suggested that the Rat Man's extension of his obsessional fears to include events in the next world "was nothing else than a compensation for these death-wishes which he had felt against his father . . . it was designed—in defiance of reality, and in deference to the wish which had previously been showing itself in phantasies of every kind—to undo the fact of his father's death" (Freud 1909, pp. 235–236).

Displacement (Verschiebung)

Early in his career, Freud (1894) referred to "the concept that in mental functions something is to be distinguished—a quota of affect or sum of excitation—which possesses all the characteristics of a quantity (though we have no means of measuring it), which is capable of increase, diminution, displacement and discharge . . . " (p. 60). Such quotas of affects, Freud believed, could be "dislodged" or "transposed" (p. 54). In short, they could be displaced.

Perhaps it was because students of the mind before Freud had themselves employed the defenses of displacement that they overlooked the importance of affects and instead cathected ideas. Defenses could not be conceptualized, however, until the defensive aspects of philosophy and theology could be surmounted and the excitement attributed to "ideas" could be returned to the instinctual sources from which it had been displaced. Even today, psychoanalysts find it easier to discuss "object relations" than love.

Freud also noted that the mechanism of displacement underlay the phenomenon of phobias. "Thus, for example," Freud wrote, "liberated anxiety, whose sexual origin must not be remembered by the patient, will seize upon the common primary phobias of mankind about animals, thunderstorms, darkness and so on . . ."(Freud 1894, p. 54). Years later he suggested that displacement was pathognomonic of the obsessive-compulsive neurotic individual: "The mechanism of psychical *displacement,* which was first discovered by me in the construction of dreams, dominates the mental processes of obsessional neurosis" (Freud 1907, p. 126).

Reaction Formation

In 1905 Freud first described reaction formation. He saw the defense as originating somewhat later in childhood than the previously mentioned defenses and being rather more adaptive. Indeed, in *Three Essays on the Theory of Sexuality,* Freud did not make a distinction between the ontogenetically related mechanisms of reaction formation and altruism. Reaction formation, Freud said, reminded him of the proverb "*Junge Hure, alte Betschwester*" ["a young whore makes an old nun"]. Freud explained that reaction formation

> begins during a child's period of latency and continues in favourable cases throughout his whole life. . . . The multifariously perverse sexual disposition of childhood can accordingly be regarded as the source of a number of our virtues, in so far as through reaction formation it stimulates their development" (Freud 1905c, pp. 238–239)

In fact, in the original edition of *Three Essays,* Freud had considered reaction formation a "sub-species of sublimation" (Freud 1905c, p. 238), and only 10 years later did he add a footnote to this original description of reaction formation and sublimation in order to suggest that, in general, it is possible to distinguish the concepts of sublimation and reaction formation as "two different processes" (Freud 1905c, p. 178, n. 2).

Ego Maturation

Thus, by 1905 Freud had already introduced the tremendously important concept of an ontogeny of defenses. Defenses such as denial and repression occur not only along a continuum of relative psychopathology but also along a continuum of ego development. If whores could become nuns, then acting out can become the parent of reaction formation and a potential grandparent of altruism. In suggesting that sublimation and reaction formation allowed the human ego to transform base instincts into noble virtues, Freud had devised a new alchemy for 20th-century psychiatry.

Later, Freud carried the possibility of a continuum of defenses further. He concluded that

> repression is not a defensive mechanism which is present from the very beginning, and that it cannot arise until a sharp cleavage has occurred between conscious and unconscious mental activity . . . before the mental organization reaches this stage, the task of fending off instinctual impulses is dealt with by the other vicissitudes which instincts may undergo—e.g. . . . "turning round upon the subject's own self." (Freud 1915c, p. 147)[1]

In his essay on narcissism, Freud (1915b) carried his tentative outline of an ego developmental continuum sequence further. "Sublimation," Freud wrote,

> is a process that concerns object-libido and consists in the instinct's directing itself towards an aim other than, and remote from, that of sexual satisfaction; in this process the accent falls upon deflection from sexuality. (Freud 1915b, p. 94)

He goes on to say: "Sublimation is a way out, a way by which those [i.e., instinctual] demands can be met *without* involving repression" (Freud 1915b, p. 95). Freud hints, then, that primitive turning against the self gives way to repression that in turn gives way to mature sublimation. In the same year Freud reiterated his belief in an ontogeny of the ego's defensive processes when he wrote that for "every transition from one system to that immediately above it (that is, every advance to a higher stage of psychical organization) there corresponds a new censorship" (Freud 1915d, p. 192). This brief discussion of ego maturation sets the stage for a group of mental mechanisms so mature and healthy that some investigators have been loath to call them defenses at all.

---

[1]Recently, Kernberg (1967, 1975) has suggested that Melanie Klein's primitive image-distorting defenses of "devaluation," "splitting," "primitive idealization," and "projective identification" must also be considered as precursors for the neurotic defenses.

Sublimation

Freud first used the term *sublimation* in a letter to Wilhelm Fliess in 1897. In discussing the fantasies of hysteria, he wrote, "They are protective structures, sublimations of the facts, embellishments of them, and at the same time serve for self-exoneration" (Freud 1897, p. 247). Eight years later Freud gave us the definition of sublimation that we use today. He suggested that sexual curiosity could "be diverted ('sublimated') in the direction of art, if its interest can be shifted away from the genitals on to the shape of the body as a whole . . ." (Freud 1905c, p. 156). Freud, then, continued to develop his concept that transformation of affects arising from sexual excitation could lead toward health as well as toward neurosis. Sublimation, Freud pointed out,

> enables excessively strong excitation arising from particular sources of sexuality to find an outlet and use in other fields, so that a not inconsiderable increase in psychical efficiency results from a disposition which in itself is perilous. . . . The multifariously perverse sexual disposition of childhood can accordingly be regarded as the source of a number of our virtues . . . (Freud 1905c, pp. 238–239)

But fuller development of this idea had to wait for the advent of ego psychology.

Altruism

Like sublimation, altruism represents another more adaptive descendant of reaction formation. Freud never discussed altruism in detail, but in his *Introductory Lectures on Psycho-Analysis* (1915–1916, 1916–1917), he at least recognized the defensive, if healthy, potential of altruism:

> The opposite to egoism, *altruism*, . . . is distinguished from it by the absence of longings for sexual satisfaction. When someone is completely in love, however, altruism converges with libidinal object-cathexis. As a rule the sexual object attracts a portion of the ego's narcissism to itself, and this becomes noticeable as what is known as the "sexual overvaluation" of the object. (Freud 1916–1917, p. 418)

Anna Freud (1937) extended the concept of altruism to cope with a far broader range of interpersonal vicissitudes than just being "in love." She memorably pointed out altruism's defensive roots when she reminded Joseph Sandler, "Altruism comes from the badness in our hearts" (Sandler 1985, p. 429).

Suppression (Unterdrückung)

Suppression is an ego mechanism of defense that can hardly be considered original to Freud. Nevertheless, before fully recognizing that ego mechanisms of defense were unconscious, Freud offered a fairly modern definition of suppression:

> These patients whom I analysed had enjoyed good mental health up to the moment at which *an occurrence of incompatibility took place in their ideational life*—that is to say, until their ego was faced with an experience, an idea or a feeling which aroused such a distressing affect that the subject decided to forget about it because he had no confidence in his power to resolve the contradiction between that incompatible idea and his ego by means of thought-activity . . .
> . . . the patients can recollect as precisely as could be desired their efforts at defence, their intention of "pushing the thing away," of not thinking of it, of suppressing it. (Freud 1894, p. 47)

As time passed, as was the case with isolation, Freud ceased to differentiate suppression from repression. In both *Jokes and Their Relation to the Unconscious* and *The Interpretation of Dreams,* Freud used "suppression" and "repression" interchangeably. He emphasized, however, that both terms referred to unconsciously defensive, not to willed, processes (e.g., "It might be said that the dream-work brings about a suppression of affects" [Freud 1900, p. 467]). In a footnote in *The Interpretation of Dreams,* Freud confessed, "For instance, I have omitted to state whether I attribute different meanings to the words 'suppressed' and 'repressed.' It should have been clear, however, that the latter lays more stress than the former upon the fact of attachment to the unconscious" (Freud 1900, p. 606, n. 2). Freud never again tried to differentiate the two terms, but he almost certainly saw suppression as far healthier than repression. Indeed, he once defined maturity as the capacity to postpone gratification. More recently, Werman (1985) has elaborated the place of the defense mechanism of suppression in psychodynamic thinking.

Humor

Humor, like sublimation and altruism, was another defense that Freud perceived as having more of an adaptive than a pathogenic quality. In *Jokes and Their Relation to the Unconscious,* Freud developed the idea of humor as a more mature defense mechanism than wit. He viewed wit as inextricably linked with the less adaptive, less mature mechanism of displacement. In contrast, Freud wrote that "humour is a means of obtaining pleasure in spite of the distressing affects that interfere with it; it acts as a substitute for the generation of these affects, it puts itself in their place . . . it arises from an economy in the expenditure of affect" (Freud 1905b, pp. 228–229). Again, hinting at a hierarchy of defenses, Freud went on to maintain that

> defensive processes are the psychical correlative of the flight reflex. . . . Humour can be regarded as the highest of these defensive processes. It scorns to withdraw the ideational content bearing the distressing affect from conscious attention as repression does, and thus surmounts the automatism of defence. (p. 233)

Freud and Ego Psychology

In his *New Introductory Lectures on Psycho-Analysis,* Freud (1932) cited only four defenses as relevant to waking behavior: repression, sublimation, displacement, and reaction formation. He wrote as if he had scant regard for the previous discoveries outlined above. One possible reason is that when Freud discussed defenses in formal language, it was in economic rather than in dynamic terms. The economic vantage point made the differentiation of individual defenses less important. In addition, Freud's discussions of defense in dynamic terms were often cloaked in clinical anecdote; thus, any reader of Freud's work learns to appreciate defensive process without requiring a formal taxonomy. Like any wise scientist, Freud put weight on phenomena rather than on semantics.

A second reason for Freud's lack of attention to a formal taxonomy was that when Freud reintroduced the concept of differentiated defenses in 1926, he already was 70 years old. Consciously or unconsciously, he preferred to delegate the need for a compendium of defenses, and so he advised the interested student of psychoanalysis that "there are an extraordinarily large number of methods (or mechanisms, as we say) used by our ego in the discharge of its defensive functions. . . . my daughter, the child analyst, is writing a book upon them" (Freud 1936a, p. 245). He was referring, of course, to what was to be his daughter Anna's 80th birthday present to him: *The Ego and the Mechanisms of Defense.*

A third possible reason for Freud's limited interest in individual defenses was that the conception of hierarchically differentiated defenses requires a highly developed appreciation of the healthy ego. Differentiated mechanisms of defense are most clear when one can study the psychopathology of healthy everyday life in detail. For example, what is the fate of a given defense as the child matures or as a patient recovers? Freud and his students had chosen to study psychologically impaired individuals. Only much later were such investigations extended so far that Schafer (1968) could suggest that every defense mechanism has some potential for pleasure. Our appreciation of the defensive nature of mature behavior awaited studies of normal populations such as those by Ernst Kris, Robert White, Heinz Hartmann, David Hamburg, and, of course, Anna Freud.

Before he died, Freud (1937) fully anticipated the future direction of ego psychology:

> The ego makes use of various procedures for fulfilling its task, which, to put it in general terms, is to avoid danger, anxiety and unpleasure. We call these procedures "*mechanisms of defence.*" Our knowledge of them is not yet sufficiently complete. Anna Freud's book (1936) has given us a first insight into their multiplicity and many-sided significance. . . .
>   . . . the mechanisms of defence serve the purpose of keeping off dangers. It cannot be disputed that they are successful in this; and it is doubtful whether the ego could do without them altogether during its development. But it is also certain that they may become dangers themselves. (Freud 1937, pp. 235–237)

Here, then, Freud leaves us with a thoroughly modern legacy. First, defenses are unconscious processes. Second, they can be distinguished one from another. Third, they serve a homeostatic function that is pathogenic in only selected instances.

In terms of a continuum of defenses from pathological to less pathological, many contributors to ego psychology (e.g., Brenner, Gill, Rapaport) have recognized the likelihood of such a hierarchy. But only by utilizing as a conceptual scheme the recovery process from schizophrenic decompensation did Elvin Semrad (1967) finally outline for psychoanalysis such a sequence of ego mechanisms.

Through a prospective 50-year study of normal adult development, I have obtained experimental confirmation of the hierarchies proposed by Freud and Semrad (Vaillant 1971a, 1971b, 1977; Vaillant et al. 1986). By using the stratagem of studying overt defense contents rather than the invisible, if theoretically more correct, mechanisms of defense, some of the problems of consensually validating choice of ego mechanism have been overcome. Such a strategy has exploited the advantage that Schafer (1968) anticipated when he suggested that

> macroscopic description is useful when one is viewing intrapsychic process from a distance. From that vantage point the observer will be impressed mainly by the regular and uniform aspects of these processes. (p. 49)

Of course, when applied to direct clinical work, such a stratagem, as Brenner (1981) reminds us, possesses many limitations.

The Need for Definition and Consensus

In order to understand ego development and in order to record dynamic formulation of clinical cases, we need a consensually validated hierarchy of defenses. Anna Freud suggested that

> defenses have their own chronology . . . they are more apt to have patho-
> logical results if they come into use before the appropriate age and are
> kept up too long after it. Examples are denial and projection which are
> "normal" in early childhood and lead to pathology in later years; and
> repression and reaction formation, which cripple the child's personality if
> used too early. (A. Freud 1965, p. 177)

But many years later she pointed out in her dialogue with Joseph Sandler that much work remained to be done:

> I was very much concerned at the time with the possibility of a chronology
> of the defenses, which was also debated then—the question of which
> comes first, of what is a primitive defense and what is a sophisticated
> defense—and I tried at one point in the book to give a vague outline as
> we had it then, in the hope that in the future we could learn more about
> this, especially as our knowledge of ego development advanced. This hope
> has not really been fulfilled up to the present day. . . . I think that in time
> we will arrive at the chronology of defenses. (Sandler 1985, p. 525)

Without consensus on terms we can never chart the ego's development or gain consensual validation as to definition. Without consensus on terminology, empirical study of defenses is hampered. Formal glossaries of defenses must be spelled out and defenses differentiated from each other with mutually exclusive definitions. Yet, in the foreword to *Defense and Resistance,* Blum (1985) wisely warns of the dangers of such oversimplification. First, defenses belong to metaphor and metapsychology. Second, all defense mechanisms, as Brenner (1981) points out, can serve other purposes. Thus, humor is also an aesthetic reaction, hypochondriasis a symptom, undoing a compromise formation, and so on. Third, in any effort to produce a comprehensive list of defenses there will be enormous disagreement. Rarely is one analyst fully satisfied with a list of defenses offered by another.

However, if psychiatry wishes further to clarify and to obtain consensus on defenses, it must recognize a dilemma. The dilemma is that to study a metapsychological construct too closely is to lose the forest for the trees. At the end of their long careers of elucidating depth psychology, the opposing positions of Charles Brenner and Anna Freud illustrate this dilemma. Brenner could write that "there are no special ego functions that are 'defenses,' functions that serve solely a defensive purpose and no other" (Brenner 1976, p. 77), and that "to discuss defense in terms of defense *mechanisms* as Freud and every analyst since has done, myself included, is wrong" (Brenner 1981, p. 561).

Anna Freud in her dialogue with Sandler takes a very different stance. In response to Sandler's suggestion that "when we begin to look microscopically at the concept [defense mechanisms], then, as with many other concepts, our theory may break down," Anna Freud replies

> You know, that applies to all defense mechanisms. . . . You will find five or six defenses compressed into one attitude. The point is that one should not look at them microscopically, but macroscopically, as big separate mechanisms . . . you have to take off your glasses to look at them[,] not put them on. (Sandler 1985, p. 176)

To put the dilemma differently, just as symphonies can never be fully understood by focus upon individual instruments, human behavior is rarely accurately reflected by focus on a single defense. However, that does not mean that understanding defenses, like understanding individual musical instruments, is not part of our understanding of the resulting behavioral complexity.

Since the failure of psychoanalysis to define defenses for the DSM-III and Brenner's disavowal of the usefulness of the concept, efforts by Meissner (1980), Vaillant (1987), and the compilers of the DSM-III-R glossary (American Psychiatric Association 1987) reflect our progress in building on the process begun a century ago by Sigmund Freud and in providing psychoanalysis with a differentiated, consensually defined hierarchy of defenses.

A continuing difficulty that has focused attention away from differentiation of the defenses has been the fact that defenses are intangible and, once recognized, difficult to validate. Methodological difficulty in this area hampered earlier efforts by Anna Freud and her Hempstead co-workers to uncover the developmental sequence of defense mechanisms. To construct such a chronological continuum requires rater reliability, which in turn means rendering ephemeral defensive processes subject to empirical study. A review of such efforts at empirical study will be a major focus of this book.

References

American Psychiatric Association: Diagnostic and Statistical Manual of Mental Disorders, 3rd Edition, Revised. Washington, DC, American Psychiatric Association, 1987

Blum HP (ed): Defense and Resistance. New York, International Universities Press, 1985

Breuer J, Freud S: On the psychical mechanism of hysterical phenomena: preliminary communication (1893), in The Standard Edition of the Complete Psychological Works of Sigmund Freud, Vol 2. Translated and edited by Strachey J. London, Hogarth Press, 1955, pp 1–17

Brenner C: Psychoanalytic Technique and Psychic Conflict. New York, International Universities Press, 1976

Brenner C: Defense and defense mechanisms. Psychoanal Q 50:557–569, 1981

Fenichel O: The Psychoanalytic Theory of Neuroses. New York, WW Norton, 1945

Feuerbach L: Das Wesendes Christentums. Leipzig, Verlag von Otto Wigand, 1841

Freud A: The Ego and the Mechanisms of Defense. London, Hogarth Press, 1937

Freud A: Normality and Pathology in Childhood: Assessments of Development. New York, International Universities Press, 1965

Freud S: Some points for a comparative study of organic and hysterical motor paralyses (1893), in The Standard Edition of the Complete Psychological Works of Sigmund Freud, Vol 1. Translated and edited by Strachey J. London, Hogarth Press, 1966, pp 160–172

Freud S: The neuro-psychoses of defence (1894), in The Standard Edition of the Complete Psychological Works of Sigmund Freud, Vol 3. Translated and edited by Strachey J. London, Hogarth Press, 1962, pp 45–61

Freud S: Draft H, Paranoia (1895), in The Standard Edition of the Complete Psychological Works of Sigmund Freud, Vol 1. Translated and edited by Strachey J. London, Hogarth Press, 1966, pp 206–212

Freud S: Draft K, The neuroses of defense (a Christmas fairy tale) (1896a), in The Standard Edition of the Complete Psychological Works of Sigmund Freud, Vol 1. Translated and edited by Strachey J. London, Hogarth Press, 1966, pp 220–229

Freud S: Further remarks on the neuro-psychoses of defence (1896b), in The Standard Edition of the Complete Psychological Works of Sigmund Freud, Vol 3. Translated and edited by Strachey J. London, Hogarth Press, 1962, pp 162–185

Freud S: Letter 61 (1897), in The Standard Edition of the Complete Psychological Works of Sigmund Freud, Vol 1. Translated and edited by Strachey J. London, Hogarth Press, 1966, pp 247–248

Freud S: The interpretation of dreams (1900), in The Standard Edition of the Complete Psychological Works of Sigmund Freud, Vols 4 and 5. Translated and edited by Strachey J. London, Hogarth Press, 1953

Freud S: The psychopathology of everyday life (1901), in The Standard Edition of the Complete Psychological Works of Sigmund Freud, Vol 6. Translated and edited by Strachey J. London, Hogarth Press, 1960

Freud S: Fragment of an analysis of a case of hysteria (1905a), in The Standard Edition of the Complete Psychological Works of Sigmund Freud, Vol 7. Translated and edited by Strachey J. London, Hogarth Press, 1953, pp 7–122

Freud S: Jokes and their relation to the unconscious (1905b), in The Standard Edition of the Complete Psychological Works of Sigmund Freud, Vol 8. Translated and edited by Strachey J. London, Hogarth Press, 1960

Freud S: Three essays on the theory of sexuality (1905c), in The Standard Edition of the Complete Psychological Works of Sigmund Freud, Vol 7. Translated and edited by Strachey J. London, Hogarth Press, 1953, pp 130–243

Freud S: My views on the part played by sexuality in the aetiology of the neuroses (1906), in The Standard Edition of the Complete Psychological Works of Sigmund Freud, Vol 7. Translated and edited by Strachey J. London, Hogarth Press, 1953, pp 271–279

Freud S: Obsessive acts and religious practices (1907), in The Standard Edition of the Complete Psychological Works of Sigmund Freud, Vol 9. Translated and edited by Strachey J. London, Hogarth Press, 1959, pp 117–127

Freud S: Creative writers and day-dreaming (1908), in The Standard Edition of the Complete Psychological Works of Sigmund Freud, Vol 9. Translated and edited by Strachey J. London, Hogarth Press, 1959, pp 143–153

Freud S: Notes upon a case of obsessional neurosis (1909), in The Standard Edition of the Complete Psychological Works of Sigmund Freud, Vol 10. Translated and edited by Strachey J. London, Hogarth Press, 1955, pp 155–249

Freud S: Formulations on the two principles of mental functioning (1911), in The Standard Edition of the Complete Psychological Works of Sigmund Freud, Vol 12. Translated and edited by Strachey J. London, Hogarth Press, 1958, pp 218–226

Freud S: On the history of the psycho-analytic movement (1914), in The Standard Edition of the Complete Psychological Works of Sigmund Freud, Vol 14. Translated and edited by Strachey J. London, Hogarth Press, 1957, pp 7–66

Freud S: Instincts and their vicissitudes (1915a), in The Standard Edition of the Complete Psychological Works of Sigmund Freud, Vol 14. Translated and edited by Strachey J. London, Hogarth Press, 1957, pp 109–140

Freud S: On narcissism: an introduction (1915b), in The Standard Edition of the Complete Psychological Works of Sigmund Freud, Vol 14. Translated and edited by Strachey J. London, Hogarth Press, 1957, pp 73–102

Freud S: Repression (1915c), in The Standard Edition of the Complete Psychological Works of Sigmund Freud, Vol 14. Translated and edited by Strachey J. London, Hogarth Press, 1957, pp 146–158

Freud S: The unconscious (1915d), in The Standard Edition of the Complete Psychological Works of Sigmund Freud, Vol 14. Translated and edited by Strachey J. London, Hogarth Press, 1957, pp 166–215

Freud S: Introductory lectures on psycho-analysis, Parts I and II (1915–1916), in The Standard Edition of the Complete Psychological Works of Sigmund Freud, Vol 15. Translated and edited by Strachey J. London, Hogarth Press, 1961

Freud S: Introductory lectures on psycho-analysis, Parts I and II (1916–1917), in The Standard Edition of the Complete Psychological Works of Sigmund Freud, Vol 16. Translated and edited by Strachey J. London, Hogarth Press, 1963

Freud S: A metapsychological supplement to the theory of dreams (1917), in The Standard Edition of the Complete Psychological Works of Sigmund Freud, Vol 14. Translated and edited by Strachey J. London, Hogarth Press, 1957, pp 222–235

Freud S: The loss of reality in neurosis and psychosis (1924), in The Standard Edition of the Complete Psychological Works of Sigmund Freud, Vol 19. Translated and edited by Strachey J. London, Hogarth Press, 1961, pp 183–187

Freud S: Inhibitions, symptoms and anxiety (1926), in The Standard Edition of the Complete Psychological Works of Sigmund Freud, Vol 20. Translated and edited by Strachey J. London, Hogarth Press, 1959, pp 77–175

Freud S: Fetishism (1927), in The Standard Edition of the Complete Psychological Works of Sigmund Freud, Vol 21. Translated and edited by Strachey J. London, Hogarth Press, 1961, pp 152–157

Freud S: New introductory lectures on psycho-analysis (1932), in The Standard Edition of the Complete Psychological Works of Sigmund Freud, Vol 22. Translated and edited by Strachey J. London, Hogarth Press, 1964, pp 5–182

Freud S: A disturbance of memory on the Acropolis (1936a), in The Standard Edition of the Complete Psychological Works of Sigmund Freud, Vol 22. Translated and edited by Strachey J. London, Hogarth Press, 1964, pp 239–248

Freud S: The Problem of Anxiety. Translated by Bunker HA. New York, WW Norton, 1936b

Freud S: Analysis terminable and interminable (1937), in The Standard Edition of the Complete Psychological Works of Sigmund Freud, Vol 23. Translated and edited by Strachey J. London, Hogarth Press, 1964, pp 216–253

Freud S: An outline of psycho-analysis (1938), in The Standard Edition of the Complete Psychological Works of Sigmund Freud, Vol 23. Translated and edited by Strachey J. London, Hogarth Press, 1964, pp 144–207

Freud S: Splitting of the ego in the process of defence (1940), in The Standard Edition of the Complete Psychological Works of Sigmund Freud, Vol 23. Translated and edited by Strachey J. London, Hogarth Press, 1964, pp 275–278

Herbart JF: Psychologie als Wissenschaft [Psychology as a Science] (1824), in Samtliche Werke, Vols V and VI. Liepzig, Voss, 1850

James W: The Principles of Psychology. New York, Henry Holt, 1890

Jones E: The Life and Work of Sigmund Freud. New York, Basic Books, 1953–1957

Kernberg OF: Borderline personality organization. J Am Psychoanal Assoc 15:641–685, 1967

Kernberg OF: Borderline Conditions and Pathological Narcissism. New York, Jason Aronson, 1975

Meissner WW: Theories of personality and psychopathology: classical psychoanalysis, in Comprehensive Textbook of Psychiatry, 3rd Edition, Vol 1. Edited by Kaplan HI, Freedman AM, Sadock BJ. Baltimore, MD, Williams & Wilkins, 1980, pp 631–728

Rush B: Medical Inquiries and Observations Upon the Diseases of the Mind. Philadelphia, PA, Grigg and Elliot, 1835

Sandler J (with Freud A): The Analysis of Defense: The Ego and the Mechanisms of Defense Revisited. New York, International Universities Press, 1985

Schafer R: The mechanisms of defense. Int J Psychoanal 49:49–62, 1968

Semrad E: The organization of ego defenses and object loss, in The Loss of Loved Ones. Edited by Moriarity DM. Springfield, IL, Charles C Thomas, 1967, pp 126–134

Vaillant GE: The evolution of adaptive and defensive behavior during the adult life cycle. Abstracted in J Am Psychoanal Assoc 19:110–115, 1971a

Vaillant GE: Theoretical hierarchy of adaptive ego mechanisms. Arch Gen Psychiatry 24:107–118, 1971b

Vaillant GE: Adaptation to Life. Boston, MA, Little, Brown, 1977

Vaillant GE: An empirically derived hierarchy of adaptive mechanisms and its usefulness as a potential diagnostic axis, in Diagnosis and Classification in Psychiatry: A Critical Appraisal of DSM-III. Edited by Tischler G. New York, Cambridge University Press, 1987, pp 464–476

Vaillant GE, Bond M, Vaillant CO: An empirically validated hierarchy of defense mechanisms. Arch Gen Psychiatry 43:786–794, 1986

Van der Leeuw PJ: On the development of the concept of defense. Int J Psychoanal 52:51–58, 1971

Wallerstein RS: Panel on development and metapsychology of the defense organization of the ego. J Am Psychoanal Assoc 15:132–149, 1967

Wallerstein RS: Defenses, defense mechanisms and the structure of the mind. J Am Psychoanal Assoc 31(suppl):201–225, 1983

Werman DS: Suppression as a defense, in Defense and Resistance. Edited by Blum HP. New York, International Universities Press, 1985, pp 405–415

Whyte LL: The Unconscious Before Freud. New York, Basic Books, 1960

Wundt W: Human and Animal Psychology. New York, MacMillan, 1894

Chapter 2

The Place of Defense Mechanisms in Diagnostic Formulation and in Modern Clinical Practice

George E. Vaillant, M.D.

Beginning with the request by Karasu and Skodol (1980) for a psychodynamic Axis VI for DSM-III (American Psychiatric Association 1980), clinicians have argued for a diagnostic axis for defense mechanisms. In his efforts to lay the groundwork for the 10th edition of the *International Classification of Diseases* (ICD-10), Norman Sartorius (Sartorius et al. 1990), the director of the Division of Mental Health of the World Health Organization, has been quite articulate in criticizing current psychiatric diagnostic nomenclature. He writes that

> psychiatric problems are responses that are not specific to causes and therefore not appropriate to a system that classifies disease entities. . . . Research during the past two decades failed to provide evidence that could help to create disease concepts and disease entities in psychiatry. . . . Most attempts to create coherent links between clinical symptoms, specific causal factors, pathogenetic models and prognostic types have failed. . . . Other ways of thinking about health and disease, mind and body, mental and physical, individual and social are needed if we are to formulate creative hypotheses and design investigations likely to result in breakthroughs in our knowledge about mental illness. . . . I believe that in selected instances a return to the allegedly outdated Meyerian reaction patterns and Freudian defense mechanisms is warranted. (p. 2)

As psychiatry moves into the 21st century, many of Freud's teachings may be discarded, but not his elucidation of defense mechanisms. In this chapter I will suggest that no mental status or clinical formulation should be considered complete without an effort to identify the patient's dominant defense mechanisms. No introductory course in behavioral medicine should be considered adequate without a full explication of defenses. Too often, so-called psychiatric disorders are only symptoms; as such they are merely the visible evidence of an unseen disease process. Many diagnoses in DSM-III-R no more reflect true diagnostic entities than does dropsy or cough. For example, hypochondriasis and somatization are treated as discrete disorders in DSM-III. The hypochondriacal individual complains of an imaginary disease, and the individual afflicted with somatization disorder complains of imaginary symptoms—as if that were an important distinction to anybody but a Thomist. It may be more useful to view both reactions as defense mechanisms, not as diseases. Hypochondriasis and its associated help-rejecting complaining often convey unconscious reproach and devaluation. In contrast, somatization often reflects a wish for secondary gain or even serves as a means of communicating an unconscious, or at least unverbalized, affective state. When the separation of somatization and hypochondriasis is made in this way, the distinction becomes clinically useful. The distinction is important both to medical education and to medical therapeutics.

In psychiatry, as in the rest of medicine, we often are dealing with *dis-ease* and not disease. Human misery is rarely caused by anything as specific as a bacillus. The insurance companies have done neither their clients nor psychiatric classification a favor by agreeing to pay only for disease and not for dis-ease. For like it or not, psychiatry *is* dynamic. Psychiatric diagnosis has more in common with the inevitable ambiguity of great drama than with the quest in DSM-III for algorithms compatible with the cold binary logic of computer science and with the reimbursable classifications of insurance carriers.

Put differently, to be maximally clinically useful, psychiatric diagnostic manuals will be enhanced by creating an axis for defenses. Indeed, in order to encompass defense mechanisms, a potential Axis VI was proposed for DSM-III; but because defense mechanisms implied unconscious etiology, and because the empirical underpinnings were not in place, the proposal was abandoned. However, for DSM-III to have ignored diagnostic concepts as well established as displacement, projection, and reaction formation and yet to have included diagnoses as vague and as poorly defined as dependent and narcissistic personality disorders may not have been justified.

Ultimately, a diagnostic axis that includes defenses may add a most valuable dimension to future diagnostic manuals. It certainly will provide a valuable teaching focus to medical education. Let me explain why this should be so. With advances in the neurosciences, clinical psychiatry in the 21st century will increasingly resemble internal medicine. To be effective, psychiatry must learn the recent lessons of internal medicine. Let me cite just a few of these lessons.

The first lesson offered to psychiatry by internal medicine is the attention of internal medicine to underlying dynamic pathophysiology rather than to static signs and symptoms. By virtue of its knowledge of specific etiologies, the rest of medicine has learned that symptoms are quite different from disease. In the 17th century, edema ("oedema") was a disease in Syndenham's (1685) atheoretical textbook of medicine. In William Osler's (1892) more modern textbook, however, edema was not a disease. Osler did not ignore edema and turgor; he simply recognized them for what they were—homeostatic physiological responses to underlying pathology. In addition, internal medicine now appreciates that so-called infectious disease is often not caused by the bacteria as much as it is a result of the idiosyncratic adaptive response of the host to the infectious agent. The same principles hold true in psychiatry. In psychiatry it is often not the stressor but the patient's idiosyncratic response that leads to disease. By deciphering defenses we can understand the underlying "pathophysiology" of our patient's disorder, and thus defenses may be viewed as the building blocks of much psychopathology. This is but one reason why defenses should be included as a diagnostic axis and as part of every diagnostic formulation.

Again, the discovery of the tubercle bacillus meant that internal medicine could understand that the very different syndromes of lupus vulgaris, tuberculous pulmonary cavitation, and tuberculous meningitis were, in fact, all one disease. On the other hand, the discovery of the tubercle bacillus also revealed that the pulmonary cavitation of coccidiomycosis, so similar radiologically and symptomatically to tuberculous pulmonary cavitation, was a quite different disease. Sometimes the symptoms of major depressive disorder reflect disordered brain amine metabolism responsive to medication, and sometimes the same symptoms reflect an integrated, neurobiologically determined cry for help.

Second, internal medicine appreciates that almost half of all visits to general physicians are made by patients with functional disorders—in other words, by patients with psychiatric illness or problems in living who have displaced, projected, repressed, or transformed these problems into serviceable medical complaints (Vaillant et al. 1970; Von Korff et al. 1987). Put differently, pain often should be used to lead us to the primary cause and not be mindlessly eradicated. In addition, recent research indicates that short-term psychotherapy—the deciphering of the somatic complaint—can significantly reduce the number of future visits to physicians by 5% to 85% (Jones and Vischi 1979). In parallel fashion, complaints of panic, of depression, and of suicidal ideation are often brought to psychiatrists to communicate distress in living. Because patients speak to doctors in such symbols, psychiatrists, like internists, must have a diagnostic means of deciphering these symbols. Of course, psychiatric complaints often do have an organic basis that needs immediate attention; so do the complaints of fully half of the patients who visit a general practitioner. But psychiatrists, like internists, still require a means of decoding their patients' chief complaints when they are only symptoms of dis-ease.

In addition, some patients turn to psychiatrists for complaints that seem to make sense to nobody, let alone to their general practitioners. Artists call such complaints metaphor; psychoanalysts call them primary process; cognitive psychologists call them hot cognition; and the patients' friends and relations regard them as *unreason*. In other words, psychiatry must concern itself with the uncertain, affective interplay between the hypothalamus, the limbic system, and the motor cortex—an interplay distorted by both the dimension of time and the alchemy of memory. As an observer says of Ophelia's melancholic, psychotic ramblings, "Her speech is nothing, yet the unshaped use of it doth move the hearers to collection." An axis of defenses provides us with a metaphorical language for discussing such complexities in our diagnostic formulations. An axis of defenses also provides a language for unreason that in turn informs our treatment plan. Walter Kaufmann (1980), the Princeton philosopher, called this language Sigmund Freud's "poetic science."

A third lesson psychiatry can learn from the rest of medicine is the internist's understanding of *referred* pain. A pain in the right shoulder may reflect cholecystitis; a pain in the left shoulder may reflect coronary thrombosis. Proper diagnosis depends upon the internist's seeing behind the symptom. Displacement is no less important in psychiatry than it is in medicine. By understanding that a task of much psychopathology is to conceal or to displace the source of conflict, we learn not to take the psychiatric symptoms too literally. Thus, it was diagnostic advances in clinical neurology that allowed Sigmund Freud to appreciate that defense mechanisms, not neural defects, underlay conversion reactions, and that conversion reactions, like edema, could reflect coping responses to trauma.

A fourth lesson that internal medicine offers to psychiatry is its understanding of the issue of compliance. When general practitioners offer effective somatic therapy to the 50% of their patients who have treatable organic disease, they appreciate that the patients' compliance in taking the prescribed medication becomes as important as the doctor prescribing the correct medicine in the first place. But the etiology of noncompliance is often not what it seems. Cognitive lecturing and rational explanation may be of no avail in getting a patient to take medicine (or, for example, to stop smoking). Unconscious defenses such as *reaction formation, turning against the self, acting out,* and *hypochondriasis* can all underlie a patient's failure to take medicine. Psychiatrists sometimes forget that understanding the dynamics of noncompliance is as important as monitoring compliance and prescribing the right drug.

Fifth, much modern medical research is focused upon Ambroïse Paré's famous dictum, "I dress the wound, God heals it." Appreciating and working in concert with the body's natural healing processes are essential to modern immunology. An adequate diagnostic system must be able to appreciate when "pathological" symptoms represent "healthy" inflammation. Experts in infectious disease regard pus as "laudable" and have learned how to facilitate, not suppress, the productive cough of chronic bronchiectasis. Surgeons know better than to relieve a lancinating pain beneath McBurney's point with paregoric. Indeed, the only psychiatrist ever to win a Nobel Prize was Julius Wagner von Jaurreg for using malaria to *give* his syphilitic patients a high fever. Thus, internists no longer thoughtlessly medicate people for cough and bellyache. Instead, they search for cause— the fish bone caught in the trachea or the inflamed appendix that needs removal. The same search for underlying cause may be necessary for understanding and working in concert with many "personality" and "major depressive" disorders.

In short, to understand defenses is to teach ourselves humility and to appreciate that the ego is wiser than we are. By understanding homeostasis, immunology, and natural healing processes, both internal medicine and surgery took giant steps forward. Only in the last half-century have the two disciplines of medicine and surgery learned how to become allies to the curative potential of the human body *instead* of its adversaries. In the same manner, understanding the homeostatic value of defense mechanisms will allow psychotherapists to appreciate that they serve as servants to, rather than masters of, psychological healing processes. The human ego, like the immune system, continues to provide human beings with better therapy than the best-trained physician or the most up-to-date pharmacy. We all must learn to understand and to work with this valuable ally.

The following is an illuminating case history of how a biologically sophisticated psychiatrist followed these principles in treating a woman with obsessions and compulsions. The case history was published by Ron Morstyn (1988), a psychiatrist who earlier in his career helped to develop use of brain electrical activity mapping (BEAM) in brain imaging. Remember, Sigmund Freud and Adolf Meyer, too, began *their* careers looking at diseased brains under the microscope.

Morstyn's case illustrates that formulating a patient's needs in terms of underlying defenses is as important as the wise understanding of objective symptomatology and biological psychiatry. "The patient," Morstyn tells us,

was a 29-year-old intelligent overseas student doing postdoctoral work in Australia. Immediately prior to presentation, she had been prescribed clomipramine continuously for 5 years for treatment of severe obsessional thoughts. The obsessions related largely to physical concerns about her bowels, to thoughts about ill-fitting clothes, and to perfectionistic concerns about her work. However, any daily concern could become an obsession. Her attempts to eradicate these intrusive and persistent thoughts included distraction, sleep, and willpower, but without much success. Her functioning was severely compromised, particularly with regard to her academic work, of which she held very high standards.

The first psychiatrist she attended told her that her obsessional symptoms were the result of a chemical imbalance and prescribed clomipramine. Every 2 or 3 months for the succeeding 5 years she saw either him or another psychiatrist for further prescriptions. She found that the clomipramine significantly controlled her obsessions without completely eradicating them. Her dose of medication had ranged up to 300 mg/day depending on the intensity of her obsessions. Some previous attempts to wean herself off the medication had resulted in relapse before cessation.

She originally presented to me [Morstyn] for a repeat prescription of her clomipramine. During the interview I discovered that she was involved in a sadomasochistic relationship with a man who controlled her every movement and was so jealous of her that she was not, for example, allowed to walk on the beach or look at other men. I found it surprising that this relationship did not ostensibly seem to bother her. Indeed, she appeared to admire her partner's strong will. Further questioning revealed that she had been brought up by a very dominant and autocratic father who did not suffer any disagreement with his authority, and an ineffectual, though intellectual, mother . . .

Morstyn certainly wondered if his patient had too little striatal serotonin. He also wondered whether her obsessions and compulsions meant that his patient had *isolated* her anger from her awareness and had *displaced* her awareness of conflict with an important person onto her more neutral obsessions over her bowels. He wondered if his patients' obsessive symptomatology meant that she had maintained a *reaction formation* against ever expressing anger.

Morstyn continues his case report:

I do not wish to discuss all the vicissitudes of her therapy, but only to focus on a very clear pattern that emerged each time her clomipramine dosage was reduced. This pattern was so obvious that it became a hidden agenda between us. Following each reduction [of clomipramine] there would be a period of intensification of her symptoms. She had usually submitted to a sadistic demand of her partner just prior to the onset of her obsessions. The greater the submission, the greater was the ferocity of her symptoms. After she had worked through this behaviour, usually by a combination of understanding its childhood origins, its transference implications, and being supported to stand up to her persecutor, she would feel better and the symptoms would abate . . .

By the time she was medication-free, she had broken off the above relationship and started dating a very different man who respected her as an equal. . . . That is not to say that her obsessions completely disappeared. On the contrary, although they were no longer crippling or inhibiting her functioning, they were still present from time to time. But now the patient almost welcomed these occasional intrusions as signals from her subconscious that there was something she was not addressing in her life—a warning that her old submissive habits were returning. (Morstyn 1988, pp. 190–191)

This case vignette illustrates that psychiatrists must learn to understand defenses as internists understand inflammation. They must appreciate that psychiatric symptom clusters may meet criteria for both Axis I diagnosis and Adolf Meyer's (1908) "reaction-types." Too often, modern diagnostic psychiatry fails to pay adequate attention to the difference between disease process, on the one hand, and homeostatic mechanisms, on the other. Too often we classify the magnitude of our patients' inflammation and ignore what lies beneath. At present, there is no place in DSM-III for encouraging physicians to concern themselves with psychological pathogenesis. Even in DSM-III-R (American Psychiatric Association 1987), ego defense mechanisms are relegated to the glossary. Our diagnostic manuals need a psychodynamic axis, and our medical curriculum needs to focus the attention of students on mechanisms of defense.

To use an axis of defensive or adaptive style in order to formulate the case history of Morstyn's patient—the biological component of her illness identified by Axis I notwithstanding—we might add the following paragraph to her medical chart:

Via the mechanism of isolation, the young woman had no conscious awareness of her angry affect or resentment; via the mechanism of reaction formation against her own wished-for independence, she admired her boyfriend's "strong will" and responded to his dominance with "willing" submission; and via the mechanism of displacement, she worried about her ill-fitting clothes rather than her ill-fitting relationship.

Clearly, until such a formulation is supported by clinical follow-up, it must remain a clinical hypothesis. Because etiology in psychiatry is uncertain, some psychiatrists believe that it is an advantage to ignore etiology altogether. Similarly, because he was uncertain of its etiology, Sydenham chose to call edema a disease. But modern psychiatrists must be expert at both descriptive and dynamic diagnosis. The effort to create a descriptive nosology that is atheoretical with regard to etiology creates a polarity between classification and explanatory formulation that is artificial. It may be that the task of an adequate diagnostic system is to appreciate the fact that most psychiatric disorders, like arteriosclerotic vascular disease, *are* the sum of multiple interacting causes. Nevertheless, etiological complexity does not mean that diagnosis can ever ignore cause.

To further illustrate the need for an adaptive axis, let me turn to the very heart of biological psychiatry: the hypothalamic-pituitary-adrenal (HPA) axis. John Mason (1968), in reviewing psychoendocrine research on the pituitary-adrenal cortical system, has suggested that we can never hope to understand human biology without taking defense mechanisms into account. "One of the interesting findings," he noted,

> in some of the chronic "low" 17-OHCS [17-hydroxycorticoid] excretors has been a tendency to *suppress* 17-OHCS levels lower on stressful days than on uneventful days. This phenomenon was seen recently in a most striking manner in a study of 17-OHCS levels in helicopter medic and combat units in Vietnam. It is thus clear that future psychoendocrine studies must take into consideration not only emotional state, but also those psychological mechanisms which are concerned with counteracting or minimizing emotional arousal. (p. 585)

Let me now turn to a hypothetical example. I wish to illustrate how by deploying different "psychological mechanisms which are concerned with counteracting or minimizing emotional arousal" to solve the same conflict, an individual might receive very different diagnoses. In each case the underlying conflict (etiology) would be the same. In each case were the conflict removed, the patient would recover. Some adaptive reactions or modes of "denial" lead to very severe psychopathology; some modes of "denial" result in no psychopathology at all. My example is analogous to the wide variety of clinical pictures that result from a tuberculous infection.

A 30-year-old Chinese-American businessman finds himself dishonored and threatened by the illegal business practices of his 65-year-old father and business partner, whom previously he has never consciously mistrusted. From his culture and upbringing, the son believes that he should continue to honor his father; but in his limbic system and amygdala he feels, "I hate my father; my father is my enemy." The young businessman is presented a reality that the father has defrauded his son's customers, a discovery for which he has had no time to prepare; but in terms of his affectional ties he finds that he can neither live with his business partner nor abandon his filial relationship with his father. In short, the young man's conflict extends well beyond a psychoanalytic model in which his culture (superego) and his emotions (id) are at war with each other. His conflict involves people as well as drives, and external reality as well as inner life. Changes in the young Chinese businessman's reality and in his personal relationships have produced *external* social conflict as dynamically important as his *internal* conflict over his patricidal impulses. Similarly, his conflicts over anger, grief, and dependency are just as salient as his conflicts might have been over forbidden libidinal conflicts had they also been present.

The son either must consciously experience both the *idea* and the *feeling* of hating his father, which will lead to profound anxiety, depression, and psychological stress; or in some way must alter his inner and/or outer reality. This process of psychological alteration may or may not lead to his being classified as mentally ill using DSM-III criteria. Table 2-1 offers a series of possible homeostatic transformations of his conflict that his ego might employ to protect him from conscious stress.

The discipline of cognitive psychology, with its attention to self-deception and to regulatory mental mechanisms, is just as well qualified as psychoanalysis to describe and offer theoretical metaphors to describe these homeostatic transformations. The only advantage of psychoanalytic concepts over cognitive psychology is that the Freudian metaphors introduced in Chapter 1 offer a more familiar language to describe integrative mental processes whose underlying neurophysiology is unknown.

Over 80 years ago Adolf Meyer was well aware of the value and promise of this approach to psychopathology. "To realize," Meyer explained,

> that such a reaction is *a faulty response or substitution of an insufficient or protective or evasive or mutilated attempt at adjustment* opens ways of inquiry in the direction of modifiable determining factors; and all of a sudden we find ourselves in a live field, in harmony with our instincts of action, of prevention, of modification, and of an understanding, doing justice to a desire for directness, instead of neurologizing tautology. (quoted in Lief 1948, p. 199)

And Meyer was trained as a neuropathologist.

To conclude, the value of a separate axis for defenses will be to separate defensive style from diagnosis. For example, although projection and schizoid fantasy are common in schizophrenia, many schizophrenic individuals in partial remission present more like individuals with a passive-aggressive character disorder. This is because during remission from psychiatric disorder, defensive patterns may change. Anger previously held in fantasy or projected now is more openly acknowledged even as it is turned against the self. Conversely, under stress, many relatively healthy individuals, like my hypothetical Chinese-American businessman, will appear as if afflicted with an Axis II disorder.

In other words, understanding defenses becomes as important to treatment as it is to diagnosis. Let me list a few of the roles that an axis for defenses could play in treatment as well as diagnostic formulation. First, defenses can serve as a shorthand for describing stereotyped "scripts" or "games people play" in stressful situations. Thus, even if we must remain unconscious of our own defenses, understanding the defenses of another person allows us to empathize rather than condemn, to understand rather than dismiss.

Second, defenses provide a way of making unreason reasonable. Defenses, like poetry, provide us a language to discuss the interplay of feelings and ideas. The image-distorting defenses (e.g., splitting, devaluation)—to be discussed in Chapters 7 and 11 by Bond and by Perry and Cooper, respectively—permit us a poetic means of discussing internalized cognitive schemata of internalized relationships in a way that allows clinicians to communicate with each other.

Third, defenses are important to treatment. If we can decipher a patient's code, we can provide a holding environment and stabilize his or her sense of self. For example, when distressed in a foreign country, we find ourselves compounding our difficulties in not being understood by shouting. As a result we not only remain misunderstood but also become increasingly unpopular. When, finally, we find someone who speaks our language, we calm down and speak reasonably. Patients are no different. When we understand the meaning behind their words, they, too, calm down.

Fourth, in psychiatry we have few ways to monitor the healing process. Ultimately, success at working and at loving may be the two best indicators that we have that a person has recovered from psychiatric disability. However, before a suitable job opening or the right lover has appeared on the scene, a shift in the maturity of defensive style may be our best clue. Thus, during recovery from psychotic decompensation, changes in defensive level can be observed that appear to parallel the healing process. In a 50-year follow-up of remitting schizophrenic individuals (Vaillant 1963), I observed that during remission the defense of intellectualization often supplanted the defenses of denial, distortion, and projection more characteristic of their psychosis. In a 12-year follow-up of individuals addicted to narcotics (Vaillant 1966), I noted that abstinent substance abusers appeared to abandon the life-styles of acting out and passive-aggressive behavior in favor of the hypothetically more mature patterns of isolation, dissociation, altruism, and reaction formation.

This pattern of defensive shift with remission of psychopathology can also be illustrated by a case history. The clinical example is taken from the Harvard Study of Adult Development (to be described more fully in Chapter 6).

> During his adolescence, Dr. Herman Crabbe, a future electronics engineer, was extremely dependent upon his eccentric, overbearingly possessive mother. He used projection and schizoid fantasy to deal with his conflicts. In college Dr. Crabbe had exhibited no desire to be with other

Table 2–1. Contrasting ways of altering the conscious representation of a conflict

Defense	Conscious representation of idea, feeling, or behavior		DSM-III phenomenological diagnosis*
No defense	I HATE (!) MY FATHER.	309.9	Adjustment reaction with mixed emotional features
Psychotic defense			
Denial	I WAS BORN WITHOUT A FATHER.	298.8	Brief reactive psychosis
Immature defenses			
Projection	MY FATHER HATES (!) ME.	301.0	Paranoid personality disorder
Passive aggression	I HATE (!) MYSELF (suicide attempt).	300.4	Dysthymic disorder
Acting out	WITHOUT REFLECTION, I HIT 12 POLICEMEN.	301.7	Antisocial personality disorder
Fantasy	I DAYDREAM OF KILLING GIANTS.	301.2	Schizoid personality disorder
Neurotic (intermediate) defenses			
Dissociation	I TELL MY FATHER JOKES.	300.1	Dissociation disorder
Displacement	I HATE (!) MY FATHER'S DOG.	300.29	Simple phobia
Isolation (or intellectualization)	I DISAPPROVE OF FATHER'S BUSINESS PRACTICES.	300.3	Obsessive-compulsive disorder
Repression	I DO NOT KNOW WHY I FEEL SO HOT AND BOTHERED.	300.02	Generalized anxiety disorder
Reaction formation	I LOVE (!) MY FATHER OR I HATE (!) FATHER'S ENEMIES.		No psychiatric disorder but may be associated with unexplained muscle tension
Mature defenses			
Suppression	I AM CROSS AT FATHER BUT WILL NOT TELL HIM.		—
Sublimation	I BEAT FATHER AT PING-PONG.		—
Altruism	I COMFORT FATHER HATERS.		—

*Diagnosis assumes that conscious representation of the conflict was carried to pathological extremes and that the other criteria for the diagnosis were met.
Source. Reprinted, with permission, from Vaillant GE: Defense mechanisms, in *The New Harvard Guide to Psychiatry.* Edited by Nicholi AM Jr. Cambridge, MA, Harvard University Press, 1988, p 205.

people. He explained to the study staff that "everyone is out to get as much as he can. It doesn't pay to pay much attention to the other fellow." The Study staff in turn described him as "solitary, stammery, unkempt and ill-bred." The Study of Adult Development's clinical psychologist, psychiatrist, and anthropologist all concurred in diagnosing him as having a schizoid personality disorder. They all believed that he should never have been included in a study of healthy adult development. Crabbe graduated from Harvard in physics with a brilliant record.

During his mid-30s his possessive mother died and his relationship with his hitherto eclipsed father improved markedly. For the first time Dr. Crabbe realized that solitary laboratory work alone would not win him everything he wanted from life. For the first time in his life, during this same period, he experienced conscious depression. He sought psychotherapy, and coincident with his therapy a change was noted in both his defenses and his life-style. Thus, in middle-life, he found himself in a safer world. When asked to describe what he liked most about his job with a West Coast electronics company, he replied, "Working with people." [He was then a research group leader.] He added that he had never imagined such a shift in his values to be possible. Schizoid fantasy was replaced by its logical successor, intellectualization. Crabbe lived his life on a strict schedule. Each event of the day was ritualized, and all his social relationships were either at work or with his wife. Although he was reserved, I was impressed as we talked by the extraordinary candor with which he discussed his own psychological workings. He described sexual problems graphically but without emotion.

Dr. Crabbe's projection also gave way to its more mature first cousin, displacement. [By this I mean that as individuals mature or recover from psychiatric decompensation, the defense of projection can be perceived to evolve into displacement and reaction formation.] When his mother died of breast cancer, he suddenly noticed pains in his own chest and wondered if he had finally developed the heart trouble that his mother had always insisted that he had. Later, as he increasingly accepted jobs that allowed him to work with people more and test tubes less, he became less preoccupied with a sense of persecution. But this previously indefatigable scientist found that this new sort of work "exhausted him." He took a vacation for his "health." But after the vacation he did not seek medical attention for "fatigue." Instead, he sought psychiatric help for "depression" (i.e., for his conflict over moving from interest in test tubes toward interest in people).

Paradoxically, as with the prior case of the obsessional woman described by Morstyn, the price of abandoning pathological defenses is often one of experiencing more conscious dysphoric emotion. For example, instead of devaluing the whole occasion of his upcoming college reunion, Crabbe displaced his reluctance to join the disturbing conviviality onto the effort that it took him to drive 400 to Cambridge and onto the dangers of a possible flu epidemic. In each case, Crabbe's ego evaded full responsibility for his fears. But whereas his earlier style had led the study staff to perceive him as mentally ill, at age 52 by the criteria that the study used to assess its members, Herman Crabbe was relatively healthy.

Of course, there are formidable problems in assessing defenses and making them part of our diagnostic formulation. Discussion of these difficulties will concern the last half of this book, but let me acknowledge a few of the difficulties here. First, it must be remembered that the whole concept of mechanisms of defense is metaphorical. In the words of T. R. Sarbin (1968), "[W]hen the metaphor turns myth, the system closes. . . . Newton's advice is worth noting here: Scientists should take their hypothetical constructs lightly" (p. 417). We will never be able to measure defenses in milligrams per cubic centimeter.

Second, because their characteristic defenses are unknown to them, patients will have difficulty in identifying and reporting their defensive style to an interested clinician. Instead, assessment of defensive style must be largely based on clinical inference from a diversity of clues. In marked contrast, the assessment of psychiatric symptoms such as phobias, sadness, and hallucinations may be apparent to all without inference. This means that rater reliability in identifying defenses will always be inferior to rater reliability in identifying the major symptoms of an Axis I disorder. Such difficulties in reliability were a major reason for not including defenses in DSM-III. However, medicine faces the same problem with referred pain. The diagnosis of anginal pain referred to an arm or chin is less certain than when it occurs over the heart but provides an equally valid clue. Clinicians must accept the fact that clinical validity and reliability are not synonymous. The polythetic criteria for diagnosing borderline personality disorder are reliable but not particularly valid (Zanarini et al. 1991). As several of the empirical chapters in this book will demonstrate, the validity of defense mechanisms often exceeds their reliability.

References

American Psychiatric Association: Diagnostic and Statistical Manual of Mental Disorders, 3rd Edition. Washington, DC, American Psychiatric Association, 1980

American Psychiatric Association: Diagnostic and Statistical Manual of Mental Disorders, 3rd Edition, Revised. Washington, DC, American Psychiatric Association, 1987

Jones K, Vischi T: Impact of alcohol, drug abuse and mental health treatment on medical care utilization: a review of the research literature. Med Care 17(12) (suppl):1–82, 1979

Karasu TB, Skodol AE: VIth axis for DSM-III: psychodynamic evaluation. Am J Psychiatry 137:607–610, 1980

Kaufmann W: Discovering the Mind, Vol 3: Freud Versus Adler and Jung. New York, McGraw-Hill, 1980

Lief A: The Common Sense Psychiatry of Dr. Adolf Meyer. New York, McGraw-Hill, 1948

Mason J: A review of psychoendocrine research in the pituitary-adrenal cortical system. Psychosom Med 30:576–607, 1968

Meyer A: The problems of mental reaction-types, mental causes amd diseases. Psychol Bull 5:245–258, 1908

Morstyn R: Clomipramine in obsessional disorders: a cautionary tale. Aust N Z J Psychiatry 22:190–194, 1988

Osler W: The Principles and Practice of Medicine. New York, D Appleton, 1892

Sarbin TR: Ontology recapitulates philology: the mythic nature of anxiety. Am Psychol 23:411–418, 1968

Sartorius N, Jablensky A, Regier DA (eds): Sources and Traditions of Classification in Psychiatry. Toronto, Hogrefe and Huber, 1990

Sydenham T: Opera Universa (1685). Translated by Swan J. London, E Cave, 1753

Vaillant GE: The natural history of the remitting schizophrenics. Am J Psychiatry 120:367–375, 1963

Vaillant GE: A twelve-year follow-up of New York narcotic addicts, IV: some characteristics and determinants of abstinence. Am J Psychiatry 123:573–584, 1966

Vaillant GE, Shapiro LN, Schmitt PP: Psychological motives for medical hospitalization. JAMA 214:1661–1665, 1970

Von Korff M, Shapiro S, Burke J, et al: Anxiety and depression in a primary care clinic. Arch Gen Psychiatry 44:152–156, 1987

Zanarini MC, Gunderson JG, Frankenburg FR, et al: The face validity of the DSM-III and DSM-III-R criteria sets for borderline personality disorder. Am J Psychiatry 148:870–874, 1991

Chapter 3

The Need for a Uniform Nomenclature for Defenses

George E. Vaillant, M.D.

One of the great obstacles to clinical acceptance of defense mechanisms, as suggested in Chapter 1, is the inability of investigators to find a means of talking about them. Not only do heterogeneous social scientists have difficulty with a common language for coping and defending, but even orthodox Freudian psychoanalysts cannot agree upon a nomenclature. One of the leading investigators of coping, Richard Lazarus, has warned that "rapid progress in the development of an adequate psychology of coping is unlikely until a theoretically based system of classification for coping responses has been evolved" (Lazarus et al. 1974, p. 307). Lazarus underscores the difficulties surrounding nomenclature in two ways. First, research in defenses will be profoundly hampered until a consensually agreed upon nomenclature is established. Second, consensus on the very nature of coping responses is lacking. By using the term "coping" rather than "defense," Lazarus illustrates the theoretical abyss that exists between the three disciplines of *psychodynamic psychiatry* (with its emphasis upon unconscious mechanisms of defense), *experimental psychology* (with its emphasis on conscious coping strategies and stress management), and *social psychology* (with its emphasis on the importance of social supports). In this chapter, which by necessity narrows the field of inquiry, our goal is to address Lazarus's challenge and to provide a theoretically based system of coping responses.

Three distinct classes of coping can be illustrated by an analogy. Consider the case of a person who has cut himself or herself badly. First, the injured individual could seek the help of a paramedic or utilize his or her health insurance for access to an emergency room. Such a response would be an example of coping via *social supports*. Second, thanks to training in emergency medicine, the injured individual could, himself or herself, place pressure on the cut artery and apply a tourniquet. This would be an example of a *conscious coping strategy*. Third, the individual could do nothing and his or her platelets, thromboplastin, fibrinogen, and factor VII would eventually stop the hemorrhage. This third possibility is an example of *unconscious, involuntary coping* and is analogous to the concept of ego mechanisms of defense. All three classes of behavior reflect broad classes of coping mechanisms. Researchers like Richard Lazarus and Albert Bandura have paid particular attention to conscious coping strategies. Such strategies—like the use of a tourniquet—have the virtue of being able to be taught with a resulting sense of increased morale and self-efficacy. This book, however, will be about the third class of coping—unconscious "ego mechanisms of defense"—which, like clotting mechanisms, are of greater interest to clinicians than to teachers and to consumers of self-help.

Even with this clarification theorists argue whether ego mechanisms of defense are not *sometimes* conscious. They also argue whether there is a meaningful distinction between unconscious *coping* and unconscious *defense* mechanisms. Finally, theorists argue whether defense mechanisms can protect against threatening *external reality* as well as against unconscious internal conflicts. Each of these three questions artificially splits psychobiological reality into black and white, when, in fact, the answer in all three cases must be gray.

First, depending on how a hypnotic subject is studied, the same phenomena can be demonstrated to be both conscious and unconscious. Defenses are no different. Second, distinction is often made between "defenses" and "coping mechanisms" (Haan 1963; Murphy 1962). Investigators making this distinction think of defense mechanisms as being more analogous to a reflex and more often associated with psychopathological disturbance (e.g., projection). They think of coping mechanisms as more conscious and closer to the flexible behavior of every day (e.g., altruism). However, I would argue that depending on the circumstances, the time frame, and one's definition of outcome, both blood clotting and projection can be classed as either adaptive or maladaptive. Defenses cope and coping defends. Third, because the perceived danger of an external threat always depends upon internal appraisal, and, conversely, because internal conflict arises from formerly external antecedents, a clear distinction cannot be made between external and internal conflict.

Let me put these questions aside and offer a working definition of this third class of coping. Ego mechanisms of defense reflect the ways in which an individual involuntarily copes with sudden changes in his or her external and internal milieu. Such changes may be produced by instinctual demands and overwhelming affects, by interpersonal conflict, by cultural taboos and unexpected pangs of conscience, or by sudden alterations in external reality. Ego mechanisms of defense differ from the other two broad classes of coping in that 1) they are relatively unconscious, 2) they often form the building blocks of psychopathology, 3) in the service of healing they often effect creative mental synthesis, and 4) they repress, deny, and distort internal and external reality and thus often appear *odd* or irrational to observers.

Some inferred "purposes" of ego mechanisms of defense are as follows:

1. To keep affects within bearable limits during sudden alterations in one's emotional life (e.g., following acute object loss or during sudden awareness of heightened intimacy *with* or dependence *upon* a taboo person)
2. To restore psychological "homeostasis" by postponing or deflecting sudden increases in biological drives (e.g., sexual awareness and "instinctual anxiety" during adolescence)
3. To obtain a "time out" to master changes in self-image or self schemata that cannot be immediately integrated (e.g., puberty, major surgery, promotion)
4. To handle unresolvable conflict with important people living or dead of whom one cannot bear to take leave (e.g., "object anxiety")

What I have said so far is not really controversial. Rather, the real difficulty arises in achieving consensual agreement on different styles of defense. The semantic difficulties in distinguishing good and bad denial, and in naming adaptive and maladaptive coping responses, are daunting. First, because defenses are metaphors, their identification reflects, as with facial recognition and interpretation of proverbs, a high order of conceptualization. Second, assigning labels to defenses is as idiosyncratic as labeling colors or perfume scents. Splitters and lumpers can argue forever, and the multiplicity of names threatens to derail the whole process of empirical validation and communication between clinicians.

Even if nomenclature of defenses is limited to relatively uniform psychoanalytic literature, the lack of a common language is striking. In 1973, Hans Sjöbäck reviewed 12 psychoanalytic authors, who among themselves had described 27 distinct mechanisms of defense, only 7 of which were noted by 11 of the 12 writers. Fifteen years later, Manfred Beutel (1988) reviewed 17 psychoanalytically informed authors (e.g., Anna Freud, Otto Fenichel) and identified 37 different terms for defense mechanisms. Only 5 of these 37 mechanisms—repression, displacement, isolation, reaction formation, and projection—were cited by 15 of Beutel's 17 authors, and only 14 of his 37 terms were cited by as many as 5 out of 17 authors. Unfortunately, psychologists employ quite different metaphors for defenses than psychoanalysts. I shall not even begin to discuss these different nomenclatures except to note that, in their exhaustive reviews, Ihilevich and Gleser (1986) and Cramer (1991) have provided the best entrées to a vast psychological literature.

Let me offer a dramatic example of the semantic difficulties surrounding nomenclature. Within a 30-mile radius of San Francisco until recently there were five groups of investigators who had each devised highly influential systems for classifying defense mechanisms. Not only was there virtually no overlap of terms among these five groups, but there was no effort by any one group to translate its own nomenclature into that of a neighboring laboratory. Such diversity of language makes the construction of Lazarus's "theoretically based system of classification of coping responses" (Lazarus et al. 1974, p. 307) as difficult as building the Tower of Babel.

It is instructive to describe these five working groups in more detail. First, Mardi Horowitz et al. (1990), at the University of California Medical School at San Francisco, has been trained in the traditional psychoanalytic approach to defenses, but he does not consider defenses fundamental processes. Instead, he considers defenses as the manifest outcome of more basic cognitive "control processes." He follows an information-processing approach to classifying defenses and has assigned these processes 29 labels drawn from cognitive psychology (e.g., "sequencing ideas by switching concepts," "sliding meanings," "altering self-schemas") (Horowitz 1988). Horowitz's ambitious and important goal reflects his effort to help psychoanalysis join the "cognitive revolution." Whether his approach is successful must depend on whether the higher intellectual activities underlying defensive mental processes can yield to the reductionistic processes used to analyze information processing. A problem is that defense mechanisms, like creativity and most personality traits, must remain metaphors.

The second nomenclature for defenses was devised by Norma Haan (1963, 1977) at the University of California at Berkeley. Like Horowitz, Haan has been influenced by psychoanalytic theory and has proposed a model of 30 linked processes. Ten processes reflect "coping," 10 reflect "defending," and 10 reflect what Haan has called "fragmentation." Of the five California models that I am describing, Haan's is the closest to the nomenclature proposed in this book. Nevertheless, only 8 of her 30 terms are the same as the 17 terms that I introduced in Chapter 1.

Third, at Berkeley, Richard Lazarus and Susan Folkman (Folkman and Lazarus 1980; Lazarus 1983; Lazarus and Folkman 1984) have developed a nomenclature of coping that has been particularly influential. Lazarus is not so much concerned with unconscious conflict as with individuals' primary cognitive appraisal of what is at stake and with their conscious appraisal of what might be done to reduce the danger. Unlike many other behavioral psychologists, Lazarus acknowledges the importance of emotionally driven responses, or what he terms "hot cognition" and "emotion based" coping. He appreciates that sometimes coping processes do not necessarily entail deliberate reflection, reason, or even awareness; but his terminology has little in common with dynamic psychiatry.

Fourth, two developmental psychologists, Jack and Jeanne Block, have been conducting a very thorough longitudinal study of ego development. Block and Block (1980) have chosen to lump all coping methods into the terms "ego brittleness," "ego resilience," and "ego control."

Finally, at Stanford, Rudy Moos, along with his colleague Andrew Billings, has worked out still another completely different language for coping. Most of the terms that Moos and Billings use refer to mental processes and behaviors under relatively voluntary control (Moos and Billings 1982). Moos and Billings list 14 mechanisms that are quite distinct from the list of 22 mechanisms provided by Lazarus and Folkman, which in turn are conceptually linked to, but semantically very different from, Haan's list of 30 and from Horowitz's list of 29 mechanisms. Not surprisingly, if one moves from the San Francisco Bay area into the international arena, semantic confusion becomes completely unmanageable.

One of the intents in this book is to help psychiatry move toward a common language for defenses. Table 3-1 summarizes my own effort 20 years ago to produce a consensually derived nomenclature of 18 ego defenses (Vaillant 1971). From the defense compendia of five well-known writers who have catalogued defenses from a psychoanalytic viewpoint— Anna Freud (1937), Percival Symonds (1945), Otto Fenichel (1945), Grete Bibring (and coworkers) (1963), and Lawrence Kolb (1968)—I tried to identify a coherent group of 18 mechanisms of defense. As indicated by the dates in brackets following the names of defenses and by the quotations given in Chapter 1, 15 of the defenses were originally described by Freud. (The terms in Table 3-1 are all defined in Appendix 3 with definitions that are simply syntheses of those from the six sources cited in the table. In constructing Table 3-1 I tried to avoid reinventing the wheel.)

Nevertheless, by the mid-1970s the nomenclature for defense mechanisms remained in semantic and conceptual disarray. This disarray was clearly illustrated by a meeting held at the New York State Psychiatric Institute in the fall of 1977 in order to plan for the *Diagnostic and Statistical Manual of Mental Disorders,* Third Edition (DSM-III) (American Psychiatric Association 1980). The meeting consisted of a group of psychoanalysts with a commitment to developing defenses as a possible axis for DSM-III. Robert Spitzer had brought us together to discuss the justification of such a step. After meeting for several hours it became clear that we were unable to agree on a common list of defenses, on consensually based definitions, or on the pathological implications of certain defenses. Each member had a different view of what constituted an important set of defenses. In addition, there appeared to be an inadequate empirical framework on which to build consensus and resolve disagreement. For that reason, among others, the decision was made not to include defenses in DSM-III.

Since the 1977 DSM-III meeting, the task of consensus building has considerably progressed (see Table 3-2). An important step in this process was made during preparation for DSM-III-R when Robert Spitzer appointed in 1984 a task force on defenses to arrive at a consensus-based set of defenses. The task force was expanded to include behavioral and cognitive psychologists. In addition, in the years that had passed since 1977, a sufficient amount of empirical work on the defenses had been accomplished so that a list of 18 defenses—or adaptive mechanisms as they are called (American Psychiatric Association 1987)—could be agreed upon and defined for the glossary of DSM-III-R. This list is presented in the first column of Table 3-2. The second column in Table 3-2 lists the nomenclature provided by William Meissner (1980) for the third edition of Kaplan, Freedman, and Sadock's *Comprehensive Textbook of Psychiatry*. The third, fourth, and fifth columns of Table 3-2 list the relatively similar nomenclatures of defenses employed by the empirical investigations to be presented in this book. Admittedly, in Table 3-2 no attempt has been made to integrate the competing languages for coping and defending that exist within American psychology and European psychiatry; however, the table does provide evidence that within American psychiatry there is increasing consensus over how to discuss defenses.

In Table 3-2 the nomenclature of defenses popularized first by Melanie Klein (1957) and then by Otto Kernberg (1967) to discuss the object relations of individuals with personality disorder has been underemphasized. These terms include splitting, omnipotence, devaluation, idealization, and projective identification. These terms are well characterized in Chapter 7 by Michael Bond as "image-distorting" defenses. Object-relations school theorists in general (see Greenberg and Mitchell 1983) suggest that such methods of defense serve to alter the mental image or schemata that control which internalized aspect of self or other person is made conscious. The question may be legitimately asked why in Tables 3-1 and 3-2 these image-distorting defenses are ignored. The reason that I offer is that these mechanisms differ only in complexity but not substantively from the terms offered by Anna Freud. Just as there were a variety of "languages" for coping processes in the San Francisco Bay area in the 1980s, there were two languages for discussing unconscious conflict in London during the 1940s and 1950s: Melanie Klein's and Anna Freud's. To oversimplify, Anna Freud focused too narrowly on conflicts produced by drives, and Klein focused too narrowly on conflicts produced by relationships. But as with other scholastic arguments over details, Melanie Klein's and Anna Freud's disagreement stemmed from trying to transform what is gray into black and

Table 3–1. A theoretical hierarchy of ego defense mechanisms

	Symonds (1945)	Bibring et al. (1963)	A. Freud (1937)	Fenichel (1945)	Kolb (1968)
Level I: "Psychotic"					
Delusional projection	0	0	0	0	0
Denial (psychotic) [1894]*	0	Denial	Denial	Denial	Denial
Distortion [1896]	0	? Depersonalization	Distortion	0	0
Level II: "Immature"					
Projection [1895]	Projection	Projection	Projection	Projection	Projection
Schizoid fantasy [1908]	Fantasy	Denial through fantasy	Denial through fantasy	0	0
Hypochondriasis [1896]	0	Falling ill	Introjection	Introjection	0
Passive-aggressive behavior [1915]	Compromise formation	Compliance	Turning against the self	0	0
Acting out	0	Acting out	0	0	0
Level III: "Neurotic"					
Intellectualizaton [1894]	Intellectualization, undoing, isolation	Intellectualization, undoing, isolation	Intellectualization, undoing, isolation	Isolation, undoing	Rationalization, restitution
Repression [1894]	Repression	Repression	Repression	Repression	Repression
Displacement [1894]	Displacement	Displacement	Displacement	Displacement	Displacement
Reaction formation [1905]	Reaction formation	Reaction formation	Reaction formation	Reaction formation	Reaction formation
Dissociation [1893]	? Regression	Affectualization, counterphobia	Reversal	0	0
Level IV: "Mature"					
Altruism [1916–17]	0	Altruistic surrender	Altruism	Sublimation	0
Humor [1905]	Regression	0	0	0	0
Suppression [1894]	0	Avoidance, withdrawal	0	0	Suppression
Anticipation	0	Control through thinking	0	0	Conscious control
Sublimation [1905]	Sublimation	Sublimation	Sublimation	Sublimation	Sublimation

*Years in brackets indicate the dates Freud first considered these defenses.

white. The human limbic system links drives and people inextricably, and so does the ego and its mechanisms of defense.

The psychiatric terms for unconscious adaptation are also completely different from those terms used by cognitive psychology. Horowitz and his colleagues (1990) have made a daring effort to bridge this gap between cognitive psychology and psychiatry but at the price of creating a new terminology. Because I wish to avoid the fate of the would-be builders of the Tower of Babel, I shall resist the paradigm shift suggested by the cognitive revolution. This book, like DSM-III-R, will retain the old Freudian metaphors. In 1865 Claude Bernard, the father of experimental medicine, wisely warned:

> Our language, in fact, is only approximate; and even in science, it is so indefinite that if we lose sight of phenomena and cling to words, we are speedily out of reality. We, therefore, only injure science by arguing in favor of a word which is now merely a source of error, because it no longer expresses the same idea for everyone. Let us therefore conclude that we must always cling to phenomena. (Bernard 1927, p. 188)

Not only does psychiatry lack an accepted nomenclature of defenses, it also lacks a glossary of mutually exclusive definitions for ego mechanisms of defense. First, analogous to the status of the planet Pluto in 19th-century astronomy, defenses cannot be directly visualized; instead, they must be appreciated by their systematic distortion of those events that we can see. It is through resistances and symptoms that we infer defenses. It is hard to provide invisible processes with mutually exclusive definitions. Second, defense mechanisms describe processes rather than discrete entities, and processes always defy exact definition or measurement. Processes must usually be defined by metaphors, which by definition can convey multiple meanings. Third, defenses are often extremely short-lived, evanescent phenomena that rarely occur in isolation. Thus, the definition of a single defense is by necessity reductionistic. It is easy to understand why Freud, like Claude Bernard (1927), preferred to discuss clinical phenomena rather than to provide discrete defenses with mutually exclusive definitions.

Nevertheless, in order that the defenses be made less elusive, consensually validated and mutually exclusive definitions of the defenses must be obtained. Without clear definition, clinical recognition of and empirical research on defenses are impossible. In an effort to achieve such definition, this book has adopted two strategies. First, each of the defenses set forth in Table 3-1 has been operationally defined in Appendixes 2–5. Hopefully, the differences found in these appendixes will be complementary rather than contradictory. Second, in Table 3-3 I have tried to outline how each defense affects the important components of Freud's so-called *topographic* and

Table 3–2. A list of common defenses and their presence or absence in several nomenclatures (as described in the appendixes)

	Nomenclature/Author				
	DSM-III-R (A1)	CTP/III* (A2)	Vaillant (A3)	Perry (A4)	Jacobson (A5)
Acting out	X	X	X	X	X
Altruism		X	X	X	X
Anticipation		X	X	X	
Asceticism		X			X
Denial	X	X	X		X
Devaluation	X			X	
Displacement	X	X	X	X	X
Dissociation	X	X	X	X	
Distortion		X	X		
Fantasy	X	X	X	X	
Humor		X	X	X	
Hypochondriasis		X	X	X	
Idealization	X			X	
Intellectualization	X	X	X	X	X
Isolation	X	X		X	
Passive aggression (turning against the self)	X	X	X	X	X
Projection	X	X	X	X	X
Projection (delusional)		X	X		
Rationalization	X	X		X	X
Reaction formation	X	X	X	X	
Regression		X			
Repression	X	X	X	X	X
Somatization	X	X			
Splitting	X			X	
Sublimation		X	X	X	
Suppression	X	X	X	X	X
Undoing	X			X	

Note. The terms *blocking, controlling, externalization, introjection, inhibition,* and *sexualization* are defined only in the CTP/III (see Appendix 2). The terms *bland denial, projective identification, omnipotence, neurotic denial, affiliation, self-observation,* and *self-assertion* are defined only by Perry (see Appendix 4). The defense termed *avoidance* is defined only by Jacobson et al. (see Appendix 5). A1, A2, A3, A4, A5 designate Appendixes 1, 2, 3, 4, 5, respectively.
*Meissner's glossary of defenses from the *Modern Synopsis of Comprehensive Textbook of Psychiatry* (see Appendix 2).

Table 3–3. Differential identification of defenses

Style of defense	Sources of conflict				Expression of impulse			
	Affects/Drives	Conscience/ Culture	Relationships/ People	Reality	Self/Subject	Idea	Affect	Object
I. Psychotic								
1. Delusional projection	Externalized	Exaggerated	Distorted	Distorted	Made object	Exaggerated	Exaggerated	Made self
2. Denial	Ignored	—	Ignored	Ignored	Omnipotent	Ignored	Ignored	Ignored
3. Distortion	Exaggerated	Ignored	Distorted	Distorted	Omnipotent	Altered	Altered	Generalized
II. Immature								
1. Projection	Externalized	—	Distorted	Exaggerated	Made object	—	—	Made self
2. Fantasy	—	Ignored	Taken inside	—	Omnipotent	—	Diminished	Within self
3. Hypochondriasis	Distorted	—	Devalued	Distorted	—	Altered	Anger becomes	displaced
4. Passive aggression	Turned on self	Exaggerated	Exaggerated	—	Made object	—	—	Ignored
5. Acting out	Disinhibited	Ignored	Altered	—	Omnipotent	Ignored	Ignored	Generalized
6. Dissociation	Altered	Altered	Exaggerated	—	—	—	Altered	—

III. Neurotic								
1. Displacement	—	—	Altered	Minimized	—	—	—	Displaced
2. Isolation/ Intellectualization	Minimized	Exaggerated	Distanced	—	—	—	Ignored	—
3. Repression	Disguised	—	—	Minimized	—	Ignored	—	Ignored
4. Reaction formation	Ignored	Exaggerated	—	—	—	Reversed	Reversed	—
IV. Mature								
1. Altruism	Minimized	Exaggerated	—	—	—	—	—	Made self
2. Sublimation	Disguised	—	—	—	—	—	Diminished	—
3. Suppression	Minimized	Minimized	Minimized	Minimized	—	—	—	—
4. Anticipation	—	—	—	—	—	Diminished	Diminished	—
5. Humor	—	—	—	—	—	Exaggerated	Altered	—

structural models of mental functioning. The purpose of exploiting these two models in Table 3-3 is to provide a schema by which each of the 18 proposed mechanisms of defense listed in Table 3-2 can be systematically distinguished from the other 17. The purpose is also to substitute in diagrammatic form Claude Bernard's phenomena for words. The same process is repeated in more explicitly phenomenological form in the clinical illustrations provided in Appendix 3.

I have represented Freud's two models of the mind: the topographic model and the structural model (Table 3-3). Freud's topographic model of the mind captures conscious and unconscious expressions of impulse. Freud suggests that an affect-laden wish can be conceived of as consisting of a subject, an object, an idea, and an emotion. This model suggests that a conflictual idea-affect complex (e.g., "I hate my father") can be retained in the unconscious and replaced in consciousness by an alternative idea-affect complex—a complex distorted by the ego in a variety of mutually exclusive ways. As the last four columns of Table 3-3 suggest, a defensive process can homeostatically distort or deny *subject, object, idea,* or *affect,* or any combination thereof. For example, in projection, the subject of "I hate my father" can be switched with the object (e.g., "My father hates me"), or via displacement the object can be altered (e.g., "I hate my father's dog"), or via isolation the affect can be denied with only the idea left in awareness (e.g., "I sometimes entertain hostile thoughts toward my father"), or via repression the idea can be denied (e.g., "I feel angry when I am in my father's house, but I don't know why"). I hope that my two uses of the term *denial* are clear. On the one hand, all defenses deny—in the broad sense—something. On the other hand, the defense of psychotic denial denies the perception of relevant external reality in the time present.

In his structural model of the mind, Freud focused more on the sources of conflict. The structural model conceptualized the *ego* as mediating between *conscience/culture* (*superego*) and *affects/drives* (*id*). To these two intrapsychic sources of conflict, as already suggested earlier in this chapter, modern psychiatrists interested in object relations and in ego psychology have added "people" and "reality." Thus, as outlined in the first four columns of Table 3-3, defenses can systematically alter or deny drives, conscience, other people, or reality, or any combination of these sources of mental conflict.

By the term *affects/drives,* I mean our emotions and our desires (hunger, grief, lust, rage, and so on). Psychoanalysts call this lodestar of conflict "id," moralists call it "sin," cognitive psychologists refer to it as "hot cognition," and neuroanatomists label it the hypothalamic and limbic regions of the brain. Freud lumped all "drives" under the term *libido,* but there are many other affects or drives. Grief, anger, and dependency all loom quite as important as sex as sources of conflict.

By the term *conscience*—the "superego" of psychoanalysis—I do not mean just those precepts that we absorbed from our mother and father before the age of 5 years. By conscience I mean our whole identification with our society, with our culture, and with our own ego ideals. Erik Erikson's view of culture—indeed, Freud's own view of civilization and its discontents—has led even the most simplistic psychoanalyst to view the superego as far more than the internalized parents of a young child. The roots of our conscience continue to grow throughout our lives.

People form the third lodestar of conflict. And by people I mean both our real-world relationships and our internalized representations of people living or dead. People become a source of conflict when we cannot live with them and cannot live without them. Death is the most obvious example, but there are many others. There are individuals to whom we are peculiarly attached but with whom we are not at peace. Obvious examples are the boss whom we strive to please but also hate, the scapegoat whom we abuse but would mourn were he or she to disappear, and the lover who terrifies us by exclaiming "Yes!" to our rather tentative proposal of marriage. Equally important are the people from our past who are incompletely "metabolized." Memories of past loves and hates live on inside.

By the term *reality,* the fourth lodestar, I mean those facets of our external environment that are capable of changing more rapidly than our ability to adapt. The drought of the Australian outback and the Amazonian damp are not stressful to those aboriginal persons for whom such drought and damp are predictable and unchanging. But five inches of snow—a mere flurry in Montreal and a blessing at Aspen or St. Moritz—can paralyze Paris or Washington, D.C. *Familiar* shifts in reality elicit conscious coping strategies and social supports, whereas *unfamiliar* shifts in reality elicit involuntary coping strategies (i.e., Anna Freud's ego mechanisms of defense).

In assessing odd and irrational behavior, clinicians can use the schema in Table 3-3 to differentiate defensive styles with much greater precision. Like a prism, by distinguishing the four lodestars of conflict, Table 3-3 can be used to refract the Platonic term "denial" into mutually exclusive processes. For example, the table notes that acting out can ignore *conscience,* reaction formation can ignore *desire,* psychotic denial can ignore *reality,* and fantasy can ignore *external relationships* by creating new ones within. As will be pointed out in Chapters 6 and 8, distinctions made on these principles are not trivial.

The lesson to be drawn from these three tables are not that they represent truth, but that they represent a process for rescuing the metaphorical but very useful concepts of ego mechanisms of defense from semantic chaos. As the subsequent empirical chapters in Section II written by different investigators will suggest, these tables are not the last word.

Rather, they represent a point of departure for the systematic empirical study of defenses and for the inclusion of defensive styles in our clinical and diagnostic formulations.

References

American Psychiatric Association: Diagnostic and Statistical Manual of Mental Disorders, 3rd Edition. Washington, DC, American Psychiatric Association, 1980

American Psychiatric Association: Diagnostic and Statistical Manual of Mental Disorders, 3rd Edition, Revised. Washington, DC, American Psychiatric Association, 1987

Bernard C: An Introduction to the Study of Experimental Medicine. New York, MacMillan, 1927

Beutel M: Bewältigungs-prozesse bei chronischen Erkrankungen. Munich, VCH, 1988

Bibring GL, Dwyer TF, Huntington DS, et al: A study of the psychological process in pregnancy and of the earliest mother-child relationship, II: methodological considerations. Psychoanal Stud Child 16:25–72, 1963

Block JH, Block J: The role of ego-control and ego-resiliency, in Development of Cognitive, Affect and Social Relations: The Minnesota Symposium on Child Psychology, Vol 13. Edited by Collins WA. Hillsdale, NJ, Lawrence Erlbaum, 1980, pp 70–87

Cramer P: The Development of Defense Mechanisms: Theory, Research and Assessment. New York, Springer, 1991

Fenichel O: The Psychoanalytical Theory of Neurosis. New York, WW Norton, 1945

Folkman S, Lazarus R: An analysis of coping in a middle-aged community sample. J Health Soc Behav 21:219–239, 1980

Freud A: The Ego and the Mechanisms of Defense. London, Hogarth Press, 1937

Greenberg JR, Mitchell SA: Object Relations and Psychoanalytic Theory. Cambridge, MA, Harvard University Press, 1983

Haan N: Proposed model of ego functioning: coping and defense mechanisms in relationship to IQ change. Psychological Monographs 77:1–23, 1963

Haan N: Coping and Defending: Processes of Self-Environment Organization. New York, Academic, 1977

Horowitz MJ: Introduction to Psychodynamics. New York, Basic Books, 1988

Horowitz MJ, Markman HC, Stinson C, et al: A classification theory of defense, in Repression and Dissociation. Edited by Singer JL. Chicago, IL, University of Chicago Press, 1990, pp 61–84

Ihilevich D, Gleser GC: Defense Mechanisms: Their Classification, Correlates and Measurement With the Defense Mechanisms Inventory. Owosso, MI, DMI Associates, 1986

Kernberg O: Borderline personality organization. J Am Psychoanal Assoc 15:641–685, 1967

Klein M: Envy and Gratitude. London, Tavistock, 1957

Kolb LC: Noyes' Modern Clinical Psychiatry. Philadelphia, PA, WB Saunders, 1968

Lazarus RS: The costs and benefits of denial, in Denial and Stress. Edited by Breznitz S. New York, International Universities Press, 1983, pp 1–30

Lazarus R, Folkman S: Stress, Appraisal and Coping. New York, Springer, 1984

Lazarus RS, Averill JR, Opton EM: The psychology of coping: issues of research and assessment, in Coping and Adaptation. Edited by Coehlo EG, Hamburg D, Adams J. New York, Basic Books, 1974, pp 249–315

Meissner WW: Theories of personality and psychopathology: classical psychoanalysis, in Comprehensive Textbook of Psychiatry, 3rd Edition, Vol 1. Edited by Kaplan HI, Freedman AM, Sadock BJ. Baltimore, MD, William & Wilkins, 1980, pp 631–728

Moos RH, Billings AG: Conceptualizing and measuring coping resources and processes, in Handbook of Stress: Theoretical and Clinical Aspects. Edited by Goldberger L, Breznitz S. New York, Free Press, 1982, pp 212–230

Murphy LB: The Widening World of Childhood: Paths Toward Mastery. New York, Basic Books, 1962

Sjöbäck H: The Psychoanalytic Theory of Defensive Processes. New York, John Wiley, 1973

Symonds PM: Defenses: The Dynamics of Human Adjustment. New York, Appleton-Century-Crofts, 1945

Vaillant GE: Theoretical hierarchy of adaptive ego mechanisms. Arch Gen Psychiatry 24:107–118, 1971

Chapter 4

The Clinical Management of Immature Defenses in the Treatment of Individuals With Personality Disorders

George E. Vaillant, M.D.

For the last century the appreciation of defense mechanisms has made a major contribution to the clinical management of neurotic disorders. Information on how to recognize and interpret the defenses underlying such disorders is widely available in texts on psychotherapy, and I do not believe that these defenses require further discussion in this book. Rather, in this chapter I wish to focus on the management of defenses most commonly deployed in personality disorders; thus, I shall focus on the immature defenses. For it is in clarifying our clinical response to the so-called "borderline" patient that I believe that a hierarchy of mutually exclusively defined defenses has the most to offer clinicians. Before narrowing the discussion, however, let me briefly mention the clinical management of defenses at the mature, the psychotic, and the neurotic levels.

First, it is important that clinicians retain as much respect for mature defenses as they do for the immune system and white blood cells. In a literal sense, the mature defenses, such as sublimation and altruism, involve the same denial, distortion, and repression of conflict that the other mechanisms do, but they accomplish this defensive task in a fashion analogous to an oyster transmuting a grain of sand into a pearl. Thus, Ludwig van Beethoven's "Ode to Joy," written at age 50, should not be dismissed as a flight into health by a once suicidal 30-year-old musician, nor should Mary Baker Eddy's founding of the Christian Science church be dismissed as denial in a once incapacitated 30-year-old hypochondriacal woman. Psy-

---

Adapted from Vaillant GE: The beginning of wisdom is never calling a patient borderline. *Journal of Psychotherapy Practice and Research* (in press)

chodynamically oriented clinicians and patients, alike, must learn to regard mature defenses with the same welcoming acceptance that Pandora must have regarded the discovery of hope within her chest of horrors. Mature defenses require no response from the clinician—other than verbal admiration. As Heinz Hartmann (1939) and others have pointed out, often such ego processes have begun as responses to conflict but over time have become autonomous, relatively conflict-free facets of character.

The psychotic defenses also require no interpretation by psychotherapists, but for a very different reason. In the case of mature mechanisms, the brain is working too well to require intervention, whereas in the case of psychotic distortion, delusional projection, and denial of external reality, the brain is not working well enough for psychotherapeutic intervention. In other words, a central nervous system incapable of testing reality is also incapable of making and maintaining a psychotherapeutic alliance.

In order to breach psychotic defenses the central nervous system must be stabilized. We can give haloperidol to the schizophrenic individual; we can wait for the young child's brain to myelinate further; and we can give physostigmine to the emergency room patient delirious from the antimuscarinic effects of Sominex or amitriptyline overdosage. In addition, we can also directly intervene in an otherwise overwhelmingly threatening environment. We can wake the dreamer. We can reduce the sensory deprivation of the patient in an iron lung; we can illuminate the room and put a calendar on the bedside table of a sundowning elderly patient. We can help opposing generals who have become delusionally prejudiced about each other's intentions through threats of nuclear terror to play golf together at Palm Springs or Yalta. In each case we are mechanically altering the brain's internal or external environment, not affecting the ego defenses themselves.

In contrast to the futility of trying to intervene in breaching defenses at the psychotic level, and to the lack of need for interpreting mature defenses, the value of interpretation at the level of neurotic defenses has resulted in an exponential growth of dynamic psychotherapy, ever since Freud wrote "The Neuro-psychoses of Defence" in 1894. The techniques involved in the interpretation of the neurotic defenses are well established. The use of dream recall, metaphor, unconditional positive regard, and a confidential confessional relationship to bring back the repressed past or to reattach affect to barren cognition is well known. The psychoanalytic strategy of free association deciphers displacement, circumvents reaction formation, and sees behind neurotic denial. The unremitting respect of psychotherapists for the validity and importance of affect and abreaction allows patients to abandon isolation of affect and to let their feelings play a role in their waking lives.

In addition, virtually all psychotherapies employ the "neurotic" defense of displacement, both to circumvent the patient's own resistance and as an intrinsic part of the therapist's own strategic intervention. The analysis of transference is but one example of the use of displacement by psychiatrists and patients to hold in consciousness an attenuated version of underlying conflicts. The child and the child-therapist live in a playroom where dolls safely substitute for parents and old wounds can be reenacted in the safety of pretend. Even the use of "desensitization" by behavior therapists involves displacement to gradually approach their patients' core phobias by initially confronting relatively less-threatening situations.

Displacement is also useful in the interpretation of reaction formations, which seldom leads to a frontal assault. To tell a pacifist directly that he really wants to punch someone is only inconsistently useful. Instead, two indirect techniques are more helpful. First, it is sometimes helpful to ask a person using reaction formation what they would say to someone else who came to them with the same complaint. For example, what would a counterdependent physician say to a colleague who had not taken a vacation in 2 years and had self-prescribed diazepam lest he bother a busy colleague? Second, if one is, for example, going to confront a pacifist on his or her use of reaction formation, it is well to point out the wish to "punch" in a positive rather than negative context. Thus, the empathic statement "I wonder if asserting yourself would feel too good for you to bear" is a more successful approach than the more negative confrontation "I wonder if you are a Quaker in order to deny your own unconscious sadism."

Management of Immature Defenses: General Principles

The treatment of personality disorders is far less easy than the treatment of neurotic conflicts. The defenses of patients with personality disorders have become part of the warp and woof of their life histories and of their personal identities. However maladaptive these defenses may be in the eyes of the beholder, they represent homeostatic solutions to the inner problems of the user. Neurotic individuals suffer from their defenses (e.g., repression, isolation, reaction formation, and displacement) and thus welcome insight and view interpretation of their defenses as helpful. In contrast, the defenses of patients with personality disorders often only make others suffer; the owners view interpretation of their defenses as an unwarranted attack (Vaillant 1977). Nevertheless, if psychiatry, psychology, and general practice are to help their most difficult patients, the immature defenses (e.g., projection, hypochondriasis, dissociation, fantasy, acting out, splitting)— the building blocks of DSM-III-R Axis II disorders—must be understood. The appreciation of immature defenses is essential to reaching the hypochondriacal help-rejecting "complainer," the wrist-cutting "borderline," the injustice-collecting litigant, the devaluing eccentric, and the noncompliant sociopath—in short the denizens of any urban emergency room on a Saturday night. However, by carelessly threatening an immature defense, a clinician can evoke enormous anxiety and depression in the patient and rupture the therapist-patient relationship. Indeed, there is the rub. Any attempts to challenge immature defenses should be mitigated by strong social supports (e.g., Alcoholics Anonymous), or the patient's defense needs to be replaced by alternative defenses—usually from the neurotic or intermediate level. For example, fantasy can evolve into isolation; projection can evolve into reaction formation; and hypochondriasis can evolve into displacement (Vaillant 1977).

Helping a patient alter defenses at the immature level, however, is easier said than done. William James spoke of character as being "set in plaster"; Wilhelm Reich, one of the early therapeutic pioneers of personality disorder, spoke of "character armor"; and Anna Freud spoke of the "petrification" of defenses. The early psychodynamic investigators of character disorder (e.g., Reich, Glover, Abraham) provided much that was of theoretical interest but little that was of practical clinical value. Advocating longer and longer psychoanalyses hardly offers a panacea to the overworked urban social worker, parole officer, or emergency room physician.

Rather, it was as psychoanalysts entered prisons (e.g., Adler and Shapiro 1969), public hospital inpatient units (e.g., Havens 1986), and general hospital wards (e.g., Kahana and Bibring 1964) that practical help was provided to our management of the immature defenses. Such help meant that the Freudian models of drive psychology and of ego psychology had to be modified. The ego and drive models are particularly well adapted to the analysis of neurotic defenses, but the analysis of immature defenses requires conceptual models that focus more on object relations. In the symptomatology of personality disorder, scripts, role-relationship models (Horowitz 1988), and internalized beloved and hated people play as crucial a part as do conflicts over forbidden desire and rage.

Each therapist-patient dyad must collaboratively develop a meaningful common language. This common language, like poetry, must lead toward a mutually understood reconstruction of the patient's inner life and his or her internalized relationships. Appreciation of the metaphors of immature defenses plays an important role in this reconstruction.

However, the therapy of personality disorders requires a broad, not a constricted, view toward competing models of defense mechanisms. Steven Cooper (1989), a Boston psychoanalyst, describes some of these competing models succinctly:

One group of theorists, including Brenner, Kernberg, Schafer, and Kris, despite important differences in their theories, define defenses within a strictly intrapsychic context. Other theorists, such as Laplanche and Pontalis (1973), Modell (1973, 1984), and Kohut (1984), emphasize that the function of some defense mechanisms is to maintain or preserve an object relation that, without it, would signify overriding anxiety. (p. 866)

Cooper goes on to point out that in contrast to Anna Freud (1937), who proposed a classification of defenses according to the source of anxiety (e.g., superego, external world, strength of instinctual pressures), many object-relations theorists have minimized drives. For example, Cooper quotes Modell (1984) as maintaining that "affects are the medium through which defenses against objects occur. Once affects are linked to objects, the process of instinct-defense becomes a process of defense against objects" (Cooper 1989, p. 879). In his efforts to help personality-disordered individuals, Kohut (1984) moved still further away from the defenses-against-drive model. He maintained that the whole concept of defense resistance is dependent on the overemphasis by classical psychoanalysis on the mechanics of mental processes to the exclusion of the patient's selfexperience.

I believe that therapists of personality-disordered patients can use help from every competent theorist they can find. Drives, people, reality, and culture are all significant. Psychoanalysis, family systems theory, cognitive therapy, and behavior modification can all play a valuable role. In this chapter, however, I wish to focus solely upon the clinical management of immature defenses in the treatment of individuals with personality disorders.

I will begin by outlining three broad principles for enabling patients to replace immature defenses with more mature defenses: stabilizing the external environment, altering the internal environment, and controlling countertransference.

Stabilizing the External Environment

An effective way to alter a person's choice of defensive style under stress is to make his or her social milieu more predictable and supportive. That is why Kohut's theories have seemed so useful to clinicians when working with personality-disordered patients. We are all a little schizoid and paranoid when among strangers who we fear may treat us harshly. We are all more adept at altruism, suppression, and playful sublimation when among friends who are empathetic toward our pain. Thus, in the consulting room, schizoid and paranoid personalities are rarely attractive, but they respond better to our empathy and forbearance than to our confrontation or rejection. Indeed, Kohut's views toward the treatment of personality disorders remind me of the old fable of the wind and the sun competing to see who can make a traveler remove his overcoat. The harder the wind blew, the more tightly the man defended himself with his overcoat. Then it was the sun's turn. When the sun shone down, of course, the man grew warm and cast his outer garments aside. Similarly, the more drive-oriented psychiatrists tug at their patients' mantle of defenses, the more they will see the immature defenses exaggerated. In contrast, the "Winnicottian" or "Kohutian" who strives empathetically to be a good enough mirror or selfobject for the patient will find his or her personality-disordered patients using more mature and less pathological defenses—until his or her patients leave the consulting room and cloak themselves once more to meet the chilly gusts of the cold outside world.

Altering the Internal Environment

Facilitating internal as well as external safety remains a cornerstone to the treatment of individuals with personality disorders. We can also help patients abandon immature defenses by altering their internal milieu. Toxic brain syndrome makes almost anyone project. Intoxication with alcohol and unlanced abscesses of grief and anger lead to fantasy, to rage turned against the self, and to acting out. We are all better at sublimation and reaction formation when we are not hungry, not tired, and not lonely. Often, adequate pharmacotherapy of affective spectrum disorders can ameliorate symptoms of Axis II disorders that are secondary to affective illness.

In addition, if we attempt to challenge patients' defenses, we must be sure that we have their permission. If in the course of examination we ask our patients to remove their protective clothing, we must protect them with something else. Psychopharmacology alone is rarely specific enough to provide such protection. Too often psychiatrists forget that the brain was designed to process information and not to act as a series of mere chemoreceptors. The limbic system was neurobiologically designed to be comforted by friendly people and not by chemistry. Either we must offer personality-disordered individuals ourselves—a luxury rarely available to busy doctors—or we must offer them alternative social systems and facilitate their use of more adaptive defenses.

Countertransference

If we are to manage our patients' immature defenses, we must manage our own countertransference. I believe that almost always the diagnosis "borderline" is more a reflection of therapists' affective response rather than their intellectual response to their personality-disordered patients. That, perhaps, is why up to 90% of patients diagnosed as "borderline" can also be assigned another, usually more discriminating, Axis II diagnosis (Angus and Marziali 1988; Fyer et al. 1988). And even when carefully applied, the DSM-III-R criteria for borderline personality disorder are extremely over-inclusive and lack specificity (Zanarini et al. 1991). For years I have demonstrated to our own residents the subjective nature of the epithet "borderline" by asking each of them to list what they considered the six most salient characteristics of the "borderline" individual. Year after year there is little consensus. As with beauty, the definition of "borderline" lies in the eyes of the beholder. For, as a function of the personality-disordered person's need to establish object constancy, his or her immature defenses have an uncanny capacity to get under the skin of some observers. To circumvent such subjectivity in working with patients who use immature defenses, it behooves the therapist to use the surgeon's favorite defense of isolation and to try to identify the patients' defensive style as precisely as possible.

When I am invited to other centers as a visiting professor, I always ask to interview a "borderline" patient. My task is to endeavor to offer an alternative, more rational diagnosis. At such clinical conferences, as an outsider, I am often impressed at how irrational the ward staff have become in the prolonged presence of their character-disordered patients' provocative behavior. Helping staff to intellectualize about the defenses of such patients allows the clinicians to appreciate the invasive, infuriating, separation/individuation–defying contagion of the immature defenses. It allows staff an opportunity to regain the sane calm reflection with which an outsider can approach "the biggest borderline" on someone else's inpatient unit.

If our inner worlds include relatively constant people toward whom in real life we have had relatively unambivalent feelings, then our external relationships will remain relatively assured, loving, autonomous, and well-demarcated. However, the internalization of stable and loving people is not the lot of individuals with personality disorders. The interpersonal relationships of such individuals remain perpetually unstable and entangled. It is often in an effort to preserve an illusion of interpersonal constancy that individuals with personality disorders unconsciously deploy immature defenses. These image-distorting defenses permit ambivalent mental representations of other people to be conveniently "split" (into good and bad) or moved about and reapportioned. Too often, clinicians unconsciously, then, label the immature defenses of such patients as perverse or taboo; for once touched, observers can rarely separate themselves completely from the immature defenses of another person.

Put differently, immature defenses are contagious. The contagion of immature defenses does much to account for the inhumanity of man to man that is seen throughout our criminal justice system. The hypochondriacal individual provokes our passive aggression, and in the presence of an acting-out substance abuser, liberals become prejudiced. When baited by their adolescent children, even the most reasonable and staid parents become hopelessly overinvolved and unreasonable. In such instances, we are hard put to distinguish "normal" countertransference and "pathological" projective identification (Brandchaft and Stolorow 1984). And yet the process by which our patients get under our skin is subtle, and, if noticed, the tumult seems quite mysterious to an outsider. Recently, I was fascinated to note that when I asked our residents to describe their own countertransference to their "borderline" patients, they collectively, but unwittingly, provided the DSM-III-R polythetic definition of borderline personality disorder. In short, the diagnosis "borderline" describes an enmeshed clinical dyad in which at least the inner experience of both participants can begin to meet the criteria for being "borderline."

I remember consulting on a very hypochondriacal patient who had been admitted to a general hospital for the 37th time. When I asked the medical resident for the patient's present illness, the resident replied mysteriously, "She was admitted for multiple stab wounds . . . inflicted in the Emergency Room." The explanation was that the patient, known to be a "hypochondriac"—which is the internist's pejorative epithet for the "borderline"—had come in complaining of chest pain. Unable to send the patient home, the exasperated staff tried to put in a subclavian intravenous line on her right side. They missed the vein and tried to insert the line on her left side and missed again. Then, furious and disgusted, they had to admit their wounded patient.

The real moral of the story, however, was that the patient greatly benefited from her week in the hospital. Her heart was healthy; it always had been. The "stab wounds" were irrelevant; she had been wounded often before in the past. But her hospitalization reduced her problem list from 20 problems to 3. What she benefited from most was her first bath in a month, the comfort of clean sheets, and the restoration of her internal milieu by intravenous fluids. For, in response to her abusive home life, she had been continuously vomiting for a week. To understand her illness it was necessary to look behind her hypochondriacal camouflage and behind her help-rejecting reproach that made her doctors so reflexively enraged. The true source of her pain was an abusive spouse who was identified nowhere in her three-volume hospital record. In her 36 prior admissions the hospital staff had been consistently misled by this hypochondriacal patient who always insisted that her social history was "noncontributory." In their anger, the staff were only too ready to remain blind to her real pain.

Only recently have psychiatrists appreciated how appropriate it may be to rediagnose many "borderlines" as having posttraumatic stress disorder (Herman et al. 1989).

By necessity, the effective therapy of a personality-disordered patient requires that the therapist avoid becoming enmeshed in the patient's own issues surrounding separation-individuation. It is well for clinicians to begin by acknowledging what the family therapists have always known—namely, separation-individuation is a lifelong process. Just as war is too important to be left up to the generals, individuation is too complex to be left up to toddlers. In other words, the purpose of the immature—or image-distorting—defenses is to manage internal and external object relations in adults as well as in children.

Just as neurotic mechanisms of defense (e.g., displacement, isolation, repression) transpose feelings, immature mechanisms (e.g., splitting, projection, hypochondriasis) magically maneuver feelings and their objects. Psychotherapists are no exception. Almost by definition, work with a personality-disordered patient creates a psychological "umbilical" link between patient and therapist. This psychic fusion, often unconscious, violates the ideal of a therapist who first provides the patient a neutral blank screen and then wisely interprets the patient's conflicts projected or transferred onto that screen. The technical, but difficult-to-define term "projective identification" (Meissner 1980) captures more abstractly the back-and-forth transfusions of affects and introjects that threaten to disrupt effective psychotherapy with patients afflicted by personality disorder.

By recognizing that the invasive, contagious quality of personality disorder "infects" and produces reciprocal "projective identifications" in the therapist (Brandchaft and Stolorow 1984), I am not saying that the phenomena that we associate with patients whom we label "borderline" are iatrogenic. For as Brandchaft and Stolorow (1991) warn, "[C]onceptualizing borderline phenomena as arising in an intersubjective field is not equivalent to claiming that the term 'borderline' refers to an entirely iatrogenic illness" (p. 1117). Rather, I am simply noting that in the presence of a patient who deploys image-distorting defenses, the therapist may unwittingly accept the patient's projections. Thus, in the blurring of ego boundaries that often accompanies the essentially dyadic process of projective identification (Goldstein 1991), the therapist may forget that "borderlines" can be stabbed by the very hand held out to feed them.

Inadvertent countertransference has led to four popular approaches for managing patients with personality disorders. These four approaches, if pursued too enthusiastically, are more likely to lead to disaster than to success. First, psychopharmacology is often overused in managing difficult borderline patients. Borderline patients seek pills; they demand pills. They abuse pills; they try to kill themselves with pills. They try to punish their therapist by taking too many or too few pills. In response, their therapists, urged on by hopeful advertising and their own frustration, try one after another of the latest pharmaceutical agents. The results of such polypharmacy, at best, are like playing roulette, and, at worst, such polypharmacy leads to iatrogenic polydrug abuse. If one takes the long view, personality-disordered patients—in sharp contrast to patients with schizophrenia and major depressive disorder—fare better as Christian Scientists or as members of any group that provides the patients a holding environment while simultaneously forbidding their use of psychopharmacological agents. By these words of caution I am not criticizing the use of carbamazepine, lithium, or low-dose neuroleptics (Cowdry and Gardner 1988; Soloff et al. 1986) to control unmanageable behavior in selected patients with personality disorders. Nor am I suggesting that antidepressants cannot play a critical role in ameliorating affective spectrum disorders (Hudson and Pope 1990) that may present as personality disorders. I am only asking clinicians to wonder each time that they reach for their prescription pads, "Will my prescription reflect scientific pharmacotherapy or countertransference?"

A second equally dangerous response to patients with personality disorders is the impulse to be "the good enough mother" that the patient never had. Responding to their idealized understanding of the wise techniques of Heinz Kohut and Margaret Mahler, such therapists try to mother, mirror, and love their patients. Borderline patients take the promise of mothering as seriously as they do the promise of a magic pill. Again, the results are often antitherapeutic. When patients really need a mother—during therapists' August vacation, at three o'clock in the morning, and on Christmas Day—would-be therapist-mothers, unlike real mothers, are never available. Such patients, often already angry and formerly abused children, take such a seeming breach of faith by an allegedly kind clinician as a justified opportunity to bite the hand that feeds them. Therapists often regard such retaliatory treatment as ungrateful and respond by condemning their patients as having too much "innate aggression" or as being afflicted with "malignant narcissism." The fight is on. Instead of finding a good mother, the patient experiences another blow to selfesteem—hardly what the doctor wished to order. This sequence of events may explain the transferential sequence of events that Gunderson and Zanarini (1987) have described as pathognomonic of a "borderline" diagnosis:

> When the borderline person senses a supportive relationship with another person (or within the structured, warm "hold" of institutional settings), he [or she] is likely to experience sustained dysphoria and a lack of self-satisfaction. When such a relationship is disrupted by the threat of separation or the withdrawal of reassuring nurturance, there is a shift to angry, hostile affect accompanied by highly characteristic manipulative, self-destructive actions. (p. 5)

Instead of helping young adults with personality disorders to find mothers, the therapist should encourage such patients to be surrogate "mothers" both to others and, equally important, to their own "inner child." Little is gained by forcing the personality-disordered person into the confining sick patient role. Rather, self-esteem is enhanced by allowing the patient to be of appropriate help to others who are more needy. Furthermore, reaction formation and altruism are less troublesome ego defenses than acting out. In other words, pill taking is rarely helpful for patients with personality disorders, but anybody's sense of object constancy, self-esteem, self-efficacy, and empowerment is helped by giving pills to others. However, such surrogate responsibility for others must occur within the matrix of a holding environment. Often this holding environment entails an "institution"; for institutions, like real mothers, remain at home during August, at three o'clock in the morning, and on Christmas Day. The "12-stepper" cares for others within the fellowship of AA; the former delinquent cares for others within the matrix of a fire department; the former narcissistic playboy, St. Francis, cares for others within the holding environment of a monastery.

Third, perceiving the need for limits in personality-disordered patients, many writers recommend a punitive, authoritarian Nurse Ratched (from Ken Kesey's *One Flew Over the Cuckoo's Nest*) approach. Once again, this approach is encouraged by the patients themselves. Many personality-disordered patients have "thrown stones at the jailhouse door" in order to obtain the limits that they feel they need. Yet to be inside a jail or a restricted psychiatric ward is as noxious for a personality-disordered patient as is too-ready access to alprazolam or to the cheat of being promised, after age 21, a "good mother."

Instead of providing limits from above, the therapist should encourage peer support. Effective, structured social supports—whether Overeaters Anonymous, group therapy, or Guardian Angels membership—render the patient's social world safer and thus reduce the need for maladaptive, image-distorting defenses. Besides, it is the presence of social support that distinguishes limits from punishment, a delicate but vitally important distinction. Although punishment is useless in mitigating personality disorders, limits, like scientific pharmacotherapy and holding environments, can be lifesaving.

Finally, a fourth popular treatment for personality disorder is "insight-oriented psychotherapy" (Kernberg 1968). Once again what seems like such a promising treatment to patient and therapist alike is often disappointing. The efforts of psychotherapists to interpret their patient's projection, splitting, and hypochondriasis may be disastrous. In response to psycho-analytic interpretation, neurotic patients are grateful and often decide to become psychotherapists themselves. In contrast, interpretation of the defenses of personality-disordered patients can make them feel disgusted, angered, or ashamed. If a therapist points out that a hypochondriacal patient's help-rejecting complaining is defensive, the interpretation will result in the patient's accusing the therapist of being heartless, unfeeling, obtuse, and stupid. To tell another person that he or she is paranoid and prejudiced results in being called a bigot yourself. To point out to patients that they use schizoid fantasy is as comforting as explaining to them that their chief defect is loneliness. To tell someone in the middle of a tantrum that he or she is "acting out" is like trying to pacify a raging ocean by flogging it. In contrast, empathy, mirroring, and what Havens (1986) calls "making contact" are most useful and allow the patient to shift from immature to neurotic defenses.

In other words, although immature defenses can be understood and managed, they can rarely be interpreted. Rather, the therapist should inquire about, and help patients to think through, the consequences of their actual or intended actions. The Socratic method stands the personalitydisordered patient in better stead than all the good advice and dynamic interpretations in the world. Thus, in the rest of this chapter I will focus on helping the psychotherapist to "manage," rather than to interpret, immature defenses.

Besides employing the Socratic method and facilitating his or her patients' discovery of peer supports, the therapist does well to empower patients toward developing more mature defenses. By this advice I mean that the therapist should help the patient evolve along a developmental continuum. For example, hypochondriasis can lead to reaction formation and then to altruism; fantasy can lead to isolation of affect and then progress to sublimation; and sadistic passive aggression can lead first to displacement and wit, and then to humor. Sigmund Freud (1905) summed the whole process up with the sexist quip, "A young whore makes an old nun."

Put somewhat differently, patients should be supported to provide the pills, the mothering, the limits, and the psychotherapy that "borderlines" seek—not receive them. We should remember that it is not an accident that Florence Nightingale and Mary Baker Eddy were once themselves severely hypochondriacal. Nor should we forget that in AA, a definition of a "pigeon" is "someone who came along just in time to keep their sponsor sober." We should not forget that, like a small child's mother, the physician's beeper is there to assert his or her value 24 hours a day. Lastly, more than one very gifted psychotherapist has met the criteria for personality disorder—once upon a time. His or her own transformation from patient to clinician was often catalyzed by his or her own individual psychotherapy—a psychotherapy that permitted projection to evolve into altruism, fantasy into sublimation, splitting into humor, and so on.

Management of Individual Defenses

If we fail to recognize and to understand the immature defensive processes of our patients, we run the risk of taking these defenses personally and of condemning our patients' use of them. Therefore, I shall shift from discussing immature defenses collectively and examine them one at a time. Readers should translate my terms into their own language. The formulations presented below will be in the language of psychoanalytic psychiatry, but the language can be translated into principles consistent with those of cognitive and behavior therapies. Because the problems presented by personality disorder are ubiquitous, I shall use examples from the emergency room and from medical and psychiatry inpatient units, as well as from psychotherapy sessions. In general, I shall use the terminology for defenses that I defined in Chapter 3 and in Appendix 3, but I will suggest instances when Kernberg's (1968) terms like "devaluation," "idealization," and "omnipotence" could be substituted.

Although patients with personality disorders may be characterized by their most dominant or most rigid mechanism, each person usually deploys several defenses. Indeed, personality-disordered patients are often called "borderline" if they tend to deploy a wide variety of immature defenses. Thus, in treating a patient with personality disorder it may seem reductionistic to focus on one or two defenses. However, sometimes in working with very provocative people, keeping it simple is helpful. Always, empathy toward immature defenses rather than countertransference is essential in creating a holding environment within the consulting room. For if the individual psychotherapist can understand the patient's defenses and avoid reactive contagion, the patient will feel empathetically understood and held. Sensitive individual psychotherapy can help to build an intrapsychic analogue to the external holding environment that is created by a receptive peer group.

Splitting

A defense mechanism commonly seen in patients with personality disorders is splitting. Instead of synthesizing and assimilating less-than-perfect past caregivers, and instead of responding to important people in the current environment as they are, the patient divides ambivalently regarded people, both past and present, into good people and bad people. For example, in an inpatient setting some staff members are idealized and others are mindlessly devalued. The effect of such defensive behavior on a hospital ward or in a therapeutic group can be highly disruptive and often provokes the staff to turn against the patient. Splitting is best mastered if the staff

members anticipate the process, discuss it at staff meetings as an intellectually interesting topic, and thus use the defense of isolation to reduce their
own irritation.

In a psychotherapy setting, to dismiss the patient's split positive and
negative affects as "just transference" is to miss the point. The therapist
must work to create an atmosphere that is conducive to letting the patient
experience simultaneously positive and negative aspects of important relationships, including his or her relationship with the therapist. Unconditional positive regard, safety, and firmness are necessary—all within the
same session. This process necessitates a psychotherapeutic "container" that
is analogous both to the metaphor of a Winnicott holding environment and
to the kind of secure containment necessary to create energy from nuclear
fusion. This is no easy task. The task necessitates the same self-restraint and
empathy that therapists use when supporting patients in acute grief, but
demands greater clarity of formulation. Splitting can evolve into its more
mature counterparts of undoing and of humor if the therapist helps the
patients recall their past loves as well as their more recent resentments.

Fantasy

Many persons—especially eccentric, frightened persons (who often are
labeled schizoid)—make extensive use of the defense of fantasy. They seek
solace and satisfaction within themselves by creating an imaginary life and
imaginary friends. Often, such persons seem strikingly aloof. One needs to
understand that such unsociability rests on a fear of intimacy. The clinician
should maintain a quiet, reassuring manner with schizoid patients and
convey interest in them without insisting on a reciprocal response. Recognition of their fear of closeness and respect for their eccentric ways are both
useful. As trust develops, the schizoid patient may, with great trepidation,
reveal a plethora of fantasies, autistic relationships, and fears of unbearable
dependency, even fears of merging with the clinician. Imaginary friends
should never be made fun of or even mentioned to the patient without the
patient's tacit permission. The patient may vacillate between fear of clinging
to the clinician and fears of fleeing through fantasy and withdrawal. Always,
therapists must beware of projecting their own loneliness that the schizoid
person may engender in them. They must remember to treat the schizoid
character as if he or she were frightened rather than lonely.

Hypochondriasis

The mechanism of defense termed *hypochondriasis*—also called "help-rejecting complaining"—is commonly seen in patients with Axis II personal-

ity disorders, especially those with a borderline or self-defeating diagnosis. Hypochondriacal patients, in contrast to the usual supposition, do not make their complaints for simple secondary gain. A moment's reflection reveals that a hypochondriacal patient's complaints can rarely be relieved. Often, his or her complaint that others do not provide help conceals bereavement, loneliness, or unacceptable aggressive impulses. In other words, hypochondriasis disguises reproach and permits the patient to covertly punish others through frustrating their desire to relieve the patient's own pain and discomfort. "Hypochondriacs" are people who bite the hands that feed them; they are not people who, like persons with conversion hysteria, gratefully bask in the warmth of special attention. The initial response of clinicians to the hypochondriacal patient is often guilt at their own failure to relieve suffering.

This response is followed by anger and rejection on the part of the clinician that only amplifies the patient's now-vindicated reproach. Depending on the medical specialty of the caregiver being reproached, the hypochondriacal patient may present unrelievable complaints of somatic pain or of suicidal ideation. The clinician's inadvertently angry response to this reproach may be polysurgery or polypharmacy, or intensive psychiatric treatment followed by abrupt discharge or transfer.

Instead of trying to gratify or to diminish the hypochondriacal patient's complaints, the caregiver should follow five rules (Brown and Vaillant 1981).

First, the clinician should acknowledge that the hypochondriacal patient's pain or insoluble dilemma is as severe as the interviewer has ever seen. Such amplification of the manifest complaint is an approach that, paradoxically, leads hypochondriacal patients to moderate their complaints. At last, someone has appreciated the pain of past trauma or unspeakable abuse that the hypochondriacal patient has been unable to reveal or to emphasize. Thus, the treatment of hypochondriasis becomes an acknowledgment of the intensity and genuineness (rather than the site) of the pain. Instead of offering reassurance, the clinician should turn the "volume" of suffering up even further. Statements such as "I don't know how you stand it" or "It must be awful to have to endure such terrible pain" are much more useful than "I hope it feels a little better today." The effect of this seemingly paradoxical approach is often startling, especially when a clinician tries it and discovers, often for the first time, the beginning of real rapport with the patient. When thus validated, the hypochondriacal patient's painful anger can again become the patient's own responsibility.

Second, the clinician should make some symbolic effort to meet the hypochondriacal patient's overall need for dependency, rather than attending to the specific complaint. For example, inexplicable complaints of abdominal pain should not be met first by reassurance and then by a covertly vindictive laparotomy. Instead, the prescription might be 3 days of strict bed rest, a special diet, and a careful, noninvasive physical examination of the whole patient. Willing offers of concern, return visits by appointment, physical therapy, and Benadryl rather than Xanax are helpful. However, hypochondriacal demands—in psychiatric practice these are often suicidal threats—will increase if the patient senses a withholding of treatment or an implication that the clinician believes that the pain is imaginary.

Third, instead of retaliating against the helplessness and anger that hypochondriacal patients engender in their caregivers, clinicians need to wonder, "Why is this patient so angry?" A careful social history may provide the answer. By including a legible psychosocial history in a prominent place in the patient's record, the clinician can remind future caregivers of the most likely source of the patient's pain. Reminding future clinicians that the patient is a survivor of Buchenwald or a victim of child abuse may be more useful than providing a chart full of negative laboratory results or of psychodynamic ruminations about the last 2 weeks of "borderline" inpatient behavior.

Fourth, as the clinician plays "detective," he or she should never regard misleading information as lying. Most hypochondriacal misinformation is as innocent and as unconscious as complaints of terrible arm pain by a patient with coronary disease. The hypochondriacal complaint is, after all, an effort by the patient to get the doctor's attention, to validate past trauma, and to displace his or her rage rather than an effort to obtain secondary gain or a quick fix. The need of Coleridge's Ancient Mariner—to repeat his tale of woe—provides an analogy. In acknowledging and validating past unspeakable trauma, the therapist will ultimately serve the so-called "borderline"—who may in fact suffer from posttraumatic stress disorder (Herman et al. 1989)—far better than if the therapist maintains too close an adherence to the theories of Mahler and Melanie Klein. Validation of past trauma is essential to the creation of a stable sense of self.

Finally, in caring for a hypochondriacal patient perhaps the most useful technique is to use the metaphor inherent in the patient's pain to link physical or self-abusive complaint to affect. A hypochondriacal patient who complains of chest pain, and who is unreassured by a normal electrocardiogram, may be comforted if the clinician says, "One thing is sure; the pain in your heart is real." Or when a patient provocatively mentions his suicidal ideation yet again, the caregiver can respond with: "I can see that things have been terribly painful for you; you must be furious that others have helped so little." In both cases the clinician, by responding with metaphor, not logic, opens the way for a broader consideration of life's pain.

These five principles permit a useful modification of the clinician's own need for omnipotence. Clinicians must become able to accept that they are not going to cure the hypochondriacal patient, just as they accept that they are not able to "cure" a mourner after a funeral. Rather, our task with hypochondriasis, as with other immature defenses, is to decipher the defense so that we may remain sensitive to the patient's pain, not so that we can abolish the defense.

Many patients who use fantasy and hypochondriasis are pejoratively labeled "narcissistic." This is because both fearfulness and poor self-esteem are shored up by a schizoid or hypochondriacal pretense of omnipotence. To the casual observer and to the unempathic clinician, such self-centered behavior may be erroneously labeled "vanity," "grandiosity," and "entitlement." An effective way of surmounting the pejorative connotations of the term "narcissism" is to translate that multisyllabic epithet into the simpler and more empathic phrase "in pain."

Patients who use splitting, fantasy, and hypochondriasis may also be unusually critical of (i.e., devalue) the clinician. Some patients may even suggest that a therapist pay for the privilege of caring for them. In response, the therapist may become defensive, contemptuous, or rejecting. Nobody likes being belittled. Clinical progress is facilitated if, instead of belittling patients or defending themselves, clinicians understand that the Kleinian defense of devaluation is a less-mature cousin of the Freudian defense of undoing. What this means is that such patients are contemptuous of their clinicians precisely because the patients also feel reluctantly loving toward or admiring of them. The paradoxical contempt and envy induced by perceiving one's therapist as lovable can only be transformed into gratitude by sustained Rogerian unconditional positive regard and by Kohutian mirroring. No easy task.

Projection

Another defense commonly encountered in patients with personality disorders is projection. Excessive fault-finding and undue sensitivity to criticism on the patient's part may seem to the observer to be prejudiced, injustice-collecting projection. But projection, however blatant, should not be met by interpretation, defensiveness, or argument. There is usually a grain of truth in most projection! Instead, even minor mistakes on the part of the clinician and the possibility of future difficulties should be frankly acknowledged. The epithet "paranoid" should be replaced with the more empathic "hypervigilant." Strict honesty, real concern for the patient's rights, and maintaining the same formal, although concerned, distance as one would with a patient using fantasy are helpful. Confrontation guarantees a lasting enemy and an early termination of the interview. Therapists need not agree with their patients' injustice collecting; instead they should ask respectfully whether they can agree to disagree.

The technique of counterprojection (Havens 1986) is especially help-ful. In that technique, the clinician acknowledges and gives paranoid patients full credit for their feelings and for their perceptions. Further, the clinician neither disputes the patients' complaints nor reinforces them; rather he or she acknowledges that the world that paranoid patients describe can be imagined. There are several components to counterprojection. First, the clinician aligns himself or herself beside, not opposite, the patient. Eye contact and confrontation are avoided and replaced with the interactive mode of a traveling companion who is trying to view the world from a similar vantage point. Both clinician and patient look out of the same bus window, as it were. Second, empathic counterprojective statements must encompass, without necessarily agreeing with, the patients' distress. Thus, Havens (1986) uses the example of a patient stubbing his toe, to which he replies, "That damned old chair!" rather than "That must have hurt." Third, the point of counterprojection is not to agree with the patient, but only to get out of the way. Thus, the therapist would not say, "The doctors in this hospital are sadists," but rather, "It must seem as if the doctors here were trying to make you suffer." In so doing the clinician distances himself or herself from the patient's tormentors. The interviewer can then talk about the patient's real motives and feelings, even though they are initially misattributed to someone else.

Fourth, unlike the case with hypochondriasis, where metaphorical speech is important, with paranoid patients precise speech is helpful. In addition, a statement—what Havens and Harry Stack Sullivan call "making marks"—is more revealing and less annoying than a question. Whereas the interrogatory "When were you born?" will meet with a rebuff, the statement "I expect that you are a Gemini (or born in June)" will elicit the response "No, I was born in September."

The clinician must remember that trust and tolerance of intimacy are troubled areas for paranoid patients. Courtesy, honesty, and respect are the cardinal rules for the treatment of any such patient. If the clinician is accused of some actual inconsistency or fault, such as lateness for an appointment, an honest apology serves better than a defensive explanation or an analytic "Mmm?"

Individual psychotherapy requires a professional and not overly warm style on the therapist's part, and argument over trustworthiness is futile. For example, consider the following dialogue:

Patient: "I am sure this room is bugged."

Therapist: "To the best of my knowledge it is not."

Patient: "I could not trust a psychiatrist who bugs his office."

Therapist: "Any sensible person would mistrust a psychiatrist who bugged his office. I expect it's a waste of time, but, if you wish, you can look for bugs. On the other hand, you may have some other topics you would rather talk about."

Too zealous a use of interpretation—especially interpretation concerning deep feelings of dependency, sexual concerns, and wishes for intimacy—significantly increases the patient's mistrust. Clinicians can often address the concerns concealed behind projection, if they wait until the patient brings these concerns up in a displaced manner. For with maturation, projection evolves naturally into displacement and reaction formation.

At times, the behavior of paranoid patients becomes so threatening that it is important to control or set limits on it. Delusional accusations must be dealt with realistically, but gently and without humiliating the patient. When disorganized by high levels of anxiety, paranoid patients can be reassured by the clinician involving security personnel. However, it is profoundly frightening for paranoid patients to feel that those trying to help them are weak and helpless. Therefore, a clinician should never threaten to take over control unless he or she is willing to and in a position to do so.

Acting Out

Antisocial personalities are especially prone to use acting out. Acting out represents the direct expression through action of an unconscious wish or conflict in order to avoid being conscious of either the idea or the affect that accompanies it. Tantrums, apparently motiveless assaults, child abuse, and pleasureless promiscuity are common examples.

To the observer, acting out often appears to be unaccompanied by guilt, but acting out is not that simple. As with conversion hysteria and its accompanying *la belle indifférence,* anxiety and pain also exist behind the "cool" indifference of acting out. In responding to such behavior, the clinician should remember the maxim "Nothing human is alien to me."

Glover has said of the sociopathic individual: "In addition to his incapacity to form deep personal attachments and his penchant to cause suffering to those who are attached to him, the psychopath is essentially a non-conformist, who in his reaction to society combines hostility with a sense of grievance" (Glover 1960, p. 128). But sociopathic individuals' "incapacity" to form attachments represents defensive process, not inability. Close relationships arouse anxiety in them. Terrified of their own dependency, of their very real "grievances," and of their fantasies of mutual destruction, sociopathic individuals either flee relationships or destroy them.

    In trying to treat the antisocial personality the clinician must remember that these persons uniformly lack benevolent, sustained relationships with their parents. They are afraid of intimacy and of assuming responsibility for it. They cannot believe that others can tolerate their anxiety, and they devoutly fear responsibility for achieving success by open competition. They can neither identify with authority figures nor accept their criticism; and they resent any thwarting of their actions, even when such intervention is clearly in their interest. Their consciences are too rigid, not too lenient; and so, rather than experience their own punitive self-judgment, they reject all moral standards and ideals. The eye-for-an-eye morality of street gangs, of terrorist organizations, and of the jailhouse subculture makes Calvinist morality seem libertine by comparison.

    Bowlby (1963) has suggested that mourning in childhood is characterized by a persistent and unconscious yearning to recover the lost object. The persistent crime and polydrug abuse of the chronic user of acting out often represent a similar quest. Bowlby tells us that in lieu of depression, bereaved children, like sociopathic individuals, exhibit intense and persistent anger that is expressed as reproach toward various objects including the self. However, Bowlby notes that such anger, if misunderstood, seems often "pointless enough to the outsider" (p. 502). Finally, sociopathic individuals, like children, often employ "secret" anodynes to make loss unreal and overt grief unnecessary. Bowlby explains that their need for secrecy is based on the fact that "to confess to another belief that the [loved] object is still alive is plainly to court the danger of disillusion" (p. 519). These defensive maneuvers, then, serve to hide the child's and the sociopathic individual's depression from our psychiatric view. Persistent, seemingly mindless delinquencies make symbolic sense if interpreted dynamically—as one might interpret misbehavior in a dream or in a child's play therapy. In short, I believe that the incomprehensible behavior of acting out is a product of a well-defended ego and of a strict, albeit primitive, conscience. I disagree with Cleckley. Acting out is no mere "mask of sanity," but it is often a mask to grief (Vaillant 1975).

    Unlike conversion hysteria, however, acting out must be controlled as rapidly as possible. First, prolonged acting out is frightening to patient and staff alike. Faced with acting out—either aggressive or sexual—in an interview situation, the clinician must recognize that the patient has lost control. Anything that the clinician says will probably be misheard, and getting the patient's attention is of paramount importance. Depending on how threatened the clinician feels, the clinician's response can be, "You have acted in this manner because you can't pull that feeling up into your head," or, "How can I help you if you keep on screaming?" If the clinician feels that the patient's loss of control is escalating, he or she can respond, "If you continue screaming, I'll leave." Or, if physical violence genuinely seems a possibility, the clinician may simply leave and ask for help, including the police. Invariably, acting out begets fear in the observer, and nobody working with psychiatric patients should bear this fear alone (Perry and Vaillant 1989).

Second, once acting out is not possible, the conflict behind the defense may be accessible. This is another reason that the clinician must find some way of limiting the patient's frightening but ultimately self-defeating behavior. To overcome the patient's fear of intimacy, the clinician must frustrate the patient's wish to run from tenderness and from the honest pain of human encounter. In doing so, the clinician faces the challenge of differentiating control from punishment and of differentiating help and confrontation from social isolation and retribution. Successful models include halfway-house residences enforced by probation, "addiction" to methadone clinics, and the kind of therapeutic community behind bars that was devised for sociopathic individuals at Utah State Hospital (Kiger 1967) and that was formerly achieved at the Patuxent Institute in Jessup, Maryland, and the Herstevester in Denmark. If those who use acting out are prevented from flight or tantrum, or if they are approached by understanding peers, instead of appearing incorrigible, inhuman, unfeeling, guiltless, and unable to learn from experience, they become only too human.

Third, chronic users of acting out should be encouraged to find alternative defense mechanisms. Play is always preferable to war. Displacement is the more mature cousin of acting out. As with a young child, the clinician should not just tell a patient with an antisocial personality to stop doing something, but should point the patient toward an affectively exciting alternative. Acting out needs to be "redirected," not forbidden.

Finally, once those individuals who have antisocial personalities feel that they are among peers, the lack of motivation for change often disappears. Perhaps that is why self-help groups have many times been more effective in alleviating these disorders than have jails and psychiatric hospitals.

Turning Against the Self

A commonly seen mechanism in patients with personality disorders is turning anger against the self. In military psychiatry and DSM-III-R, such behavior is called passive-aggressive behavior; in psychoanalytic terminology such behavior is most often described as masochism. "Long suffering" and "self-sacrificing" comprise more empathic adjectives than masochism, which implies that the patient suffers because it is fun. The defense of turning against the self includes failure, procrastination, silly or provocative behavior, and self-demeaning clowning, as well as more frankly self-destructive behavior. The hostility in passive aggression and masochism, however, is never entirely concealed. Indeed, behaviors like wrist cutting engender such anger in others that these individuals feel that they themselves have been assaulted, and thus they come to view the wrist slasher as a sadist, not a masochist. In Massachusetts, attempted suicide used to be classified as a felony.

The best way to deal with turning against the self is by helping the patient to ventilate anger and to direct his or her assertiveness outward rather than against the self. It is important to treat the suicide gestures of passive-aggressive patients as one would any covert expression of anger and not as one would treat grief or primary depression. Antidepressant medications should be prescribed only when clinical indications are pressing and the possibility of overdose has been seriously weighed.

However, just as it is seldom wise to respond to angry suicidal patients as though they were simply depressed, it is seldom wise to isolate such patients in seclusion rooms for their angry gestures. As in the management of hypochondriasis, the therapist's task is to help patients acknowledge their anger, not to act out the patients' anger for them. The relief of tension that some patients obtain from repeatedly cutting or burning themselves should be accepted as matter-of-factly by the clinician as the clinician would tolerate equally dangerous two-pack-a-day smoking in a colleague. Rather than treating self-inflicted cigarette burns as perverse or dangerous, staff members should say gently, "I wonder if there's some other way you could make yourself feel better. Can you put what you are feeling into words?" The clinician must continually point out the probable consequences of passive-aggressive behavior as they occur. Questions such as "What do you really want for yourself?" may help to change the patient's behavior more than would a corrective interpretation, or, as is all too common, instituting retaliatory suicidal restrictions.

Therapeutic techniques that help channel the patient's anger away from passive resistance and into more productive expression are very helpful. One means is to recognize that passive aggression can be channeled into displacement and humor. Wit, parody, caricature, even "guerilla theatre—"instead of self-deprecatory clowning and sadistic hotfoots—offer more acceptable ways of redirecting anger formerly turned against the self.

Behavior therapy techniques such as assertiveness training and the explicit setting of limits are often useful. If stubborn, passive-aggressive patients are reluctant to help themselves, it is sometimes useful to take a "time out." Leaving the room or postponing the next appointment breaks the pattern of struggle and underscores the point that passive-aggressive struggles result in less, rather than more, attention. After a short time out, the interviewer, too, is able to continue the relationship in a less angry and covertly sadistic manner (Perry 1989).

Recovery may be usefully presented to the long-suffering patient as a special additional task. Sometimes long-suffering, self-sacrificing patients are more able to cooperate in a medical regimen because of their readiness to add to the burdens that they carry rather than because of their anticipation of the benefits that might accrue to themselves. In every interaction with self-defeating patients, however, it is important to avoid humiliating comments about foolish, inexplicable behavior. Nobody's pride is easier to wound than a person who continually shoots himself or herself in the foot.

Dissociation/Neurotic Denial

The defense (or defenses) of dissociation and neurotic denial involves the patient's replacing unpleasant affects with pleasant ones. In its most extreme form dissociation is manifested by multiple personality disorder. In childhood and for short periods in adult life, such denial can serve to mitigate an otherwise unbearable affect. For example, if honest self-awareness and expression repeatedly brought down abuse from caretakers, dissociation allows abused children to remain separated from their emotional experience; but, of course, dissociation does not make problems disappear. Whereas the six defenses previously discussed tend to contaminate the intersubjective field by eliciting negative affects in the therapists, the danger of dissociation within the intersubjective field is countertransferential seduction. Dependent longing and unacknowledged grief are misperceived as sexual excitement or counterphobic exuberance.

Persons using dissociation often proclaim that they feel fine, although their underlying anxiety, depression, or resentment may be obvious to others. Because their troubling affects, impulses, and wishes are disavowed and actively pushed out of consciousness, users of dissociation have a tendency to feel accused and devalued if anyone points out their troubles. They are often seen as dramatizing, theatrical, and emotionally shallow. Although they may often be labeled correctly as "histrionic" personalities, "captivating" is a less pejorative adjective. Their behavior is reminiscent of the stunts of anxious adolescents who, to erase anxiety, carelessly expose themselves to exciting danger. To accept such patients as enthralling and enthralled is to become blind to their pain and neediness, but to confront them with their vulnerabilities and defects is to make them more defensive still.

Because patients who use dissociation seek appreciation of their attractiveness and courage, and because they need some expression of prohibited impulses, the clinician should not be too reserved—only calm and firm. Reframing vulnerabilities as opportunities or potential strengths is often more effective than confronting such patients with their defects. Rather than lecture a "macho" coronary care patient, "Mr. Jones, you have had a very severe heart attack. You may die if you do not follow unit regulations," a better approach may be, "Mr. Jones, it takes real guts to put up with inactivity and the CCU routines, but remember, every day that you can tough out the pain of bedrest, your heart is getting stronger."

Such patients are often imaginative, if inadvertent, liars, but they benefit from having a chance to ventilate their own anxieties. In the process of free association they often "remember" what they "forgot," and through psychotherapy their self-serving lies can evolve into the acknowledgment of painful truths. Therefore, dissociation and neurotic denial are best dealt with if the clinician uses displacement and talks with the patient about the same affective issue but in a less-threatening context. Empathizing with the denied affect, without directly confronting the patient with the facts, may allow the patient himself or herself to reintroduce the original painful topic.

Final Suggestions

What follows are four final suggestions of how to use an understanding of immature defenses in individual psychotherapy.

First, defenses, especially immature (i.e., image-distorting) defenses, occur in a rich and complex interpersonal, intersubjective context. Such defenses encompass real past relationships as well as present, if primitive, transferences, in addition to the realities of the current doctor-patient relationship. The simplified techniques outlined above for managing these defenses are offered only as suggestions and guides to the complexities of individual psychotherapy. Like all suggestions for managing intimate and intense interpersonal relationships, such suggestions must be carried out with sensitivity to context and mutuality.

Second, the greater the variety of immature defenses that patients have, the more likely these patients are to be labeled "borderline." I believe, therefore, that using that term will always obscure differential diagnosis. Worse yet, such name calling leads to perceiving such patients' defenses as attacks on the clinician. If readers believe that they can use the epithet "borderline" while maintaining clinical objectivity, let me invite them to try the experiment of imagining that they found themselves described in their own therapist's notes as a "borderline."

Instead of resorting to name calling, therapists should always find something to admire in their patients' attempts to master past pain. In their formulations, if not in their diagnoses, therapists need to reframe the DSM-III-R Axis II labels so that paranoid becomes "hypervigilant," narcissistic becomes "in pain," hysterical becomes "captivating," masochistic becomes "long suffering," schizoid becomes "independent," and "borderline" becomes "posttraumatic stress disorder" or "that patient who sure knows how to push my buttons."

Third, therapists should also always find something to admire in their patients' attempts to change and grow. Taking genuine pleasure in a patient's attempts to try out new, more adaptive behaviors is very rewarding for patient and clinician alike. Therapists must remember that the personality disorders are dynamic. Like adolescents, patients with personality disorders can outgrow their difficulties with a little help from time and their friends: paranoid individuals can become reformers; hypochondriacal persons can become healers; and once sociopathic individuals can become enforcers of the law or department chairmen. In short, the therapy of personality disorder always proceeds more smoothly if we can remember our own recovery from adolescence.

However, no defense can be abruptly altered or abandoned without an acceptable substitute. For example, abstinence from drugs is achieved through a process analogous to mourning: slowly the depended-upon substance is replaced with other loves. In similar fashion, successful treatment of personality disorder demands that the clinician try to help the patient develop a substitute for each defense.

Finally, in treating personality disorder we have to modify the conventional doctor-patient model. One-to-one therapeutic relationships, by themselves, are rarely sufficient to change individuals with severe personality disorder. Immature defenses repel, wound, and overwhelm the efforts of individuals; burnout is common. Only an extended family or self-help group can withstand such assault. In addition, the "borderline" patient needs to absorb more of other people than one person, no matter how loving, can ever provide. Nor can we look to help from drugs. There is no drug that can teach us Chinese or that can replace parents who were abusive or inconsistent throughout our childhoods. Like adolescents, individuals with personality disorders need opportunities to internalize fresh role models and to make peace with the imperfect familial figures who are already within. A clinician, even seen five times a week, is not enough to satisfy an orphan. Especially, at the start of the recovery process, only a "church," a self-help residential treatment, or addicting drugs provide relief for a borderline patient's pain; all three provide an external holding environment 24 hours a day. On the other hand, individual psychotherapy, with its capacity to provide selfobjects and mirroring, may be more effective in modifying and enhancing those psychic structures that maintain an internal holding environment.

In other words, some form of self-help group is a useful adjunct to psychotherapy in the treatment of personality-disordered individuals. To begin with, individuals with personality disorders, like the rest of us, need to find groups to which they can belong with pride. They often know only too well that they have harmed others; but they can meaningfully identify only with people who feel as guilty as themselves. They can abandon their defenses against grief only in the presence of people equally bereaved. Only acceptance by peers or by a "higher power" can circumvent their profound fear of being pitied. Only acceptance by "recovered" peers can restore their defective self-esteem. A therapist's "love" is not enough.

There is another reason for combining peer groups with one-on-one therapy. Intensive individual psychotherapy seems most useful for people who (like many clinicians) have had too much parenting and for people who have learned from society not wisely but too well. In contrast, patients with personality disorders have experienced inconsistent or too little parenting. Because of defects in genes, socialization, and maturation, personality-disordered individuals have had difficulty learning what society wished to teach them. Thus, individuals with personality disorders often need care that is very similar to the care required by adolescents. Indeed, adolescents do not need therapy at all; they need a social group that offers them the time, space, and safety to internalize the valuable facets of their parents and their society and to extrude the chaff. They need mentors and loves in order to catalyze the developmental transmutation whereby adolescent envy becomes adult gratitude. Object constancy—as defined by Kernberg, not Piaget—is an essential ingredient of maturity, and object constancy is lacking both in adolescents and in individuals with personality disorders. The task of therapy for personality-disordered individuals, then, is to create such object constancy. For adults, groups and institutions sometimes provide this constancy and the opportunities for fresh identifications more consistently than can a single individual a few hours a week. At the same time, individual psychotherapy can play a vital role in the treatment of personality disorder. It is easier to walk with two crutches than with one.

References

Adler G, Shapiro LN: Psychotherapy with prisoners, in Current Psychiatric Therapies, Vol 9. Edited by Masserman J. New York, Grune & Stratton, 1969, pp 99–105

Angus LE, Marziali E: A comparison of three measures for the diagnosis of borderline personality disorder. Am J Psychiatry 145:1453–1454, 1988

Bowlby J: Pathological mourning and childhood mourning. J Am Psychoanal Assoc 11:500–541, 1963

Brandchaft B, Stolorow R: The borderline concept: pathological character or iatrogenic myth, in Empathy, Vol 2. Edited by Lichtenberg J, Bernstein M, Silver D. Hillsdale, NJ, Analytic Press, 1984, pp 333–357

Brandchaft B, Stolorow RD: The borderline concept. J Am Psychoanal Assoc 38:1117–1119, 1991

8

Brown HN, Vaillant GE: Hypochondriasis. Arch Intern Med 141:723–726, 1981

Cooper S: Recent contributions to the theory of defense mechanisms: a comparative view. J Am Psychoanal Assoc 37:865–893, 1989

Cowdry RW, Gardner DL: Pharmacotherapy of borderline personality disorder. Arch Gen Psychiatry 45:113–119, 1988

Freud A: The Ego and the Mechanisms of Defense. London, Hogarth Press, 1937

Freud S: The neuro-psychoses of defence (1894), in The Standard Edition of the Complete Psychological Works of Sigmund Freud, Vol 3. Translated and edited by Strachey J. London, Hogarth Press, 1962, pp 45–61

Freud S: Three essays on the theory of sexuality (1905), in The Standard Edition of the Complete Psychological Works of Sigmund Freud, Vol 7. Translated and edited by Strachey J. London, Hogarth Press, 1953, pp 130–243

Fyer MR, Frances AJ, Sullivan T, et al: Comorbidity of borderline personality disorder. Arch Gen Psychiatry 45:348–352, 1988

Glover E: The Roots of Crime. New York, International Universities Press, 1960

Goldstein WN: Clarification of projective identification. Am J Psychiatry 148:153–162, 1991

Gunderson JG, Zanarini MC: Current overview of the borderline diagnosis. J Clin Psychiatry 48 (no 8, suppl):5–11, 1987

Hartmann H: Ego Psychology and the Problem of Adaptation. New York, International Universities Press, 1939

Havens L: Making Contact. Cambridge, MA, Harvard University Press, 1986

Herman JL, Perry JC, van der Kolk BA: Childhood trauma in borderline personality disorder. Am J Psychiatry 146:490–495, 1989

Horowitz MJ: Introduction to Psychodynamics. New York, Basic Books, 1988

Hudson JI, Pope HG: Affective spectrum disorder: does antidepressant response identify a family of disorders with a common pathophysiology? Am J Psychiatry 147:552–574, 1990

Kahana RJ, Bibring GL: Personality types in medical management, in Psychiatry and Medical Practice in a General Hospital. Edited by Zinberg N. New York, International Universities Press, 1964, pp 108–123

Kernberg O: The treatment of patients with borderline personality organization. Int J Psychoanal 49:600–619, 1968

Kiger RS: Treatment of the psychopath in the therapeutic community. Hosp Community Psychiatry 18:191–196, 1967

Kohut H: How Does Analysis Cure? Chicago, IL, University of Chicago Press, 1984

Laplanche J, Pontalis JB: The Language of Psychoanalysis. New York, WW Norton, 1973

Meissner W: A note on projective identification. J Am Psychoanal Assoc 28:43–67, 1980

Modell A: A narcissistic defense against affects and the illusion of self-sufficiency. Int J Psychoanal 56:272–282, 1973

Modell A: Psychoanalysis in a New Context. New York, International Universities Press, 1984

Perry JC: Dependent personality disorder, in Treatments of Psychiatric Disorders, Vol 3. Washington, DC, American Psychiatric Assoc, 1989, pp 2762–2770

Perry JC, Vaillant GE: Personality disorders, in Comprehensive Textbook of Psychiatry, 5th Edition, Vol 2. Edited by Kaplan HI, Sadock BJ. Baltimore, MD, Williams & Wilkins, 1989, pp 1352–1387

Soloff PH, Anselm G, Swami NS, et al: Progress in pharmacotherapy of borderline disorders. Arch Gen Psychiatry 43:691–697, 1986

Vaillant GE: Sociopathy as a human process. Arch Gen Psychiatry 32:179–189, 1975

Vaillant GE: Adaptation to Life. Boston, MA, Little, Brown, 1977

Zanarini MC, Gunderson JG, Frankenburg FR, et al: The face validity of the DSM-III and DSM-III-R criteria sets for borderline personality disorder. Am J Psychiatry 148:870–874, 1991

Section II: Empirical Studies

Chapter 5

The Struggle for Empirical Assessment of Defenses

George E. Vaillant, M.D.

I t is no coincidence that Freud's decision to redifferentiate the ego mechanisms of defense and to abandon nonspecific terms like "countercathexis" occurred simultaneously with the birth of ego psychology. As noted in Chapter 1, in 1926 Freud formally suggested that the concept of defense be reintroduced as a broad term under which specific defense mechanisms like "repression" and "isolation" would be subsumed. Ten years later, Freud (1936) advised the student interested in "the extraordinarily large number of methods (or mechanisms, as we say) used by our ego in the discharge of its defensive function" (p. 245) to seek out Anna Freud's *The Ego and the Mechanisms of Defense* (1937), which to this day remains one of our definitive texts on the subject.

However, neither Sigmund nor Anna Freud provided mutually exclusive definitions of defenses or guidelines for their empirical study. In spite of the ambitious goals of Anna Freud's Hampstead Index (A. Freud 1965) in systematically cataloging the defenses of children in analysis, no substantive empirical publications on defenses have emerged from the Hampstead Clinic (now the Anna Freud Clinic). Anna Freud and her Hampstead coworkers attempted, but failed, to achieve rater reliability in identifying defenses. By tradition, Anna Freud is said to have described 10 defense mechanisms. However, if one reads *The Ego and the Mechanisms of Defense* with care, one can find at least 20 different labels for defenses. Such vagueness of definition could not help but hinder empirical studies.

The quest for a reliable nomenclature of defenses has been reviewed in Chapter 3. In order to do empirical research on defenses, we not only need to have mutually exclusive definitions, we also need to arrange the defenses in some sort of theoretical hierarchy. Clearly, recognition of hierarchically differentiated defenses requires a highly developed appreciation of the healthy ego. Freud and his early followers had chosen to study children and psychologically impaired individuals. Thus, they paid relatively less attention to the fate of a given defense as the child matured and as the patient recovered. This trend limited psychoanalysts' appreciation of healthy ego function, for differentiated mechanisms of defense become clearest when one can study the psychopathology of everyday life in detail. In terms of recognizing a continuum of defenses from pathological to less pathological, many early contributors to ego psychology—for example, Glover (1956), Gill (1963), and Rapaport (1960)—recognized the likelihood of such a hierarchy. But none provided specific hierarchical outlines or empirical evidence for such a hierarchy. Thus, 30 years ago, Brenner (1955) observed that the wish to establish a chronology of defenses, "which seems like such a stimulating one, has not so far been followed up" (p. 101).

It was not until World War II that psychoanalytically trained individuals began to study healthy adaptation in normal populations (e.g., Grinker and Spiegel 1945). Although a complete list of the influential postwar clinical investigators of defense mechanisms is beyond the scope of this chapter, Percival Symonds, Ernst Kris, Heinz Hartmann, George Engel, Robert White, David Hamburg, John Mason, Irving Janis, Lois Murphy, and Karl Menninger belong on the list of those individuals who deserve credit for underscoring our need to define a hierarchy of defense mechanisms. Each of these investigators provided mutually exclusive definitions *or* sought rater reliability *or* provided empirical evidence of defense utilization beyond clinical anecdote, but none achieved all three goals. Only George Engel (1962) had published a formal developmental hierarchy of defenses. Unfortunately, his hierarchy was not subjected to clinical validation. The efforts of many others at centers like the Menninger and Hampstead clinics to obtain a clinically valid hierarchy have been frustrated in large part by problems of definition and inter-rater reliability.

One of the most ambitious, important, and illustrative research studies during the postwar period was the 1964 investigation by Carl Wolff, John Mason, and co-workers on the relationship between psychological defenses and urinary corticoid excretion rate in the parents of fatally ill children. Their work illustrated, however, that even though they had access to one of the most sophisticated stress laboratories in the country, the issues of reliably rated and operationally defined terms had not been solved.

After the war there also arose outside of clinical psychiatry a parallel experimental literature on defenses. Unlike the work undertaken on clinical populations by investigators like David Hamburg and John Mason, this effort was based in the psychology laboratory and not the clinic. The difficulty, of course, with the psychological laboratory is that often validity is sacrificed in order to obtain reliability and experimental control. Exhaustive reviews by Moos (1974) and Kline (1972) have summarized findings from several hundred empirical studies of defenses prior to 1980. In contrast to clinical investigations, many of these studies achieved operational definition of terms, rater reliability, and reproducible assessment strategy. But the price paid for such reliability and experimental control was that the results had very limited relevance to real life. Unfortunately, the controlled setting of the psychology laboratory, the uniform stimuli of the pencil-and-paper tests, and the revealing insights from projective tests failed to provide any systematic basis for understanding defenses in the real world.

For example, in a sample of 100 nonpatient college graduates, I contrasted their defensive style in everyday life with defenses identified from results obtained by rating their responses to thematic apperception tests. No correlation was found (Vaillant 1977). One of the tasks of the ego, after all, is to distinguish reality from simulation. By way of less-anecdotal evidence, Kline (1972) summarized his review of the experimental literature: "It is clear from our discussion of the empirical studies reported in this chapter that methodological difficulties, not unexpectedly, have proved too much for most investigators" (p. 192). In short, if the clinical studies were unsatisfactory methodologically, the satisfactory methodological studies from the laboratory were unsatisfactory clinically.

In addition, contemporary social psychology and personality theorists have often tried to integrate the three contrasting coping models of 1) social supports, 2) conscious cognitive strategies, and 3) "unconscious" mechanisms of defense (Kobasa et al. 1982; Lazarus et al. 1974). But by mixing apples and oranges, these efforts have sometimes confused, rather than synthesized, the three models. I believe that for progress in research to be made, conscious cognitive coping strategies (i.e., health practices) have to be distinguished from ego defensive styles (i.e., personality dispositions), and for this reason in this book I will focus only on the latter.

In recent years the efforts by experimental psychologists to study defenses empirically have been more fruitful. Ihilevich and Gleser (1986), Paulhus et al. (1992), and Cramer (1991) have produced exhaustive reviews of this literature. Although Cramer identifies 58 different empirical methods for assessing defense, I shall review only a few of the more important empirical efforts by psychologists to study involuntary ego adaptation.

One effort has been the study of attributional styles that can lead to performance deficits and to labeled psychopathology (Abramson et al. 1978). These styles have been termed "self-deceptive" and "emotional coping" by Lazarus (1983). In expanding on this theme, Shelley Taylor (1989) has suggested that there are three basic illusions (i.e., involuntary ways of coping with stress): self-enhancement, exaggerated belief in one's personal control, and unrealistic optimism. *Self-enhancement* involves the perception of one's self, one's past behavior, and one's enduring attributes as more positive than is actually the case. *Exaggerated belief in one's personal*

control involves the perception that one is personally responsible for bringing about primarily positive but not negative outcomes. *Unrealistic optimism* involves perceptions that the future holds an unrealistically bountiful
array of opportunities and a singular absence of adverse events. Taylor
examines how such an attributional style of high self-esteem, personal
self-efficacy, and optimistic belief in the future may lead to both physical
and mental health.

Kobasa, Maddi, and Kahn (1982) have undertaken empirical study of
a second trio of more or less involuntary cognitive styles—commitment
(approach not avoidance), internal locus of control, and challenge (integrated, effective appraisal of incongruent events)—that are used to describe
hardiness. Their terms of *hardiness* and *transformational coping* have much
in common with the mature defenses discussed in Chapter 3 (see Tables
3-1 and 3-2), but Kobasa et al.'s language and frame of reference are very
different. Similarly, what I call in this book immature defensive styles have
much in common with what Kobasa et al. term *regressive coping*. For 2 years,
Kobasa and her associates (1982) monitored the physical health of healthy
business executives who were under high stress but who did not become
physically ill. Kobasa et al. observed that those men who at the start were
identified as manifesting the traits of *commitment, control,* and *challenge*
were less likely to become ill. The difficulty with their research is that it
failed with certainty to distinguish the cart from the horse. *Challenge*
(perceiving changes as an opportunity rather than a disaster) is a reflection
of both absence of depression and presence of a resourceful ego. *Control*
(reflecting mastery of life and competence) likewise is powerfully interfered
with by low self-esteem that can result from both depression *and* alcoholism, neither of which was controlled in Kobasa et al.'s study. Thus,
undiagnosed depression or alcoholism could have explained their findings.
Nevertheless, their study still represents a model of an effort to combine
methodological rigor and reliability with clinical validity.

In the late 1960s, Gleser and Ihilevich (1969) developed a psychological instrument, the Defense Mechanisms Inventory (DMI), to test response
to conflict. They classified subjects' responses to threat using five defensive
categories: turning against the self, projection, principalization, turning
against the object, and reversal. In addition, Ihilevich and Gleser (1986)
have provided perhaps the best bibliography on defenses extant. Their DMI
test has generated a great deal of empirical work, but, unfortunately, the
test has demonstrated higher retest and inter-item reliability than it has
clinical validity (Cramer 1988).

The Berkeley Stress and Coping Project has been well summarized by
Lazarus and Folkman (1984). They have focused more on conscious
appraisal and cognitive coping than on unconscious mechanisms of defense.
Their Ways of Coping (WOC) Scale (Folkman and Lazarus 1980) contains

68 items in a yes/no format and has been widely used. Like other pencil-and-paper tests, its advantages are convenience and reliability rather than validity. The WOC Scale, which has been widely employed with healthy populations, has generated a great deal of empirical data, but it may have less applicability to psychiatric populations.

Daniel Weinberger, a psychologist, has successfully identified a form of denial or repression that could be appreciated by behaviorists as well as psychoanalysts. He has used an elegant paradigm. By means of a self-report scale (Weinberger et al. 1979), he identified individuals who *reported* very low levels of state anxiety (tension) even when participating in stressful tasks. Unlike less defensive, overtly anxious individuals, these so-called "repressors" saw remaining cheerful as essential to their self concept. However, when these "repressors" were given a stressful task, many of them exhibited elevated forehead muscle tension (on the electromyogram), increased sweating, and accelerated heart rate to the same degree as subjects who on the same self-report tests identified themselves as *more* anxious than usual. Thus, Weinberger identified physiologically anxiety-prone subjects whose low scores on anxiety measures were due to their lack of awareness of emotional states. These unaware but anxious subjects could be reliably distinguished from true "low-anxious" subjects who on the same tasks neither reported anxiety nor experienced it physiologically. Weinberger (1990) notes that such "repressive" personality was not found in hysterical subjects but rather in excessively rational subjects. In other words, in the language employed in Chapter 3 (see Table 3-3), what Weinberger called "repression" would be termed isolation and reaction formation.

In the last 25 years there have been three important scientific advances that have provided a means of overcoming the issue of rater reliability and of allowing the metaphorical nature of defenses to become tangible to serious investigators. The first of these advances has been the availability of data from prospective longitudinal studies of adult development. The second advance is the availability of low-cost, but technically excellent, videotapes of clinical interactions. The third advance is that the cognitive revolution and advances in artificial intelligence have allowed academic psychologists to appreciate and to study the phenomena that psychoanalysts have labeled defense mechanisms under terms like "self-deception" and "competing cognitive schema." The expanding discipline of cognitive psychology brings with it both a greater intellectual rigor and an opportunity to link the neurosciences to the discipline of psychoanalysis.

In the 1960s an important advance in the empirical study of defense mechanisms came through the study of longitudinal life history by both Norma Haan, a psychologist at the Institute of Human Development (IHD) at Berkeley, and Elvin Semrad, a professor of psychiatry at the Massachusetts Mental Health Center at Harvard Medical School.

Haan (1963) originally described a set of 20 adaptive styles with explicit definitions (most unusual in the literature up to that time). She divided these styles into two groups: 10 styles were described as *coping* (healthy) and 10 adaptive styles—first cousins to the other 10—were described as *defending* (pathological). On the basis of interviews, two IHD raters judged 99 members of the Oakland Growth Study for Haan's coping/defending styles and achieved generally acceptable rater reliability. The value of Haan's work was that it 1) explicitly defined a hierarchy of defenses according to pathological significance, 2) provided mutually exclusive definitions, and then 3) demonstrated validity by correlating the assessment of defenses with important longitudinally derived measures of mental health. Haan's efforts have spawned a number of empirical studies, many of which are summarized in her book *Coping and Defending* (Haan 1977). Two limitations of Haan's study were that, first, her data were based on a unique longitudinal study and, second, as suggested in Chapter 3, many of her definitions of defenses were idiosyncratic. A third limitation was rater reliability. Haan obtained inter-rater reliability on all of the 20 mechanisms for both men and women. For seven mechanisms, rater reliabilities were under .4.

Simultaneous with Haan's work, Elvin Semrad, a psychoanalyst, studied defenses in a developmental longitudinal context through scrutiny of the recovery process in acute schizophrenia. Semrad (1967) suggested that if, consequent to unbearable loss, a patient experiences schizophrenic decompensation, he or she regresses to the defenses of denial, projection, and distortion. Then, during convalescence the patient employs progressively less pathological defenses: first, hypochondriasis and ritual, then dissociation and somatization. Finally, during recovery, the patient learns to experience relatively unmodified depression and anxiety. For 20 years Semrad elucidated for his psychiatric residents the recovery process in schizophrenia by ordering defenses along a continuum of psychopathology. Over the years Semrad's students have generalized his schema to other clinical populations (Vaillant 1971; Ablon et al. 1974; Meissner 1985; Jacobson et al. 1986).

Semrad and his co-workers (1973) also outlined a finite list of defenses arranged hierarchically and developed a rating scale for the empirical study of defenses during the remission process in schizophrenia. Leopold Bellak and his co-workers (1973) have also attempted to develop an ego profile scale as a means of studying schizophrenia. Neither rating scale has ever been adequately validated.

Since 1966, in order to understand maturational changes in personality observed in a "normal" sample of men, I have tried to synthesize both Semrad's and Haan's models of ego development. To achieve this goal, I took advantage of a longitudinally observed cohort of men from a then 30-year prospective study of adults: the Harvard Study of Adult Development started by Arlie Bock and Clark Heath in 1938 with support from W. T. Grant (Heath 1945). This investigation, often called the "Grant Study," was an investigation of the development of college sophomores. In a subsample of 95 college men, I observed that mature defenses correlated positively and immature defenses correlated negatively with a 32-item scale reflecting objective success in working and loving (Vaillant 1976). Problems of rater reliability that seemed insurmountable in written transcripts of therapy hours could usually be overcome when inconsistencies in human behavior were observed for three decades or more (see Chapter 9). Put differently, the very phenomena that had been impressing psychoanalysts in the fantasy life of their patients were made tangible through the longitudinal psychobiographical studies of lifetimes. Using an inner-city sample of 307 47-year-old men also followed for 30 years, I replicated my previous findings (Vaillant et al. 1986). Mental health was assessed by using the Health-Sickness Rating Scale (HSRS; Luborsky 1962). The methodology for rating defenses is described in Chapter 8.

Much progress has been made since 1977 in the empirical study of defense mechanisms. Table 5-1 depicts the hierarchy of defenses that was defined and given wide currency by Kaplan, Freedman, and Sadock's *Comprehensive Textbook of Psychiatry* (1980) (see Appendix 2). The table demonstrates the general agreement of six recent studies, each of which correlated defensive style with a different measure of mental health. In addition to my own two studies, Haan (1963, 1977) demonstrated that the mechanisms which she called "coping" were significantly correlated with upward social mobility, adult increases in IQ, and three other measures of positive midlife outcomes. Mechanisms that she called "defending" were negatively correlated with such outcomes. Jacobson et al. (1986), using Loevinger's (1976) Sentence Completion Test as a measure of ego maturity, came to similar conclusions, as did Battista (1982), who assessed the defensive style of 78 psychiatric inpatients by means of an ego function inventory rated on a 5-point Likert scale and rated patients' outcome by means of the Global Assessment Scale (GAS; Endicott et al. 1976).

Bond et al. (1983) used a self-administered questionnaire of self-perception of defensive style with 209 patients and nonpatients. Factor analysis revealed four clusters of defenses that Bond et al. correlated with independent questionnaire measures of ego adaptation. Questions reflecting projection, passive aggression, dissociation, and acting out all loaded highly in the cluster that correlated most *negatively* with estimates of ego strength and maturity. Questions reflecting humor, suppression, and sublimation all loaded highly in the cluster that correlated most *positively* with estimates of ego strength and ego maturity.

Perry and Cooper (see Chapter 11; not shown in Table 5-1) utilized the GAS to assess mental health and used videotaped interviews scored by

Table 5–1. Correlation of selected defense mechanisms with global assessment of mental health

Defense[a]	Haan (1977)	Vaillant (1976)	Battista (1982)	Vaillant et al. (1985)	Bond et al. (1983)	Jacobson et al. (1986)
Mature defenses						
Anticipation (objectivity)	Coping	++	+	++	Not rated	Not rated
Suppression (suppression, concentration)	Coping	++	+	++	+	++
Altruism	Coping	NS	NS	++	Not rated	++
Sublimation (substitution, sublimation)	Coping	NS	NS	++	+	Not rated
Humor (playfulness)	Coping	Not rated	Not rated	++	+	Not rated
Asceticism	Not rated	Not rated	Not rated	Not rated	Not rated	NS
Neurotic (intermediate) defenses						
Intellectualization (isolation)	Defending	NS	+	NS	NS	++
Repression (repression)	Defending	NS	NS	NS	NS	–
Reaction formation (reaction formation)	Defending	NS	Not rated	NS	NS	Not rated
Displacement	Defending	NS	NS	+	NS	NS

Defense[a]							
Externalization, inhibition, sexualization, somatization, controlling, rationalization	Not rated	Not rated	Not rated	Not rated	Not rated	Not rated	Not rated
Immature defenses							
Passive aggression or masochism (repression)	Defending	NS	NS	NS	–	–	NS
Hypochondriasis	Not rated	NS	NS	–	–	Not rated	Not rated
Acting out	Not rated	–	NS	–	–	–	–
Dissociation (denial)	Defending	NS	–	–	–	–	–
Projection (projection)	Defending	–	NS	NS	–	–	–
Schizoid fantasy	Not rated	–	–	–	–	Not rated	Not rated
Blocking, introjection, regression	Not rated	Not rated	Not rated	Not rated	Not rated	Not rated	Not rated

Note. + or − = Positive or negative correlation (*P* ≤ .05; Pearson product-moment coefficient) or *r* > .25. ++ or −− = Positive or negative correlation (*P* < .001). NS = Not statistically correlated with mental health.

[a]Defense terms used in table are from Kaplan HI, Sadock BJ (eds): *Modern Synopsis of Comprehensive Textbook of Psychiatry*, 3rd Edition. Baltimore, MD, Williams & Wilkins, 1981, pp. 137–138. Psychotic or "narcissistic" defenses (e.g., denial of external reality, delusional thinking, distortion [hallucinations])—that is, mechanisms associated with frank psychosis—have been excluded. Terms in parentheses are Haan's (1977) terms for equivalent mental processes.

Source. Adapted, with permission, from Vaillant GE: Defense mechanisms, in *The New Harvard Guide to Psychiatry.* Edited by Nicholi AM Jr. Cambridge, MA, Harvard University Press, 1988, p 205.

multiple observers to assess defenses. The authors noted the same negative correlation of the immature defenses with mental health as did Bond et al., but also found a significant *positive* association of mental health with intellectualization, isolation, and undoing. This may have been because a patient population was being studied.

In summary, the so-called immature defenses listed in Table 5-1 correspond to those inferred intrapsychic mechanisms commonly observed in adolescents and in the Axis II disorders of DSM-III (Vaillant 1987). Such immature defenses, which are consistently and negatively correlated with global assessment of mental health, profoundly distort the affective component of interpersonal relationships. In contrast, the so-called mature defenses identified inferred intrapsychic mechanisms that have been consistently associated with successful psychological adaptation. These mechanisms allow the individual to experience the affective component of interpersonal relationships but in a tempered fashion. The intermediate defenses reflect mechanisms proposed by psychoanalytic theory to identify neuroses. Across studies these defense mechanisms show little positive or negative correlation with mental health. In Chapters 7–12 the different methodologies underlying the empirical evidence for this hierarchy will be described.

The second methodological breakthrough in the study of defense mechanisms is the use of videotape. One can search for what one seeks where the light is good, or one can search for what one seeks where one thinks it may be hidden. Those who have sought to search for defense mechanisms where the methodological light is brightest—with psychological instruments and in the laboratory—have found good reliability but relatively little clinical value (Kline 1972; Moos 1974). For example, in reviewing earlier experimental laboratory research efforts to demonstrate repression, Ericksen and Pierce (1968) documented a large number of studies that did not produce clinically useful results. The alternative is to study defense mechanisms where their importance may be greatest—that is, in the clinical setting. In such situations the problems of obtaining reliability have been formidable and labor intensive. By using videotapes of psychotherapy, Horowitz (1987) has documented regular patterns of intrusions and omissions in the short-term therapy of individuals coping with traumatic stress. Further exploitation of clinical videotapes has continued in his laboratory. David Spiegel (1990), Perry and Cooper (see Chapter 11), and Leigh McCullough and co-workers (1991) have also found that the use of videotapes in clinical samples provides a promising and valid means of capturing the subtle phenomena of defensive distortion for consensual agreement.

The third methodological advance has been the progress in cognitive psychology. Since 1975, steady progress has been made in the laboratories of experimental psychology in understanding the cognitive processes underlying defenses. First, students of "learned" coping strategies (e.g., cognitive restructuring, social skills training) have begun to realize that mental mechanisms of denial and self-deception could reduce cognitive dissonance and allow individuals to minimize sudden changes in internal and external environments by altering how these changes are perceived (Breznitz 1983). This pioneering work on self-deception, some of which is found in Taylor and Brown (1988), Quattrone and Tversky (1984), Horowitz (1988a), and Lockhard and Paulhus (1988), entails talking of ego mechanisms of defense in very different metaphors. These newer metaphors use the framework of artificial intelligence, neurolinguistics, and computer science. Under the direction of Mardi Horowitz, the Program on Conscious and Unconscious Mental Processes of the John D. and Catherine T. MacArthur Foundation has been the most promising center for integrating the two fields of psychoanalysis and cognitive psychology. A book edited by Horowitz (1988b), *Psychodynamics and Cognition,* is the first summary of this important area of bridge building.

Clearly, there is still no fully satisfactory way of assessing defenses. Perhaps analogous to subatomic particles, defenses can be studied only with great difficulty, uncertainty, and expense. But I believe that understanding, appreciating, and even measuring defenses are central to the scientific study of psychopathology. It is in that spirit that defenses were tentatively in-cluded in DSM-III-R (American Psychiatric Association 1987).

In the following chapters several different empirical approaches are used to study defenses. It is hoped that these chapters will provide a useful starting point for future investigators attempting to assess and study defenses. I shall summarize the chapters here in a somewhat different order than they occur in the text.

Just as in biography dominant personality traits become evident by repetition, just so defenses can be identified by the frequency with which they are noted. This is the method illustrated in Chapter 9 by Leigh McCullough. Such clinically based biographical rating procedures can be improved by using the techniques of psychobiography. We cannot measure a mountain from top to bottom, but we can assess its height through triangulation (i.e., by integrating two indirect and oblique views of its peak). So it is with defenses. In the case of psychobiography, defenses can be identified by combining biography, autobiography, and the subject's symp-toms and/or creative products. This is the methodology used by myself and Caroline Vaillant in Chapter 6. Such clinically based procedures can be methodologically further improved by using videotape and teams of raters as is illustrated in Chapter 11 by J. Christopher Perry and Steven Cooper. Next, there are self-report measures that have the advantage of not requiring an observer's clinical judgment. These measures, which can be inexpensively administered and objectively scored, are used by Michael Bond as reported in Chapter 7. Clinically based procedures can also be improved by the use of the Q-sort, which permits subjective judgment and clinical data to be reliably and quantitatively rated. This method is based on a system of rank ordering a set of cards with simple statements that describe aspects of the domain of study. This is the method described by Diane Roston and Kimberly Lee in Chapter 12.

Yet another way of bringing empirical order to rating defenses is to use convergent validity and apply more than one scientific methodology to the same clinical sample. In Chapter 8, Bond's self-report instrument and my own different psychobiographical method of evaluating defenses on the same sample are contrasted. Roston and Lee, in Chapter 12, contrast the Q-sort technique with the Bond self-report method outlined in Chapter 7 and the psychobiographical method described by Vaillant and Vaillant in Chapter 6. As illustrated by Perry and Cooper in Chapter 11, defenses can be identified by using both observer-rated interviews and raters' evaluations of self-reported responses to stress. Readers will need to judge for themselves which methods provide the most adequate starting point for their investigations.

References

Ablon SL, Carlson GA, Goodwin FK: Ego defense patterns in manic-depressive illness. Am J Psychiatry 131:803–807, 1974

Abramson LY, Seligman MEP, Teasdale J: Helplessness in humans: critique and reformulation. J Abnorm Psychol 87:49–74, 1978

American Psychiatric Association: Diagnostic and Statistical Manual of Mental Disorders, 3rd Edition, Revised. Washington, DC, American Psychiatric Association, 1987

Battista JR: Empirical test of Vaillant's hierarchy of ego functions. Am J Psychiatry 139:356–357, 1982

Bellack L, Hurvich M, Gediman HK: Ego Functions in Schizophrenics, Neurotics, and Normals: A Systematic Study of Conceptual, Diagnostic, and Therapeutic Aspects. New York, John Wiley, 1973

Bond M, Gardner ST, Christian J, et al: Empirical study of self-rated defense styles. Arch Gen Psychiatry 40:333–338, 1983

Brenner C: An Elementary Textbook of Psychoanalysis. New York, International Universities Press, 1955

Breznitz D (ed): The Denial of Stress. New York, International Universities Press, 1983

Coelho GV, Hamburg DA, Adams JE: Coping and Adaptation. New York, Basic Books, 1974

Cramer P: The Defense Mechanisms Inventory: a review of research and discussion of the scales. J Pers Assess 52:142–164, 1988

Cramer P: The Development of Defense Mechanisms: Theory, Research and Assessment. New York, Springer, 1991

Endicott J, Spitzer RL, Fleiss JL, et al: The Global Assessment Scale: a procedure for measuring overall severity of psychiatric disturbance. Arch Gen Psychiatry 33:766–770, 1976

Engel GL: Psychological Development in Health and Disease. Philadelphia, PA, WB Saunders, 1962

Ericksen CW, Pierce J: Defense mechanisms, in Handbook of Personality Theory and Research. Edited by Norgatta EF, Lambert WW. Chicago, IL, Rand-Mc-Nally, 1968, pp 1007–1040

Folkman S, Lazarus RS: An analysis of coping in a middle-aged community sample. J Health Soc Behav 21:219–239, 1980

Freud A: The Ego and the Mechanisms of Defense. London, Hogarth Press, 1937

Freud A: Normality and Pathology in Childhood: Assessments of Development. New York, International Universities Press, 1965

Freud S: A disturbance of memory on the Acropolis (1936), in The Standard Edition of the Complete Psychological Works of Sigmund Freud, Vol 22. Translated and edited by Strachey J. London, Hogarth Press, 1964, pp 239–248

Gill MM: Topography and Systems in Psychoanalytic Theory. Psychological Issues, Monograph 10. New York, International Universities Press, 1963

Gleser GC, Ihilevich D: An objective instrument for measuring defense mechanisms. J Consult Clin Psychol 33:51–60, 1969

Glover E: On the Early Development of Mind. New York, International Universities Press, 1956

Grinker RR, Spiegel JP: Men Under Stress. Philadelphia, PA, Blakiston, 1945

Haan N: Proposed model of ego functioning: coping and defense mechanisms in relationship to IQ change. Psychological Monographs 77:1–23, 1963

Haan N: Coping and Defending: Processes of Self-Environment Organization. New York, Academic, 1977

Heath C: What People Are. Cambridge, MA, Harvard University Press, 1945

Horowitz MJ: States of Mind, 2nd Edition. New York, Plenum, 1987

Horowitz MJ: Introduction to Psychodynamics: A New Synthesis. New York, Basic Books, 1988a

Horowitz MJ: Psychodynamics and Cognition. Chicago, IL, University of Chicago Press, 1988b

Ihilevich D, Gleser GC: Defense Mechanisms: Their Classification, Correlates, and Measurement With the Defense Mechanisms Inventory. Owosso, MI, DMI Associates, 1986

Jacobson AM, Beardslee W, Hauser ST, et al: Evaluating ego defense mechanisms using clinical interviews: an empirical study of adolescent, diabetic and psychiatric patients. J Adolesc 9:303–319, 1986

Kaplan HI, Freedman AM, Sadock BJ (eds): Comprehensive Textbook of Psychiatry, 3rd Edition. Baltimore, MD, Williams & Wilkins, 1980

Kline P: Fact and Fantasy in Freudian Theory. London, Methuen, 1972

Kobasa SC, Maddi SR, Kahn S: Hardiness and health: a prospective study. J Pers Soc Psychol 42:168–177, 1982

Lazarus RS: The costs and benefits of denial, in Denial and Stress. Edited by
   Breznitz S. New York, International Universities Press, 1983, pp 1–30
Lazarus RS, Folkman S: Stress, Appraisal and Coping. New York, Springer, 1984
Lazarus RS, Avrill JR, Opton EM Jr: The psychology of coping: issues of research
   and assessment. in Coping and Adaptation. Edited by Coehlo GV, Hamburg
   DA, Adams JE. New York, Basic Books, 1974, pp 249–315
Lockhard JS, Paulhus DL (eds): Self-Deception: An Adaptive Mechanism? New
   York, Prentice-Hall, 1988
Loevinger J: Ego Development. San Francisco, CA, Jossey-Bass, 1976
Luborsky L: Clinicians' judgments of mental health. Arch Gen Psychiatry 7:407–
   417, 1962
McCullough L, Winston A, Farber BA, et al: The relationship of patient-therapist
   interaction to psychotherapeutic outcome in brief psychotherapy. Psychother-
   apy 28:525–533, 1991
Meissner WW: Theories of personality and psychopathology: classical psychoanaly-
   sis, in Comprehensive Textbook of Psychiatry, 4th Edition, Vol 1. Edited by
   Kaplan HI, Sadock BJ. Baltimore, MD, Williams & Wilkins, 1985, pp 337–418
Moos RH: Psychosocial techniques in the assessment of adaptive behavior, in
   Coping and Adaptation. Edited by Coelho GV, Hamburg DA, Adams JE. New
   York, Basic Books, 1974, pp 334–399
Paulhus DL, Fridhandler B, Hayes S: Psychological defense: contemporary theory
   and research, in Handbook of Personality Psychology. San Diego, CA, Aca-
   demic, 1992
Quattrone GA, Tversky A: Causal versus diagnostic contingencies: on self-decep-
   tion and the voter's illusion. J Pers Soc Psychol 46:236–248, 1984
Rapaport D: The Structure of Psychoanalytic Theory. Psychological Issues, Mono-
   graph 6. New York, International Universities Press, 1960
Semrad E: The organization of ego defenses and object loss, in The Loss of Loved
   Ones. Edited by Moriarty DM. Springfield, IL, Charles C Thomas, 1967,
   pp 126–134
Semrad E, Grinspoon L, Feinberg SE: Development of an ego profile scale. Arch
   Gen Psychiatry 28:70–77, 1973
Spiegel D: Hypnosis, dissociation and trauma: hidden and overt observers, in
   Repression and Dissociation. Edited by Singer JL. Chicago, IL, University of
   Chicago Press, 1990, pp 121–142
Taylor S: Positive Illusions: Creative Self-Deception and the Healthy Mind. New
   York, Basic Books, 1989
Taylor SE, Brown J: Illusion and well-being: a social psychological perspective on
   mental health. Psychol Bull 103:193–210, 1988
Vaillant GE: Theoretical hierarchy of adaptive ego mechanisms. Arch Gen Psychia-
   try 24:107–118, 1971
Vaillant GE: Natural history of male psychological health, V: the relation of choice
   of ego mechanisms of defense to adult adjustment. Arch Gen Psychiatry
   33:535–545, 1976
Vaillant GE: Adaptation to Life. Boston, MA, Little, Brown, 1977
Vaillant GE: A developmental view of old and new perspectives of personality
   disorders. Journal of Personality Disorders 1:146–156, 1987

Vaillant GE, Bond M, Vaillant CO: An empirically validated hierarchy of defense mechanisms. Arch Gen Psychiatry 43:786–794, 1986

Weinberger DA: The construct validity of the repressive coping style, in Repression and Dissociation. Edited by Singer JL. Chicago, IL, University of Chicago Press, 1990, pp 337–386

Weinberger DA, Schwartz GE, Davidson RJ: Low-anxious, high-anxious, and repressive coping styles. J Abnorm Psychol 88:369–380, 1979

Wolff CT, Friedman SB, Hofer MA, et al: Relationship between psychosocial defenses and mean urinary 17 hydroxycorticoid excretion rates, I: a predictive study of parents of fatally ill children. Psychosom Med 26:576–591, 1964

Chapter 6

Empirical Evidence That Defensive Styles Are Independent of Environmental Influence

George E. Vaillant, M.D.
Caroline O. Vaillant, M.S.S.W.

I f the status of defense mechanisms is to be shifted from the realm of quaint psychoanalytic folk belief to the realm of scientific medicine, there are three questions that must be answered in the affirmative. First, can *defenses* be reliably identified outside of a psychoanalytic setting? Inter-rater reliability is a critical means of validating a science that depends on metaphor. For example, can defenses be reliably identified by unsophisticated clinicians in working-class men with modest verbal skills who have never been in psychotherapy? Second, if defense mechanisms can be reliably identified, do they have predictive *validity*? Can a causal link be forged between choice of defense and future psychopathology? Third, can maturity of defenses be demonstrated to be independent of environment? Can defensive style be shown to be relatively independent of education, ethnicity, gender, and social privilege and thus more similar to the body's other homeostatic mechanisms such as blood clotting and the immune system?

In this chapter we will try to address these three questions telescopically, not microscopically. Conventionally, the social sciences in general and psychoanalysis in particular have tried to examine human behavior under ever higher magnification. In understanding personality, however, the use of high magnification has often been as unrewarding as the use of a magnifying glass in the study of geography or of Monet paintings. If we study landscapes with a microscope, the forest becomes lost in the trees. To study defenses—and Monet—we need to view our subject from a distance. Thus, to answer the three questions we will depend on prolonged prospective study of the three heterogeneous groups of adults included in the Study of Adult Development.

The Study of Adult Development

The Study of Adult Development incorporates three separate longitudinal studies: one located at Harvard University, one at Dartmouth Medical School, and one at Stanford University. In an effort to study healthy human lives, the Study of Adult Development was begun in 1938 at Harvard University Health Services. The study was eventually expanded to include three cohorts of individuals, each prospectively studied for over half a century: the Harvard (COLLEGE) sample was made up of individuals who were born about 1920; the Glueck (CORE CITY) sample, about 1930; and the Stanford (TERMAN women) sample, about 1910.

The Samples

   The COLLEGE sample.   The Grant study (COLLEGE sample) was begun at Harvard University Health Services in 1938 by Arlie Bock and Clark Heath (see Heath 1945; Vaillant 1977). In the selection process about 40% of the students in each Harvard class were arbitrarily excluded because there was some question as to whether they would meet the academic requirements for graduation. (Usually this meant that their freshmen grade average was C or lower.) The health services records of the remaining 60% of each class were then screened, and half of the students were excluded because of evidence of physical or psychological disturbance. Each year the names of the remaining 300 sophomores were submitted to college deans who selected about 100 boys whom they recognized as "sound." About 80 of the 100 students selected each year agreed to participate in the study.

   Over four years, 1939 to 1942, 268 sophomores were selected for study. In college 12 of these students dropped out, and since then 8 more men have withdrawn from the study. For half a century, the rest of the men have continued to participate with remarkable loyalty. They have received questionnaires about every 2 years, physical examinations every 5 years, and interviews about every 15 years.

   As measured by their scholastic achievement tests (SATs), the academic achievement of the students fell in the top 5% to 10% of high school graduates; but their average score of 584 did not put them beyond the reach of many other able college students. Although they were no more intellectually gifted than their fellow classmates, 61% of the men chosen for study were graduated with honors in contrast to only 26% of their classmates, and 76%, a higher percentage than was found in their classmates, went on to graduate school. Half of the men were either the oldest in the family or an only child.

Socioeconomically, the COLLEGE sample men were drawn from a privileged group but not exclusively so. A third of the men's fathers had some professional training, but half of their parents never graduated from college. Almost half of the men had some private education, but during college almost half of the men were on scholarship and/or had to work during the academic year.

The physical and mental health of the COLLEGE sample was clearly better than that of the population at large. Only a seventh as many of the COLLEGE men as expected were rejected for military service on physical grounds; only a twelfth, as many as would have been expected by chance, were rejected for psychiatric reasons (Monks 1957). By age 65 the mortality of the COLLEGE sample was only half that expected of white males of the same birth cohort; it was only two-thirds as great as that of their college classmates.

At age 47 the average earned income of the COLLEGE sample would have been about $90,000 in 1989 dollars, yet they were Democrats more often than Republicans. In short, they had the incomes and social status of corporate managers, yet they drove the battered cars and pursued the hobbies, politics, and life-style of college professors.

The CORE CITY sample.   The 456 men of the Glueck study (CORE CITY sample) represented a very different cohort. In junior high school they were chosen as the controls for a prospective study conducted by Sheldon and Eleanor Glueck at Harvard Law School that led to a landmark book, *Unraveling Juvenile Delinquency* (Glueck and Glueck 1950). Between 1940 and 1944, the Gluecks selected the CORE CITY men from Boston inner-city schools on the basis of their not being known to be seriously delinquent. Like the COLLEGE men, the CORE CITY men were studied originally by a multidisciplinary team of physicians, psychologists, psychiatrists, social investigators, and physical anthropologists. The CORE CITY men were interviewed at ages 14, 25, 32 (Glueck and Glueck 1968), and 47 (Vaillant 1983). Over the first 35 years of the study, attrition due to dropping out was held at 5%, and only 4 subjects (1%) could not be located after age 40.

In order to match the CORE CITY sample with delinquent youths, the Gluecks had used four criteria in their selection. The CORE CITY subjects had to be of the same age, to be of the same intelligence, to be of the same ethnicity, and to reside in a Boston community with the same neighborhood crime rate as was found among the Glueck's 500 delinquents whose misdemeanors (and social disadvantage) were sufficiently severe to send them to reform schools. The boys' average IQ was 95, and 61% of their parents were foreign born. In childhood, half of the CORE CITY men had lived in clearly blighted slum neighborhoods. Half came from families known to five or more social agencies, and more than two-thirds of their families had recently been on welfare. Half of their childhood homes had no tub and shower, and only 30% of their homes had hot water, central heat, electricity, *and* a tub and toilet.

Unlike brighter children from the inner city, the CORE CITY men's low average intelligence had denied them access to Boston's elite public high schools. Nevertheless, as the men matured during the 1950s and 1960s, they showed marked upward social mobility. If only 10% of their parents had belonged to the middle class (i.e., social classes II and III [Hollingshead and Redlich 1958]), 51% of the CORE CITY sample themselves at age 47 met such criteria. At age 47, the CORE CITY men's mean income would have been about $30,000 in 1989 dollars, or one-third that of the COLLEGE sample.

The TERMAN women sample.   The 90 women of our TERMAN women sample are a representative subsample of the 672 women in Terman's study of gifted California public school children. Between 1920 and 1922 Terman had attempted to identify all of the children in urban California with an IQ of 140 or over (Terman 1925). He had chosen to focus on three metropolitan areas in California: greater Oakland, greater San Francisco, and greater Los Angeles. Terman tested the most promising children individually with the Stanford-Binet Intelligence Test. In this fashion he identified 1,000 children with an IQ of 140 or above—the brightest 1% of California's urban public school children. Children who attended either private schools or schools in which Chinese was spoken were arbitrarily excluded. Over the next few years, Terman rather impulsively added additional cases of very bright children to his sample. Ultimately, he ended up with 672 women and 856 men.

Twenty percent of the TERMAN women's fathers were in blue-collar occupations, and 29% of the TERMAN women had fathers in "the professions." This figure was 10 times that of their public school classmates who served as control subjects; however, Terman's definition of "the professions" was broad and included high school teachers.

The TERMAN women were precocious. They had walked 1 month earlier than their schoolmates, and they had talked 3 months earlier (Terman 1925). Their average IQ was 151. Twenty percent of the women learned to read before age 5, and 60% had graduated from high school at

16 or younger. Their mental health was demonstrably better than their classmates' (Terman 1925). Their physical health was also better. Compared with their classmates they had better nutrition, better mental stability, fewer headaches, and fewer middle ear infections. Their siblings had suffered only half the childhood mortality experienced by the siblings of their classmates, and, up to the age of 78, the mortality of the TERMAN women has been only half what would be expected for white American women in their birth cohort.

From 1922 to 1986, Lewis Terman (1922–1956), and then his successors, first Melitta Oden (1956–1970), and then Robert Sears (1970–1989), followed these 1,528 gifted children by questionnaire (every 5 years) and by personal interview in 1940 (Terman 1925; Terman and Oden 1959; Oden 1968; Sears 1984). In 1940, 20 years after the initial study, Terman made his second concerted effort to interview and retest all of his subjects. Besides death, attrition at that time amounted to 2%. In 1986, after 65 years of follow-up, attrition for reasons other than death was still less than 10%.

In 1987, we selected a representative subsample of 90 women from Terman's original sample of 672 and reinterviewed 40 of the survivors who consented to an interview. Their average age was 78, and all had been born between 1909 and 1913. The process by which the 90 women in our subsample were chosen is illustrated in Table 6-1. Because of withdrawal,

Table 6–1. The representative sample of TERMAN women: the selection process

(1)	**Original sample**	$N = 672$
	Died before age 41	– 39 women
	Dropped/lost* 1920–1987	– 68 women
(2)	**Still active in 1950 (eligible for study)**	$N = 565*$
	Died after age 40 but before 1987*	– 182 women
(3)	**Eligible for interview in 1987**	$N = 383$
(4)	**16% of sample with birthdate 1909–1913 and address in selected area**	$N = 61$
(5)	**Addition of 16% of the 182 women who died prior to 1987**	$N = 29$
(6)	**Total**	$N = 90$
	Declined interview	–13 women
	No 1986 questionnaire	– 8 women
(7)	**Personal interview in 1987**	$N = 40$

*Because the numbers of subjects in lost and dropped categories have shifted over time due to new information, these figures may differ slightly from other published figures.

loss, and early death, the sample still eligible for study in midlife totaled 565. From this sample, in order to make their age as uniform as possible, we selected all women with birthdates between 1909 and 1913. In order to reduce travel time and sample size, we selected only those women who lived within two California telephone areas codes. These procedures reduced the sample to 61 (16%) of those women who survived until 1987. To this group we added an equal proportion—29 (16%)—of the 182 women who had died prior to our visit to California. Thus, there were a total of 90 women whose records we read and evaluated. We did not interview 8 of the 61 surviving women because they had not returned their 1986 questionnaires, which was our evidence of informed consent to request interview. In addition, 13 women refused reinterview, usually due to poor physical health. (An additional reason may have been because they had not been interviewed for almost 50 years.)

Because most of the 50 women that we did not interview had been followed for half a century, they could be included in most data analyses. In general, except for inferior physical health, these 50 women did not differ significantly from the 40 women that we interviewed.

Comparison of the Three Samples

Thirty percent of the COLLEGE men's fathers, but none of the CORE CITY men's fathers, were in social class I (physicians, successful lawyers, and businessmen); 31% of the CORE CITY men's fathers, but none of the COLLEGE men's fathers, were in social class V (unskilled laborers without 10 grades of education). The parents of the TERMAN women were largely middle class or skilled laborers (social classes III and IV). Among the TERMAN women's fathers there was only one unskilled laborer.

The mean education of the TERMAN women's fathers was 12 years, which is in contrast to 8 years for the fathers of their public school classmates, 8 years for the fathers of the CORE CITY men, and 16 years of education for the COLLEGE men's fathers. Fifteen percent of the TERMAN women's mothers had gone to college compared with 32% of the mothers of the COLLEGE men. The mean (Binet) IQ of the TERMAN women was 151; the mean (WAIS) IQ of the CORE CITY men was 95; the estimated mean IQ of the COLLEGE men was between 130 and 135. Perhaps the most convincing evidence that the TERMAN women's high intelligence was not an artifact of environmental privilege but based on biological potential was the fact that 75 times as many of their children as would be expected by chance had IQs over 170. Their children were clearly more "gifted," as defined by standardized IQ tests, than the children of the socially and economically more privileged COLLEGE men. Whereas negative environmental factors can profoundly lower tested IQ scores, positive environmental factors can elevate tested IQ by only a few points.

Sixty-seven percent of the TERMAN women were college graduates, in contrast to 99% of the COLLEGE and 10% of the CORE CITY men. Thirty-five percent of the CORE CITY men had completed fewer than 10 grades of education. Twenty-four percent of the TERMAN women and 76% of the COLLEGE men attended graduate school.

Taken individually, none of the three samples can be viewed as representative of the general population. However, the three samples do have the virtues of being vastly different socially from each other, and each sample represented a quite different historical birth cohort. Yet *within* each sample there was considerable homogeneity. Thus, the between-group *similarities* and the consistent within-group *differences* may be generalizable to other American Caucasian samples.

If, as was suggested in Chapter 5, some defenses are hypothesized to be more mature (more "healthy") than other defenses, can these distinctions in adaptiveness be reliably made? To address the first question of reliability I shall focus on the CORE CITY men, because, for them, the available information was the least rich and thus the methods used for those men can be most easily generalized to other samples. The methods used to assess the somewhat richer clinical records of the TERMAN women and of the COLLEGE men were essentially the same (Vaillant 1977; also see Chapter 9).

Working definitions of defenses were provided to each rater (see Appendix 3). The raters were first trained on interview protocols that had been rated by many others and then given a 20- to 30-page summary of the CORE CITY men's 2-hour semistructured interview obtained at age 47. The raters—a medical social worker and a recent college graduate in psychology—were deliberately chosen because they had not been psychoanalytically trained. These raters were blinded to both the CORE CITY men's childhood records and to the independent adult ratings of outcome.

Interview protocols were prepared by the interviewer from verbatim notes taken during a 2-hour interview of each of the CORE CITY men. These interviews had been designed to focus on difficulties in the individuals' relationships, physical health, and work. Numerous direct quotations were included in the interview protocols, but the methodology embodied both the scientific limitations and the advantages of journalism. The purpose was to use the interviewer's summary as the first step in data reduction and to retain interview emphases that are often lost in transcripts and tape recordings. In writing the interview summary to be used by the blind rater, the interviewer was instructed to elucidate, but not label, the behaviors by which the individuals had coped with their difficulties.

For each interview protocol, the raters were asked to note all possible instances of each of the 18 defensive styles discussed in Chapter 3. However, the three "psychotic," or level I, defenses listed in Table 3-3—delusional projection, denial, and distortion—were noted so seldom as to be irrelevant. The rater paid attention to both known past behaviors and alleged style of adaptation to past difficulties, as well as to the special vicissitudes of the interview interactions. Clinical inference was allowed. In this way, in each of the interviews obtained from the CORE CITY men, the raters identified from 10 to 30 defensive vignettes.

Once an individual's defensive styles were identified, the following procedure was used in order to wrestle clinical intuition into the computer (in order to transform metaphors into numbers). Because a critical question for reliability and validity was the distinction between "good denial" (mature defenses) and "bad denial" (immature defenses), the 15 individual defenses used frequently enough to count were clustered into three groups: *mature* (sublimation, suppression, anticipation, altruism, and humor), *intermediate or neurotic* (displacement, repression, isolation, and reaction formation), and *immature* (projection, schizoid fantasy, passive aggression, acting out, hypochondriasis, and dissociation).

In order to control for marked variation across subjects in the frequency of identified defensive vignettes, ratios of defenses at different levels of maturity rather than absolute numbers of defenses were employed. By this I mean that suppression as a style of defense received the same weight if it were noted three times in someone for whom 10 vignettes were counted and nine times in someone for whom a total of 30 vignettes were counted.

The relative proportion (i.e., the ratio) of defense vignettes in each of the three general categories (mature, intermediate, immature) was thus determined. In order to obtain a 9-point scale of maturity, the ratio between immature and mature defenses was used to distribute a total of 8 points. Of these 8 points, 1 to 5 points could be assigned to each of the three categories of maturity, but the total had to be 8, and every category had to be assigned at least 1 point. For example, someone who manifested 10 examples reflecting sublimation and suppression, 4 examples reflecting displacement and reaction formation, and *no* examples of immature defenses would be assessed a score of mature defense = 5, immature defenses = 1, and intermediate defenses = 2. If someone exhibited 6 examples reflecting mature, 8 examples reflecting intermediate, and 9 examples reflecting immature, he or she would be scored mature = 2, intermediate = 3, and immature = 3. Subtracting the rating (1–5) for mature defenses from the rating (1–5) for immature defenses provided a total score of +4 to –4 (i.e., a 9-point scale). For purposes of computation the score for overall maturity of defensive style for each individual was transformed into a 1-to-9 scale by adding 5 points to the total. Thus, a score of 1 reflected the most mature style and a score of 9 reflected the least mature adaptive style.

This procedure produced a normal (i.e., bell curve) distribution of scores, with a rater reliability of .84 for the CORE CITY men and .87 for the TERMAN women. Expressed less mathematically, the 9-point global ratings of maturity of defense assessed by two independent raters differed by more than 2 points in only 23 of 307 CORE CITY subjects rated and by more than 1 point in only 7 of the 37 TERMAN women so rated. In short, independent raters could consistently agree on whether an individual's dominant defensive style was mature (adaptive) or immature (maladaptive).

Are Defense Mechanisms Valid?

Maturity of Defenses and Mental Health

Having demonstrated that maturity of defenses can be reliably rated, the next question becomes validity. Does the maturity of persons' defenses tell us any more about their lives than would their handwriting or their astrological sign? As illustrated in Table 6-2, maturity of defenses is significantly associated with mental health, with maturity, and with the

Table 6–2. Association of maturity of defense and the major outcome variables

	TERMAN women (*n* = 37)	COLLEGE men (*n* = 186)	CORE CITY men (*n* = 307)
Life satisfaction (age 60–65)	.44	.35	NA*
Psychosocial maturity (Erikson [1950] stage)	.48	.44	.66
Mental health (GAS or HSRS)	.64	.57	.77
Job success (age 47)	.53	.34	.45
Marital stability (age 47)	.31	.37	.33
Job enjoyment (age 47)	.51	.42	.39
Percent of life employed	.37	NA	.39

Note. Pearson correlation coefficient was the measure of association used in this table. GAS = Global Assessment Scale (Endicott et al. 1976); HSRS = Health-Sickness Rating Scale (Luborsky 1962).
*Variable not available for this sample. Except for the three lowest correlations for the TERMAN women, all Pearson correlations are significant at *P* < .001.

capacity to work and to love. When roughly comparable variables were compared for our three samples, the associations remained equally strong, suggesting that the positive associations between maturity of defense and mental health were independent of social class, education, and gender. Prior work by Norma Haan (1963) also confirmed that maturity of psychosocial adaptation and mental health were correlated with maturity of defenses for both men and women.

A measure called *life satisfaction* (age 60–65) suggested that happiness in the TERMAN women predicted their maturity of defenses. Life satisfaction was assessed by asking the TERMAN women at age 60 to rate their satisfaction with their lives in five areas—friendships, family life, community service, cultural life, and joy in living—each on a 5-point scale. Their scores were summed and correlated with the assessed maturity of their defensive style 15 years later by a rater who was blind to their earlier self-reports.

It might be argued that joy in living allows the user the luxury of mature defenses. Thus, it is more important to demonstrate that maturity of defensive style has *predictive* validity rather than just the *face validity* suggested by most of the correlations shown in Table 6-2.

Predictive validity was assessed in two ways. First, life satisfaction for the COLLEGE sample at age 60–65 was assessed as follows: having reviewed the COLLEGE sample's biennial questionnaires from age 50–65, raters blind to the past scored (on a 5-point scale) how they would feel about having the same adjustment at that age. Mature defensive styles assessed from ages 20–47 predicted a subsequent life that others would view as satisfactory ($r = .35$; $P < .001$).

Second, the data in Table 6-3 suggest that maturity of defense predicts mental health as well as life satisfaction. Raters who knew nothing of the COLLEGE men's lives before age 50 assessed their joy in working, their use of psychiatrists and tranquilizers after age 50, the stability of their marriages, and whether their careers had progressed or declined since age

Table 6–3. Relation of maturity of defensive style with late midlife adjustment in the COLLEGE sample 15 years later

Psychosocial adjustment at 65	Defensive style (age 20–47)	
	Most mature ($n = 37$)	Least mature ($n = 31$)
Top quartile	19	1
Middle half	17	13
Bottom quartile	1	17

Note. $r = .42$; $P < .0001$.

47 (Vaillant and Vaillant 1990). Only one man assessed as using immature defenses before age 47 was doing relatively well at age 65. Only one man who used mature defenses before age 47 was doing relatively badly 18 years later.

The defenses of the 23 COLLEGE men who at some point in their adult lives were clinically depressed were contrasted with those of the 70 least-distressed COLLEGE men (i.e., men who in 30 years of observation never used tranquilizers, visited psychiatrists, *or* ever appeared to merit a psychiatric diagnosis). There is a marked difference in the overall maturity of defenses of the most-depressed men contrasted with the least-distressed (see Table 6-4). First, 61% of the least-distressed and only 9% of the most-depressed men exhibited generally mature defenses, whereas 47% of the most-depressed men and only 7% of the least-distressed men consistently favored less mature defensive styles. Stoicism (suppression) was relatively less common among the depressed men. Although altruism was used by many men and women with unhappy childhoods to master adult life, sustained use of altruism was never noted among those COLLEGE men who were ever found to manifest severe depression as adults. Instead, the most-depressed men were most likely to use displacement, dissociation (i.e., neurotic denial), reaction formation, and passive aggression (i.e., turning anger against themselves).

However, suspicions are still warranted, because simple association does not prove cause. For example, immature defenses are associated with, but do not cause, alcohol abuse and brain damage; however, both alcohol

Table 6–4. Difference between the most common defenses deployed by the least-distressed and the most-depressed COLLEGE men

	Percent using selected defenses as a major coping style	
	Most depressed ($n = 23$)	Least distressed ($n = 70$)
Suppression	26	53
Altruism	0	19
Reaction formation	17	4
Displacement	39	6
Dissociation	26	7
Passive aggression	30	16
Most mature (score = 1–3)	9	61
Least mature (score = 6–9)	47	7

Note. Differences significant at $P < .05$.

abuse and brain damage can *cause* regression in defense maturity. The association of immature defenses with depression is most likely not a simple horse-and-cart relationship. In some people severe depression probably leads to a regression in maturity of defenses. In other people immature defenses predispose them to depression. In still others, depression and immature defenses both reflect complementary aspects of a beleaguered ego. Much more evidence must be provided to clarify the relationship between affective disorder and maturity of defenses.

Maturity of Defenses and Physical Health

Using the COLLEGE sample, a final question was asked to test predictive validity for our assessment of defenses. Could we demonstrate that the assessment of defenses in young adulthood predicted future physical health? Unfortunately, evidence for prediction of physical health is not quite as convincing as the evidence for prediction of psychosocial adjustment at age 65.

In Figure 6-1 the declining physical health of 79 COLLEGE men with relatively mature defenses (white bars) is contrasted with the declining physical health of 61 COLLEGE men with relatively immature defenses (black bars). Maturity of defenses was assessed on the basis of the men's adaptive style between the ages of 20 and 47. For each 5-year period prior to age 60, men with immature defenses were much more likely to develop irreversible illness than were men with mature defenses. In other words, for at least 10 years after the defensive style was assessed, the health of the men with mature defenses continued to deteriorate less quickly. Thus, at least for a while, adaptive choice of defense mechanisms may have provided some kind of immunization against unsuccessful living. By age 65, however, this association of mature defenses with continued good health could no longer be discerned.

Expressed differently, when the five competing predictors of *physical* health at age 65 shown in Table 6-5 were controlled, other variables such as chronic alcoholism and clinical depression replaced maturity of defenses as the premorbid variables that distinguished COLLEGE men who would remain physically healthy from those who would not. However, if immaturity of these men's defenses made no unique contribution to prediction of physical health, neither did their blood cholesterol, obesity, or exercise and smoking habits at age 50.

Table 6-5 tells a different story for the predictors of psychosocial adjustment at age 65. When all of the other five variables affecting physical health in late midlife are controlled, maturity of defenses before age 50 still predicts an important amount of the observed differences in mental health

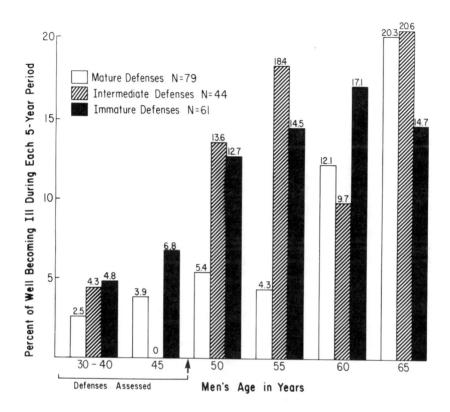

Figure 6-1. Comparison of physical health of COLLEGE men (*n* = 79) with relatively mature defenses (the white bars) with that of COLLEGE men (*n* = 61) with relatively immature defenses (the black bars). Maturity of defenses was assessed on the basis of the men's adaptive style between the ages of 20 and 47. The bars of the graph show only the percent of men *still in good health* ("excellent" or "minor problems") at the start of each 5-year period.

at age 65. Unfortunately, the size of the data set provides too little statistical power to allow the estimated variance contributed by *external* manifestations of mental illness (i.e., prior clinical diagnosis of depression and anxiety, and prior use of mood-altering drugs) on mental health to be dissected from the estimated variance contributed by the highly correlated style of inferred *intrapsychic* homeostasis (i.e., ego mechanisms of defense). Perhaps

Table 6–5. Unique variance of predictor variables in explaining physical
health and adult adjustment of COLLEGE men in late midlife

| | Partial correlation of each predictive variable with the other five variables controlled | |
	With physical health at age 63	With adult adjustment age 50–65
Use of mood-altering drugs before age 50	− .39***	− .28***
Maturity of defenses (age 20–47)	.04	.32***
Childhood environmental strengths	.21***	.08
Alcohol abuse before age 50	− .16*	− .18*
Vigorous exercise in college	.11	.22**
Ancestral longevity	.07	.01

Note. N = 164 (not 186) due to missing variables for some subjects.
*P < .05; **P < .01; ***P < .001.

immaturity of defenses and vulnerability to anxiety and depression may
simply reflect two sides of the same coin, but such circularity can still be
used to argue the power of the concept of maturity of defenses.

Is Maturity of Defensive Style Independent of Gender, Education, and Social Privilege?

A major task of psychiatry is to try to divorce the homeostatic mechanisms
by which human beings maintain mental health from sociocultural artifact.
In biological medicine the task is easier. For example, blood clotting factors
are distributed in an egalitarian fashion. Thus, the Romanov and Hapsburg
royal families died young from hemophilia, but their peasants did not.
Hopefully, biology has been as democratic in its distribution of ego strength
as it has been in distributing clotting factors and immune mechanisms, but
there is room for doubt.

Certainly, many parameters of mental health *are* clearly a function of
social class, of societal bias toward gender, and/or of education and IQ.
For example, the extent of psychiatric utilization is an index of mental illness
only among socially homogeneous groups. Thus, about 40% of the COL-
LEGE men sought help from outpatient psychiatrists, and approximately
3% of the CORE CITY men did so; yet, if anything, the mental health of
the less highly selected CORE CITY men was worse. Again, in a *within-*

cohort comparison of CORE CITY men, income correlated with mental health. In a *between*-cohort comparison, however, the equally mentally healthy TERMAN women earned only a third of what the intellectually less gifted and only modestly better-educated COLLEGE men earned. The responsibility for this difference lies more with society than with mental health. Finally, the undereducated CORE CITY men (and the least verbally gifted COLLEGE men) scored a full ego development stage lower on Loevinger's Sentence Completion Test than did verbally fluent COLLEGE men (Vaillant and McCullough 1987). In short, socioeconomic status and gender can make a big difference in many variables that we may use to measure mental health.

However, maturity of defensive style seemed to be unaffected by such demographic variables (see Table 6-6). True, the COLLEGE men originally selected for mental health look a little better, and the CORE CITY men deliberately matched with delinquents for social disadvantage look a little worse. But considering the vast difference in intelligence, social privilege, and education between the two samples, these differences in defensive maturity are inconsequential and easily explained by original sampling bias. The COLLEGE sample was selected to be mentally healthier than their Harvard classmates; the CORE CITY men were selected to be as similar as possible to their delinquent classmates.

A less-distorted view of the effect of privilege on defensive style is achieved by comparing the members of each group with each other. In this way initial selection bias is circumvented. The effect of social class, IQ, and education on within-group differences in defensive maturity has been examined (see Table 6-7). The association is insignificant. Even the relationship of a warm childhood environment upon maturity of defense is less strong than one might expect. Such independence from social environment is what one would expect for biological differences (e.g., blood groups or immunological competence).

Table 6–6. Relative maturity of defensive style among the three samples

Maturity of defense score	TERMAN women (*n* = 50)	COLLEGE men (*n* = 187)	CORE CITY men* (*n* = 203)
1–3	44%	42%	29%
4–6	36%	47%	46%
7–9	20%	11%	25%

*Men with IQs less than 80 and alcohol abuse were excluded to avoid the confounding effects of possible brain damage.

Table 6–7. Association of defensive maturity with biopsychosocial antecedents

	TERMAN women (n = 37)	COLLEGE men (n = 186)	CORE CITY men (n = 277)[a]
Parental social class	−.07	.04	−.02
IQ	.18	−.05	.10
Years of education	.09	NA	.17*
Warm relations with father	.24	.23*	.01
Warm child environment	.39*	.36*	.10
Warm relations with mother	.22	.18*	.04
Parental longevity	.02	.10	NA

Note. Pearson correlation coefficient was the statistic used in this table. NA = not available or not applicable.
[a]Thirty men with IQs of less than 80 excluded.
*$P < .01$

Are there individual defensive styles more favored by women than men? Certainly, everybody we have asked "knows" that women deploy different defensive styles than men. But their knowledge has been based on intuition, not on data. In the Study of Adult Development, in order to obtain a numerical score for the individual defenses, weighting was achieved through frequency of observed use. Each rater scored each defense 0 if absent, 1 if noted once or twice, and 2 if it was the most frequently used defense or noted 3 times or more in the 2-hour interview for the TERMAN women and the CORE CITY men. For the more intensively studied COLLEGE sample, the 0, 1, 2 rating was made on all data gathered between ages 20 and 47. The two raters did not always agree. Indeed, depending on the defense, in 4% to 20% of the cases, one rater could see a defense as major when the other rater had scored it as absent. The two raters' ratings for each subject in each sample were summed. This provided an individual rating for each defense that ranged from 0 (if both raters agreed it was absent) to 4 (if both agreed it was major). What were the differences in choice of defensive style among the three groups? The answer, as suggested by Tables 6-8 and 6-9, was that the differences were surprisingly small.

In Table 6-8 we ordered by rank the frequency with which each defense was used as a major style by each sample. (Relative differences in ranking are underlined to help the reader follow the text, but underlining does not reflect statistical significance.) Displacement and projection were used as major defenses relatively more by CORE CITY men, whereas sublimation was noted more often among the highly educated groups. Because displace-

Table 6–8. Relative frequency of a given defense being a major defensive style

	CORE CITY men (*n* = 203)		TERMAN women (*n* = 40)		COLLEGE men (*n* = 188)	
	Rank order	Percent	Rank order	Percent	Rank order	Percent
Isolation	1	52	2	38	1	46
Displacement	2	47	6	13	4	18
Suppression	3	34	1	43	1	46
Repression	4	16	11	5	5	17
Dissociation	5	15	6	13	6	13
Altruism	6	12	3	33	6	13
Reaction formation	7	10	5	20	9	11
Passive aggression	8	10	8	10	3	23
Projection	9	9	14	3	13	2
Sublimation	10	7	4	30	6	13
Fantasy	11	5	8	10	11	3
Anticipation	11	5	11	5	10	4
Humor	11	5	10	8	14	1
Hypochondriasis	14	3	11	5	11	3
Acting out	15	1	15	0	15	0

Note. Underlined values indicate relative (but not necessarily significant) differences in the use of defenses by the three samples.

ment evolves into sublimation, the difference in the rater's perception of less graceful, less mature attenuation of impulse among the CORE CITY men may be real or it may be an artifact of education or of rater bias. For example, in mastering conflict, writing graffiti on subway cars would be classified as displacement and writing that would appear in *The New Yorker* would be classified as sublimation; however, the difference may rest more on the artist's education and IQ than upon his or her ego maturity.

The TERMAN women were somewhat more likely to use fantasy, altruism, and reaction formation. This finding may reflect their special adaptation to the social injustices that they experienced throughout their lives, rather than the influence of biology. But in view of the different methods used and the number of comparisons made, it would be hard to argue that any of the differences in the data shown in Tables 6-8 and 6-9 were statistically significant. Of greater interest perhaps is that two defenses, passive aggression (masochism) and repression—sometimes thought to be more common among women—were, if anything, more common among the men.

Table 6–9.   Relative frequency of **never** using a given defensive style

	CORE CITY men (n = 203)		TERMAN women (n = 40)		COLLEGE men (n = 188)	
	Rank order	Percent	Rank order	Percent	Rank order	Percent
Hypochondriasis	1	73	4	70	1	76
Humor	2	68	9	33	5	57
Fantasy	3	60	5	65	4	68
Acting out	4	57	1	95	2	72
Anticipation	4	57	2	78	6	44
Sublimation	6	56	9	33	11	30
Projection	7	51	2	78	3	69
Altruism	8	47	12	20	8	34
Passive aggression	9	34	6	58	7	38
Reaction formation	10	26	13	18	10	32
Dissociation	11	17	7	55	8	34
Suppression	12	15	14	13	14	8
Repression	13	13	8	53	13	20
Isolation	14	5	14	13	15	6
Displacement	15	1	11	28	12	25

The frequency with which members of each sample were *never* observed to use a given defensive style was ordered by rank in Table 6-9. The only difference not already remarked upon was the that TERMAN women were more likely to use humor and less likely to use its less mature first cousin, dissociation. Whether this difference is an artifact of the effect of the women's intelligence and sophisticated verbal repartee upon the rater's judgment or a reflection of the maturity of the TERMAN women's ego function is uncertain. Certainly, the boundary that divides the denial and self-deception of humor from the denial and self-deception of dissociation is fuzzy and susceptible to observer bias. However, given the modest reliability of assessment of the individual defenses, the most noteworthy finding drawn from these two tables is that none of the differences is more than suggestive. Far more careful experimental control would be required to validate the differences. The main lessons to be taken away from the data presented in Tables 6-8 and 6-9 are the similarities. In short, defensive style did not seem to be an artifact of social class, education, or gender.

If gender and social class are not important in shaping maturity of defensive style, what about ethnicity? Because of the subtle nuances in idiomatic language and difficulties in exactly matching samples, it is very difficult to draw valid conclusions about differences in defensive styles between residents of different countries. Serendipitously, however, the CORE CITY sample provided a way around this difficulty. Sixty-one percent of the CORE CITY men had had parents who had been born in a foreign country; and yet all of the subjects had grown up in Boston schools, were fluent in English, and had been sampled and studied in the same way. In some facets of adult life, parental ethnic differences had a profound effect. For example, men of white Anglo-Saxon Protestant and Irish extractions were five times as likely to develop alcoholism as were men of Italian extraction (Vaillant 1983); but, at least in this sample, parental ethnicity did not appear to exert a significant effect on defensive style.

When 55 men with parents born in Italy were contrasted with 100 men with parents born either in Great Britain or in anglophone Canada or of old Yankee stock, the similarities were extraordinary (see Table 6-10). As with gender, the differences in defensive style that we intuitively ascribe to culture may be more apparent than real. Dissociation was the one defensive

Table 6–10. Effect of ethnicity on the use of selected defenses as a major style among CORE CITY men

	Italian (*n* = 74)	White Anglo-Saxon Protestant* (*n* = 100)
Mature defenses		
Suppression	25%	30%
Altruism	10%	12%
Sublimation	6%	6%
Anticipation	4%	5%
Humor	6%	11%
Intermediate defenses		
Reaction formation	8%	14%
Isolation	50%	45%
Repression	16%	20%
Displacement	37%	50%
Immature defenses		
Dissociation	16%	39%
Projection	12%	12%
Passive aggression	19%	18%
Hypochondriasis	7%	4%
Fantasy	3%	4%
Acting out	4%	5%

*Men of old American or English or anglophone Canadian parents.

style noted significantly more often $(P < .01)$ among the men's white Anglo-Saxon Protestant parentage. This difference could not be ascribed to the greater frequency of alcohol abuse among this group. Even among the men who were not alcohol abusers, dissociation was still twice as common among the white Anglo-Saxon Protestant men as among men of Italian extraction. Clearly, the question of ethnic differences in defensive styles requires more research, but with improving research on personality, cultural anthropologists have come to similar conclusions. With proper control for observer bias, personality differences appear to be relatively independent of ethnicity (Kleinman 1986; Levine 1973).

However, if culture exerts little effect on defensive style, biology exerts a profound effect. The central nervous system of some men in the study had been impaired by chronic alcoholism. (We are not discussing acute intoxication, for most men were relatively sober when interviewed.) Some men also had *possible* cognitive impairment as suggested by an IQ of less than 80. In both groups defensive styles were significantly less mature. As can be seen in Table 6-11, all the immature defenses were two to four times

Table 6–11. Effect of cognitive impairment and alcohol abuse on the use of mature and immature defenses as a major defensive style among CORE CITY men

	Unimpaired CORE CITY sample ($n = 203$)	IQ < 80 ($n = 29$)	Chronic alcoholism ($n = 24$)
Mature defenses			
Suppression	34%	34%	11%**
Altruism	12%	7%	0%
Sublimation	7%	3%	0%*
Anticipation	5%	3%	0%
Humor	5%	3%	4%
Immature defenses			
Dissociation	15%	45%**	83%**
Projection	9%	10%	29%*
Passive aggression	10%	31%	46%**
Hypochondriasis	3%	17%**	21%*
Fantasy	5%	0%	13%*
Acting out	1%	10%	8%**

Note. In order to compute statistical significance, the full sample of 307 men was used and years of alcoholism and IQ were correlated with the full range (0–4) rating for each individual defense. Pearson correlation coefficient was the statistic used in this table.
*$P < .01$; **$P < .001$.

as common in the two groups with compromised central nervous systems as in the unimpaired sample. Because of the small numbers of individuals in the samples, the differences could not always be demonstrated to be statistically significant. Also, postponement of gratification (suppression) was much more common among CORE CITY men with normal (IQ in the 80–120 range) intelligence than among those afflicted with alcoholism.

These findings confirm and expand on those reported by Vaillant et al. (1986). Although maturity of defensive style differs greatly among adults, the sources of this variance appear to be more biological than psychosocial.

References

Endicott J, Spitzer RL, Fleiss JL, et al: The Global Assessment Scale: a procedure for measuring overall severity of psychiatric disturbance. Arch Gen Psychiatry 33:766–770, 1976

Erikson E: Childhood and Society. New York, WW Norton, 1950

Glueck S, Glueck E: Unraveling Juvenile Delinquency. New York, Common Wealth Fund, 1950

Glueck S, Glueck E: Delinquents and Non-Delinquents in Perspective. Cambridge, MA, Harvard University Press, 1968

Haan N: Proposed model of ego functioning: coping and defense mechanisms in relationship to IQ change. Psychological Monographs 77:1–23, 1963

Heath C: What People Are. Cambridge, MA, Harvard University Press, 1945

Hollingshead A, Redlich FC: Mental Health and Mental Illness. New York, John Wiley, 1958

Kleinman A: Social Origins of Distress and Disease. New Haven, CT, Yale University Press, 1986

Levine RA: Culture, Behavior and Personality. Chicago, IL, Aldine Publishing, 1973

Luborsky L: Clinicians' judgments of mental health. Arch Gen Psychiatry 7:407–417, 1962

Monks JP: College Men at War. Boston, MA, American Academy of Arts and Sciences, 1957

Oden MH: The fulfillment of promise: 40-year follow-up of the Terman gifted group. Genetic Psychological Monographs 77:3–93, 1968

Sears RR: The Terman Gifted Children Study, in Handbook of Longitudinal Research, 9th Edition. Edited by Mednick SA, Harway M, Finello KM. New York, Praeger, 1984

Terman LM: Genetic Studies of Genius, Vol 1: Mental and Physical Traits of a Thousand Gifted Children. Stanford, CA, Stanford University Press, 1925

Terman LM, Oden MH: Genetic Studies of Genius, Vol 5: The Gifted Group at Midlife. Stanford, CA, Stanford University Press, 1959

Vaillant GE: Adaptation to Life. Boston, MA, Little, Brown, 1977

Vaillant GE: Natural History of Alcoholism. Cambridge, MA, Harvard University Press, 1983

Vaillant GE, McCullough L: A comparison of the Washington University Sentence Completion Test (SCT) with other measures of adult ego development. Am J Psychiatry 144:1189–1194, 1987

Vaillant GE, Vaillant CO: Natural history of male psychological health, XII: a forty-five year study of predictors of successful aging at age 65. Am J Psychiatry 147:31–37, 1990

Vaillant GE, Bond M, Vaillant CO: An empirically validated hierarchy of defense mechanisms. Arch Gen Psychiatry 43:786–794, 1986

Chapter 7

An Empirical Study of Defensive Styles: The Defense Style Questionnaire

Michael Bond, M.D.

The concept of defense mechanisms has been a clinically useful metaphor that can be used to explain certain speculated intrapsychic processes. However, the accurate empirical measurement of defense mechanisms has been confounded by lack of inter-rater reliability, validity, and conceptual clarity. In March 1983, I, along with Susan T. Gardner, Ph.D., John Christian, Ph.D., and John Sigal, Ph.D., reported on our research with a questionnaire, the Defense Style Questionnaire (DSQ), designed to eliminate the problem of inter-rater reliability (Bond et al. 1983). In a follow-up study, with Jacqueline Sagala Vaillant, M.D., we reported our findings on the relationship between defense style and diagnosis (Bond and Sagala Vaillant 1986). Currently I am trying to establish the validity of the DSQ by comparing the results of patients' self-reports with raters' judgments of defense mechanisms while watching videotaped clinical interviews. In this chapter all our research to date is brought together.

The concept of defense mechanisms is pervasive in the psychiatric and psychoanalytic literature, but there is confusion and inconsistency about what defense mechanisms are and how they relate to diagnosis. Laplanche and Pontalis (1973) defined defense mechanisms as

> different types of operations through which defense may be given specific expression. Which of these mechanisms predominate in a given case depends upon the type of illness under consideration, upon the developmental stage reached, upon the extent to which the defensive conflict has been worked out, and so on.
>
> It is generally agreed that the ego puts the defense mechanisms to use, but the theoretical question of whether their mobilization always presupposes the existence of an organized ego capable of sustaining them is an open one. (p. 109)

Laplanche and Pontalis continued: "Freud's choice of the word mechanisms is intended, from the outset, to indicate the fact that psychical phenomena are so organized as to permit scientific observation and analysis" (p. 109). However, the scientific examination of defense mechanisms has proved to be a difficult and confused exercise. Our primary purpose was to develop a questionnaire for the experimental study of defense mechanisms that did not rely on the rater's subjective judgment. Our achievement was more modest. We devised a self-administered questionnaire, the DSQ, that taps possible conscious derivatives of defense mechanisms.

Within the definition of Laplanche and Pontalis, one can see some of the confusing facets of defense mechanisms associated both with "illness" and with "an organized ego capable of sustaining them [the defense mechanisms]." These mechanisms can be seen both as a constricting influence that limits growth and as an adaptive process that protects the person and enables him or her to function. This theme runs throughout the writing of Freud (1926), A. Freud (1937), and Kernberg (1967), even as they link defense mechanisms with illness. Vaillant (1976), Haan et al. (1973), and Semrad et al. (1973) are more explicit in describing the adaptive aspects of defense or coping mechanisms as well as the regressive aspects. We wanted to investigate whether there is, as Freud (1926) suggested, "an intimate connection between special forms of defense and particular illnesses" (pp. 163–164), or whether there is a factor other than specific illnesses that is more closely correlated with specific groupings of defense mechanisms.

This focus brought us to certain crucial questions. Which phenomena can be labeled defense or coping mechanisms? Can these phenomena be measured? Do defense or coping mechanisms cluster into defense styles? Can defenses be measured? Along with function, are defense styles organized? Can defense styles be related to the developmental stage reached or other unique information about ego functioning?

Defense Mechanisms

To answer the first question regarding which phenomena can be called defenses, we began with Freud (1926), who listed regression, repression, reaction formation, isolation, undoing, projection, introjection, turning against the self, and reversal. A. Freud (1937) described sublimation, displacement, denial in fantasy, denial in word and act, identification with the aggressor, and altruism. Kernberg (1967) and Klein (1973) described splitting, omnipotence with devaluation, primitive idealization, projective identification, and psychotic denial.

Vaillant (1976) substituted some overt behaviors for intrapsychic processes in his study, claiming that "such substitution permits the examination of ego function in operational rather than in theoretical terms" (p. 54). In so doing, he added to the list of defenses fantasy, passive aggression, hypochondriasis, acting out, suppression, humor, and anticipation.

It seems timely to try to bring some order into such a bewildering array of proposed defenses. We set out to see whether current statistical methods—specifically, factor analysis—could serve this purpose.

Several investigators have attempted to answer the question of whether and how these phenomena can be measured. In trying to develop an experimental method for the study of defense mechanisms, both Vaillant (1976) and Haan et al. (1973) used psychiatric interviews in combination with other measures, such as psychological tests, questionnaires, and autobiographical reports. Vaillant pointed out that the clinical judgment required in his study limited the objectivity and reliability of the ratings. He went on to emphasize the need to make intrapsychic processes operational so that defenses can be studied experimentally.

Bellak et al. (1973) attempted to determine empirically the extent to which defense mechanisms in general maladaptively affect ideation, behavior, and the adaptive level of other ego functions, and the extent to which defenses succeed or fail in controlling dysphoric affects. The difficulty with this approach was that it did not provide a means for identifying and examining individual defense mechanisms.

Semrad et al. (1973) created an ego profile scale that they used to empirically measure different types of ego functioning. The items for the questionnaire were generated by two of the authors and then categorized into nine ego defense categories by 25 senior psychiatrists. An item was accepted as indicative of a particular ego defense if a sufficient number of raters independently agreed on its assignment to that category. The ego profile scale was filled out by patients' therapists on a weekly basis. The creation of this scale, as well as the scoring of the scale, depended solely on therapist's opinions and observations. An instrument that does not depend on therapists' subjective opinions for predetermining defense grouping or for making individual ratings is still needed.

Measurement of Defense Mechanisms: An Empirical Study of Defense Styles

The problem of measuring intrapsychic phenomena that are often unconscious is immense. The method that we developed for this study is merely an attempt to approach the measurement of defense mechanisms through self-appraisals of conscious derivatives. Although this method does not directly measure defense mechanisms, it may relate to them.

In this chapter, the term *defense mechanism* is used to describe not only an unconscious intrapsychic process but also behavior that is either consciously or unconsciously designed to reconcile internal drives with external demands. It would be impossible to conclude anything about isolated defense mechanisms, but we hoped that we could approximate the measurement of groups of defense mechanisms that collectively we call *defense style*.

We hypothesized that defense styles might identify aspects of a person's stage of development and render other information about ego functioning independent of diagnosis. Vaillant (1975, 1976), who divided defenses into narcissistic, immature, neurotic, and mature groups, demonstrated that this theoretical hierarchy of defenses correlated with empirical definitions of mental health. Haan and co-workers (Haan 1969; Haan et al. 1973) divided ego processes into coping, defensive, and fragmentation, placing emphasis on different styles and not only on level of development. Semrad et al. (1973) also proposed a hierarchy of ego functioning, specifically with regard to defense styles.

Shapiro (1965) used neurotic styles to refer to "a form or mode of functioning . . . that is identifiable, in an individual, through a range of his [or her] specific acts" (p. 1). He outlined four major neurotic styles—obsessive-compulsive, hysterical, paranoid, and impulsive—but used no empirical data.

Linking defenses with specific illnesses can create confusion. The term *defense* should refer to a style of dealing with conflict or stress, whereas the term *diagnosis* should refer to a constellation of symptoms and signs. Separating the examination of defenses from the issue of diagnosis would allow the concept of defense to be used more precisely during investigation of fluctuations in a person's style in dealing with a particular stress at a particular time and under particular circumstances. The use of that style would also reveal something about the level of psychosocial development.

A description follows of our preliminary attempt to contribute to the search for an objective, empirical method of studying the relations among defense mechanisms, diagnosis, level of maturity, and other ongoing psychological phenomena.

Subjects

In our study, 209 volunteers participated: 111 nonpatients and 98 patients. The persons in the nonpatient sample, from their own point of view, were functioning adequately and at the time of testing were not undergoing psychiatric treatment. The patient sample consisted of 98 persons drawn from the psychiatric wards or psychiatric outpatient departments of three university teaching or affiliated hospitals.

The nonpatient sample comprised 10 high school students, 5 students at a junior college, 36 university students, 57 subjects actively employed in socially recognized occupations or as homemakers, and 3 retired persons. Ages ranged from 16 to 69 years (mean = 31 years); 48 of the subjects were male and 63 were female.

The patient sample included 42 inpatients and 56 outpatients. According to the simple, forced-choice evaluation sheet, the following diagnoses were made by the attending psychologist or psychiatrist: psychotic, 39; borderline, 26; neurotic, 22; having personality disorder, 6; and other, 5. Ages ranged from 25 to 64 years (mean = 27 years); 48 were male and 50 were female. The mean ages in the three major diagnostic categories of psychotic, borderline, and neurotic were 29.3 (SD = 11.2), 25.1 (SD = 7.3), and 24.0 (SD = 11.4) years, respectively.

Methods

Questionnaire measuring self-report of defense styles

In the classical psychoanalytic sense, defense mechanisms are an unconscious process. A self-report thus may not detect a phenomenon of which a subject is unaware. Our approach to this objection was based on the following premises. There are times when defenses fail temporarily, and at those times a subject may become aware of the unacceptable impulses and his or her usual styles of defending against them. In addition, others often point out defense mechanisms to the person. A statement such as "People tell me that I often take my anger out on someone other than the one at whom I'm really angry" might tap displacement even if the subject is unaware of defensive behavior at the time that it is happening. A statement such as "When I have a close friend, I need to be with him all the time" can tap clinging behavior because the subject may have had this behavior pointed out to him or her, or the subject may have noted anxious or depressed feelings when unable to use this defensive behavior. The DSQ was designed to elicit manifestations of a subject's characteristic style of dealing with conflict, either conscious or unconscious, based on the assumption that persons can accurately comment on their behavior from a distance. Only a clinical examination could identify unconscious processes as they are happening.

With this rationale, statements were designed to reflect behavior suggestive of the following 24 defense or coping mechanisms: acting out, pseudoaltruism, as-if behavior, clinging, humor, passive-aggressive behavior, regression, somatization, suppression, withdrawal, dissociation, denial, displacement, omnipotence-devaluation, inhibition, intellectualization, identification, primitive idealization, projection, reaction formation, repression, splitting, sublimation, and turning against self. These statements were subjected to an initial test of face validity by asking two psychologists and one psychiatrist (two of the three are psychoanalysts), independently, to match up each statement with its relevant defense or coping mechanism. Only the statements on which they all could agree formed our initial 97-statement questionnaire. The entire revised questionnaire can be found in Appendix 6. Below are some representative examples.

1. "If someone mugged me and stole my money, I'd rather he be helped than punished." [Reaction formation]
2. "There's no such thing as finding a little good in everyone. If you're bad, you're all bad." [Splitting]
3. "If my boss bugged me, I might make a mistake in my work or work more slowly so as to get back at him." [Passive-aggressive behavior]
4. "I always feel that someone I know is like a guardian angel." [Primitive idealization]

Subjects were asked to indicate their degree of agreement or disagreement with each statement on a 9-point scale: 1 indicated strong disagreement and 9 indicated strong agreement. All scales were constructed so that a high score on any one defense measure indicated that the defense was being used by that subject.

In a pilot project, we tested 30 patients on the first version of our DSQ, which consisted of the statements measuring self-appraisal of defense style randomly interspersed with statements from a parallel research project (R. D. Brown, M.D., and S. T. Gardner, Ph.D., personal communication, January 1980) designed to measure ego functioning. Internal consistency among statements that were designed to measure the same defense was assessed through item-to-total correlations. Only statements correlating with their parent group at a significance level of greater than .001 were retained.[1] We thus kept 81 of the initial 97 statements measuring possible conscious derivatives of defense mechanisms and have added 7 more statements.

---

[1]The number of statements in each category ranged from one to six. Thus, the item-to-total correlation procedure was satisfactory for only some of the defenses. The face validity criterion mentioned earlier can be considered a complement, for item selection purposes, to the item-to-total correlation method when the latter would yield spuriously high correlations.

Our hypotheses were that 1) factor analysis would demonstrate separate clusters of defense mechanisms—that is, defense styles, and 2) defenses thought to be immature (such as acting out, projection, withdrawal, and passive-aggressive behavior) would cluster at the end opposite from defenses thought to be more mature.[2]

Ego development

The following measures of ego development were correlated with data from the DSQ to determine if there was a hierarchy of defense mechanisms.

Ego Function Questionnaire.   In an attempt to cross-validate Bellak et al.'s (1973) conclusion that ego functioning is multidimensional, Brown and Gardner (personal communication) constructed a questionnaire designed to measure a number of different ego functions. Because only one factor was found, Brown and Gardner argued that a subject's total score on the questionnaire, which is referred to as the "ego strength score," reflected the person's general level of adaptation.

Sentence Completion Test.   The second measure of ego development was a sentence completion test consisting of 36 items—23 from Loevinger (1976) and Loevinger and Wessler (1970) and 13 from Aronoff (1971). Subjects completed items in whatever way they wished. Two of Loevinger and Wessler's original raters rated one-third of the Loevinger protocols according to the Loevinger-Wessler method of rating. The inter-rater reliability coefficient was .84 ($P < .001$). The remaining protocols were scored by one rater. Ego development scores computed on the basis of the sentence completion test are referred to herein as the "ego development score."

Several questions can be raised concerning the validity of Loevinger and Wessler's Sentence Completion Test. First is the question of *discriminant validity*—that is, whether the test is measuring qualities or characteristics that are different from those measured by other tests. Because several criteria for scoring the test concern cognitive differentiation or complexity, it is important to establish that the test is not simply measuring the intelligence level or IQ. Blasi (1970) reported correlations of between .46 and .50 between scores on the Sentence Completion Test and the

---

[2]This approach differs from that of Semrad et al. (1973) in that it does not cluster defenses into preconceived categories; it relies on factor analysis to determine the clusters. Our approach also differs from that of Semrad et al. in that the data come from subjects' responses to a questionnaire rather than clinicians' ratings.

Large-Thorndike Intelligence Test. Thus, only 21% to 25% of ego development level variance is accounted for by IQ.

Second, there is the question of *predictive validity*—that is, how effective the test is in predicting an external criterion. Hauser (1976) argued that while a single external criterion would be unlikely to be related to any particular ego development stage, patterns or constellations of behavior should serve as suitable criteria. In this regard, Cox (1974) considered helping behavior in relation to ego development, Blasi (1972) considered responsibility, and Hoppe (1972) looked at conformity behavior in relation to ego development. The findings are generally extremely complex, frequently because situational cues were not adequately taken into account.

Finally, a closely related question is one that concerns *construct validity*—that is, if the construct of ego development (Loevinger 1966) is accurate, then certain phenomena should be expected to follow. Hauser (1976) has reviewed the numerous phenomena that may be related to the construct, but a few basic assumptions about interpersonal behavior can be mentioned here. For instance, Frank and Quinlan (1976) reported that subjects who scored at the lower ego developmental levels (impulsive and self-protective) showed significantly ($P < .05$) more fighting incidents and running away than adolescents from all other stages. Blasi (1972) found that the relation between the degree to which sixth-grade boys and girls behaved responsibly (rated by these observers) and their ego development scores was statistically significant, the correlation being .56 for girls and .54 for boys.

The Loevinger-Wessler (1970) conception of ego development postulates that the tendency to conform increases through the early stages of development (impulsive and self-protective), peaks at the middle stages (conformist), and declines with later development (conscientious, autonomous, and integrated). Using a variety of techniques, Hoppe (1972) rated conformity behaviors and found the predicted relationship: maximum values of conformity were associated with subjects scoring high in the conformist range of the ego development test ($P < .05$). Although some of Loevinger's postulates, such as the invariant sequence of stages, have yet to be thoroughly investigated, an increasing body of research suggests that the Sentence Completion Test is based on a construct that is basically sound and relates well with the constellations of behavior that are described by or can be inferred from Loevinger's account of each stage.

Results

As in the pilot project, item-to-item correlations were carried out for each question, and then for the total score of the questions attributed to each defense mechanism in relation to the factor to which it belonged, to ensure that reliability had been retained and that the statements still correlated with the other statements in the relevant defense category. All correlations remained significant at a greater that .001 level.

Principal component (type PA1, quartimax rotation) (Nie et al. 1975, pp. 484–485) factor analyses were carried out on the sets of statements on the 24 postulated defenses for the entire sample and for the patient and nonpatient samples taken separately. The size of the eigen values indicated that a four-factor solution provided an adequate representation of the data for the combined group and for the nonpatient and patient samples taken separately (see Table 7-1; other data obtainable on request). In the factor analysis carried out on the combined group, and in that on the nonpatient and patient samples taken separately, the same defenses clustered together.

Table 7–1. Factor loadings on defenses (combined sample)

Defense	Factor 1	Factor 2	Factor 3	Factor 4
Acting out	.76	.11	−.10	−.23
Regression	.67	−.01	−.09	−.29
Passive-aggressive behavior	.74	.10	−.02	−.09
Withdrawal	.75	−.17	.11	.05
Projection	.69	.31	.02	−.41
Inhibition	.69	−.20	.17	−.01
Omnipotence-devaluation	.17	.70	−.10	.21
Splitting	.38	.60	−.05	−.20
Primitive idealization	.36	.54	.36	.15
Pseudoaltruism	.33	−.08	.62	.06
Reaction formation	.36	−.07	.56	.06
Sublimation	−.09	.12	.17	.64
Humor	−.14	.02	−.27	.63
Suppression	−.10	.02	.00	.62
As-if behavior	.62	.05	.07	.32
Clinging	.64	.34	.04	.02
Denial	.33	.04	.52	−.05
Displacement	.49	.15	−.19	.05
Dissociation	.63	.22	.15	−.17
Identification	.45	.32	.19	.29
Intellectualization	.49	−.12	−.11	.33
Repression	.53	−.08	.05	−.17
Somatization	.56	.19	.11	.10
Turning against self	.61	−.26	.02	−.03

Note. Type PA1, quartimax rotation (25).
Source. Reprinted from Bond et al. 1983, with permission from the American Medical Association. Copyright 1983, American Medical Association.

Defense style 1 (factor 1) consisted of apparent derivatives of defense mechanisms usually viewed as immature—namely, withdrawal, regression, acting out, inhibition, passive aggression, and projection. All of the above produced factor loadings greater than .65 on the combined analyses and loadings greater than .55 on the separate analyses, except for regression, which only loaded at .40 for the nonpatients.

Defense style 2 (factor 2) consisted of apparent derivatives of omnipotence, splitting, and primitive idealization. All three defenses loaded greater than .50 on all three of the factor analyses.

Defense style 3 (factor 3) consisted of apparent derivatives of only two defense mechanisms: reaction formation and pseudoaltruism. There was some question as to whether to include denial within defense style 3, since it loaded fairly highly on both the factor analysis of the combined sample and that of the patient sample taken separately. However, denial was eliminated because it loaded negatively on this factor when the analysis was carried out on the nonpatient sample alone.

Defense style 4 (factor 4) consisted of apparent derivatives of suppression, sublimation, and humor, all of which loaded at a level greater than .50 on all three factor analyses, with the exception of sublimation, which loaded at the .47 level when factoring was done on the nonpatient sample alone. Projection showed a strong negative loading on factor 4 for the patient sample, whereas regression had a strong negative loading on factor 4 for the nonpatient population.

The level of development of these four defense styles was assessed in a number of ways. Defense style 1 has a significant negative correlation with style 4 (see Table 7-2). The correlations of the four defense styles with the two measures of maturity—namely, ego strength score and ego development score—are presented in Table 7-3. The relative relations of these correlations indicate that defense styles 1 through 4 can be ranked in that order—that is, the ego strength score has a high negative correlation with style 1, a lower negative correlation with styles 2 and 3, and a significantly

Table 7–2.   Intercorrelations of defense styles

	Style 2	Style 3	Style 4
Style 1	.39*	.37	−.28*
Style 2		.18**	.07
Style 3			−.02

*P < .001. **P < .01.

Source. Reprinted from Bond et al. 1983, with permission from the American Medical Association. Copyright 1983, American Medical Association.

positive correlation with style 4. The same pattern holds for the ego development score (i.e., the Loevinger test).

When the ego strength and ego development scores were factor analyzed (type PA1, quartimax rotation) (Nie et al. 1975) along with the separate defenses that constitute the four defense styles, a four-factor solution resulted, with the ego strength and ego development scores loading negatively with style 1 defenses and positively with style 4 defenses.

The mean scores on defense styles 1–3 were higher for the patients than for the nonpatients (132.7 vs. 9.7, 36.9 vs. 30.3, and 25.8 vs. 22.6), whereas the score on defense style 4 was higher for the nonpatients (28.2 vs. 24.4).

This difference between the nonpatient and the patient samples in the use of defense styles is again borne out if one examines the defense styles used by individual subjects. If a subject's score was 0.5 SD above the mean on a particular factor, we considered that that subject used that corresponding defense style. A cutting point of 0.5 SD provided the best discrimination here. Of those with computable scores, 60% of the patients used defense style 1 in conjunction with other styles, and 16% used it exclusively. In contrast, 11% of the nonpatients used style 1 in conjunction with other styles, and only 3% used it exclusively. With regard to defense style 4, 48% of the patients used it in conjunction with other defense styles, and only 9% used it exclusively. In contrast, 90% of the nonpatients used defense style 4 in conjunction with other defenses, and 42% used it exclusively.

The following clinical example illustrates how scores on our scales might be related to clinical information:

> The patient had a diagnosis of an acute schizophrenic episode and borderline personality at different times. At the time that she was tested, she was an outpatient. At her worst, she showed signs of regression, withdrawal, and primitive projection. She had delusions of persecutions, influence, and grandiosity; however, by structuring her life and by encouraging her activity in the creative arts and music, she was helped to cope.

Table 7–3. Correlations of defense styles with the ego strength measures of Brown and Gardner and Loevinger's ego development measure

	Style 1	Style 2	Style 3	Style 4
Ego strength	−.91*	−.37*	−.38*	.32*
Ego development	−.42*	−.22	−.29*	.19**

*$P < .001$. **$P < .01$.

Source. Reprinted from Bond et al. 1983, with permission from the American Medical Association. Copyright 1983, American Medical Association.

This patient had high scores on defense styles 1, 2, and 4. We believe that style 1 reflected her regressive behavior, style 2 reflected her omnipotence and primitive idealization, and style 4 reflected her adaptive coping mechanisms. The fact that a subject used multiple styles might provide clues as to why he or she would receive different diagnoses at different times. If this patient was using styles 2 and 4 most strongly and her regressive behavior was under control, then she would seem borderline to some clinicians.

Comments

Questionnaire. A questionnaire has some important advantages over the clinical interview for the assessment of defensive functioning. It saves time, it does not require highly trained and highly paid professionals to administer it, it eliminates problems of inter-rater reliability, it can provide a measure of the degree to which defenses are present on a standardizable continuum, and it provides an opportunity to gather normative data. As a result, it permits the development of cutting points that may be used to discriminate between impaired and unimpaired functioning.

Our results demonstrate that the construction of such a questionnaire is feasible. We have produced an instrument that has desirable statistical properties. Even more important, the factors make clinical sense. We do not presume, however, that the present questionnaire is complete. It does not measure all the possible conscious derivatives of defense mechanisms. Nonetheless, it does provide a frame to which questions measuring other defenses or more items measuring the same defenses can be added. It must be stressed, however, that we are measuring only self-appraisals of defense styles and not actually measuring defense mechanisms. A further study is needed to validate the relationship between what we are measuring and the traditional notion of defense.

A number of findings lend support to the validity of the questionnaire. The internal consistency of the questionnaire was demonstrated by two experimental findings. First, the item total correlations on the questions and the defenses that they were supposed to represent were all significant ($P < .001$). Second, the defenses clustered in the factor analysis along lines that make theoretical sense. Thus "immature" defensive maneuvers (e.g., regression, acting out) clustered together on factor 1. It is possible to think of the defenses of factors 2 and 3 (e.g., splitting, primitive idealization, pseudoaltruism) as intermediate in nature, and the defenses clustered in factor 4 (sublimation, suppression, and humor) are commonly associated with the idea of maturity. Further, the high negative correlation of the expected primitive defenses with the expected higher-level defenses provides additional evidence for internal consistency.

The criterion validity of the questionnaire was supported in two ways. First, the defense styles related to other indices of ego development, as expected. That is, the relative correlations of styles 1 through 4 with the scores on the Loevinger and ego strength tests indicate that these styles can be ranked, in that order, on a continuum of development or adaptation. Second, the fact that patients tend to use the less mature defenses and nonpatients the higher-level defenses adds credence to the questionnaire. The patient sample had significantly higher mean scores than did the non-patient sample on defense styles 1, 2, and 3. The nonpatient sample had a significantly higher mean score on style 4 defenses. When factor scores were computed for individual subjects, the patients tended to use style 1 defenses much more and the style 4 defenses much less than did the nonpatients.

Clusters of self-perceptions of characteristic defenses. From our data it was clear that subjects' perceptions of their own characteristic behaviors clustered into what we call defense styles. It is interesting to speculate, for each style, about what the common elements might be that applies to all the inferred defenses associated with that style. For the six defenses that clustered on factor 1—withdrawal, acting out, regression, inhibition, passive aggression, and projection—immaturity may not be the best term, because these defenses can sometimes be found in well-functioning persons. Perhaps the common feature of this factor is that all these behaviors indicate the subjects' inability to deal with their impulses by taking constructive action on their own behalf. The subject who is acting out requires controls. The withdrawn or inhibited person needs to be actively drawn out. The passive-aggressive person acts to provoke anger in the person with whom he or she is involved. The regressed person requires someone to take over and do something for him or her. The projecting person puts the blame and responsibility on others instead of accepting his or her own impulses. Thus, this defense style might be labeled "maladaptive action patterns."

The essence of the inferred defenses that clustered on factor 2—splitting, primitive idealization, and omnipotence with devaluation—is splitting of the image of self and other into good and bad, strong and weak. This style clearly differs from the defenses of style 1 in that it is image-oriented rather than action-oriented. Although style 2 could interfere with object relations, it need not necessarily affect achievement and accomplishment. The defenses of this style could be invoked in the service of constructive adaptation in situations of stress by persons who do not use them habitually. For example, one way of dealing with a severe physical illness may be to trust in the omnipotence of the physician. These defenses may also be used nonadaptively by persons who have chronic difficulty in forming mature relationships. In the literature, this style is associated with narcissistic and borderline personality disorders (Kernberg 1967). These clustered defenses, then, can be described as the "image-distorting" style.

The items designed to test the two inferred defenses constituting style 3—reaction formation and pseudoaltruism—reflect a need to perceive one's self as being kind, helpful to others, and never angry. This is characteristic of martyr types and "do-gooders." It is our impression that these people are often involved in stable but not necessarily healthy (often masochistic) relationships and that they are usually able to function adequately. They often come to the attention of psychiatrists when they suffer a loss and their characteristic defense pattern cannot contain their anger and anxiety. They then become depressed. Style 3 can be characterized as consisting of "self-sacrificing" defenses. (We suspect that with a larger sample or with a greater number of questions, more defenses could have been grouped on this factor. It could evolve into an obsessive-compulsive factor with the addition of intellectualization and the related defenses of undoing and isolation.)

The inferred defenses for style 4—humor, suppression, and sublimation—are clearly associated with good coping. Suppression allows an anxiety-producing conflict to be put out of awareness until the individual is ready to deal with the issue. Humor reflects a capacity to accept a conflictual situation while taking the edge off its painful aspects. Sublimation uses the anxiety-provoking impulse in the service of creative response. All three defenses are associated with a constructive type of mastery of the conflict. Style 4 can be labeled the "adaptive" defense style.

For the most part, the defense styles are different from the "neurotic styles" that Shapiro (1965) outlined by means of theoretical construction from psychoanalytic descriptions rather than by using empirical data. He described the obsessive, paranoid, hysterical, and impulsive styles. Our maladaptive action patterns probably correspond to his impulsive style, but the other "neurotic styles" seem to be organized along factors different from our defense styles. It is interesting to compare these different results obtained from different methods, but it is also possible that Shapiro had a different population in mind when constructing his styles.

Maturity and defense styles.   The correlations of each of the defense styles with two measures of maturity—ego strength and ego development (i.e., Loevinger tests)—indicate that in developmental terms there is a progression from the maladaptive action patterns, through the image-distorting defenses and the self-sacrificing defenses, to the adaptive defenses, along the line of increasingly constructive ways of dealing with the vicissitudes of life.

The least mature people have behavior problems. Those in the image-distorting group have a problem in realistically viewing themselves and others, which lends itself to relationship problems. The self-sacrificing persons have more stable relationships but cannot fulfill their creative potential. The adaptive defenses reflect less preoccupation with relationships and allow more creative expression of one's inner self. Thus, the defense styles reflect a shift from preoccupation with control of raw impulses, to preoccupation with all-important others, to creative expression of oneself.

Other studies also reflect this shift. With a clinical population, Semrad et al. (1973) suggested that as patients improve, their defenses become less primitive and more mature. One patient in their study moved from what they labeled as narcissistic patterns to affective defensive patterns to neurotic defensive patterns as therapy progressed. Vaillant (1976), in his 20-year follow-up study of a normal male college-age population, found an increasing use of more-mature defenses over time. Mature defenses not only enhanced the men's ability to work but also enhanced their ability to love. Thus, the results from Vaillant's study of normal subjects, the study of patients by Semrad et al., and our study of both patients and nonpatients indicate that defenses can be arranged in a hierarchy of maturity that relates to a person's successful adaptation to the world.

Follow-up on the Relationship Between Diagnosis and Defense Style

Methodology. In order to determine how the scores on the DSQ related to diagnosis, it was necessary to use uniform, valid, and reliable diagnostic classification. Diagnoses recorded in the patient's charts were inadequate for this purpose because the attending psychiatrists and psychologists did not all use the same diagnostic criteria and because they did not all distinguish between principal and secondary diagnoses. For these reasons, patients were rediagnosed using their charts, which provided data gathered from subsequent contacts. Two independent raters (a staff psychiatrist and a senior psychiatry resident) applied DSM-III criteria and rated defense styles used by the patients. Charts were available for 74 of the patients who had completed the DSQ. These patients were diagnosed on Axes I and II by both raters, who recorded principal and secondary diagnoses. Axis IV was used by only one rater, in cases ($n = 48$) for whom there was adequate information about psychosocial stressors. Axes III and V were not used because of a lack of sufficient information in the charts.

Because of small sample size, the Axis I and Axis II diagnoses were grouped as suggested by Treece (1982). Axis I diagnoses were grouped into the following four categories: psychotic disorders (including schizophrenia, paranoia, and schizoaffective disorder), major affective disorders (bipolar and unipolar), anxiety disorders, and other Axis I disorders (including adjustment disorder and dysthymic disorder). Axis II diagnoses were grouped into the following four categories: type A (schizoid, schizotypal, paranoid), type B (histrionic, narcissistic, antisocial, borderline), type C (avoidant, dependent, compulsive, passive-aggressive), and other personality disorders. Raters compared principal diagnoses and reached agreement in 93.2% of the cases (n = 69). Cases about whom there was disagreement (n = 5) were excluded from the analysis. Inter-rater reliability, calculated by the kappa coefficient (Spitzer et al. 1967), was .98. This result is higher than those in literature reports on inter-rater reliability using Axis I (.78) and Axis II (.61 or less) (Mellsop et al. 1982; Spitzer et al. 1979), probably because our data came from charts instead of clinical interviews and because we used broader categories of diagnoses designed to increase the number of cases on whom we agreed. It is unlikely that the limitations of case record data (problems with missing data, conflicting descriptions, and differing evaluations of the degree to which a particular behavior is pathological) would affect the value of statistical analysis (Strauss and Harder 1981).

Follow-up results: defense styles and Axis I and Axis II diagnoses.   Relationships between defense styles and Axes I and II were analyzed in this reduced sample of 69 patients, which did not differ from the original total patient sample (N = 98) in terms of age, sex, patient status, chart diagnosis, and defense styles.

The original patient group had already been compared with the control group for the number and the types of defense styles used as described previously. Then, each of the different diagnostic categories was compared with the reduced patient sample in terms of the number and the types of defense styles used (see Table 7-4).

The majority of our 69 patients were in one of the following three diagnostic categories: psychotic disorders (n = 22), affective disorders (n = 16), and personality disorders–type B (n = 20). Hence, for calculation purposes, we paired anxiety disorders (n = 2) with other Axis I disorders (n = 5), and personality disorders–type A (n = 2) with personality disorders–type C (n = 2). Calculations were done using the chi-square statistic.

Within the patient group, the most striking finding was that, except for affective disorders, no diagnosis was associated with the reported use of any particular number or type of defense style. For patients with affective disorders, the questionnaire responses resulted in a description of "no defense style" more often (44%) than in other patients, such as psychotic individuals (5%) and those with personality disorders–type B (20%). Patients with affective disorders reported multiple styles (25%) less often than other

Table 7–4. Percentage of subjects within diagnostic categories (DSM-III Axes I and II) reporting the use of each defense style

Principal diagnosis	Percentage (number) of subjects				
	No style	Style 1	Style 2	Style 3	Style 4
Psychotic disorders (*n* = 22)	5 (1)	36 (8)	36 (8)	41 (9)	36 (8)
Affective disorders (*n* = 16)	44 (7)	19 (3)	13 (2)	25 (4)	31 (5)
Anxiety and other Axis I disorders (*n* = 7)	0 (0)	29 (2)	29 (2)	14 (1)	43 (3)
Personality disorders, type B (*n* = 20)	20 (4)	40 (8)	45 (9)	30 (6)	30 (6)
Personality disorders, types A and C (*n* = 4)	0 (0)	75 (3)	50 (2)	50 (2)	25 (1)
Total patient group (*n* = 69)	17 (12)	35 (24)	33 (23)	32 (22)	33 (23)
Total control group (*n* = 111)	42 (47)	6 (7)	16 (18)	16 (18)	37 (41)

Note. Because many subjects reported testing multiple defense styles, the sum of percentages in any row may exceed 100.
Source. Reprinted from Bond et al. 1983, with permission from the American Medical Association. Copyright 1983, American Medical Association.

patients (X^2 = 29.4, df = 2, P < .001). Patients with affective disorders reported using the "adaptive" defense style 4 (31%) more often than style 1 (19%), style 2 (13%), and style 3 (25%). This pattern of style use was significantly different from that of other patients, who for the most part reported using styles 1, 2, and 3 as often as or more frequently than style 4 (X^2 = 28.1, df = 4, P < .001).

Discussion. Although styles 1, 2, and 3 are associated with patient status, defense style could not be used to predict diagnostic category, nor could Axis I, II, or IV diagnoses be used to accurately predict defense style. Most of the patients with major affective disorders used either no style that could be detected or style 4, a combination that resembled the defense pattern of control subjects more than of patients. I will offer several possible explanations for this later in this section. However, a minority of patients with affective disorders reported defense patterns typical of those of other patients, using styles 1, 2, and 3. Our results suggest that diagnosis and defense style may be two independent dimensions. Diagnosis is related to symptoms and pathological behavior, but defense style is related to the way in which one deals with a given situation, whether consciously or unconsciously.

The data from these studies reflect the complexity of human psychology and the wide range of human potential. Chodoff and Lyons (1958) showed that conversion reactions occur in many personality types, not only, and not even more frequently, in histrionic personalities. This finding is consistent with the notion that Axis II cannot predict Axis I and vice versa. Such findings challenge the linear thinking that implies that certain symptoms are a direct outgrowth of a certain personality structure.

Several limitations to our study have to be resolved before our conclusions can be accepted without question. First, we did not measure defense mechanisms directly. Cross-validation with clinicians' ratings of defense mechanisms would be necessary to prove that our factors *actually* represent clusters of defenses. This is a project that we in fact went on to do and will report on later in this chapter.

Second, we may not have enough questions to tap all the defenses that our subjects used. An insufficient number of appropriate statements on the DSQ or a poorly chosen cutting point may yield too many false negatives (Meehl and Rosen 1955). In individuals for whom no consistent style was detected, it is possible that the defense or coping mechanisms that these people used were not reflected in the DSQ items. We made no effort to tap the more adaptive processes (e.g., self-assertion, self-observation, anticipatory problem solving) that might be common among nonpatients.

A related point is that some people may not be aware of their defenses as coping mechanisms and thus may not acknowledge them in their responses to the questionnaire. It may be that this type of person is overrepresented among people who have not sought psychiatric help or among those with major affective disorders. at this point we have no way of proving or disproving this hypothesis.

Third, because we examined broad diagnostic categories rather than specific diagnoses, we might have overlooked significant relationships, particularly between defenses and the Axis II diagnosis. For example, one might expect an obsessive-compulsive personality to use isolation, undoing, reaction formation, and intellectualization. In our factor analysis, only reaction formation loaded strongly on one of the four factors—factor 3, together with pseudoaltruism. Thus, we did not find a clear-cut obsessive-compulsive defense style.

Our sample might have similarly limited findings. For example, we had only one patient with obsessive-compulsive personality disorder and two with obsessive traits. The former was rated as having no clear defense style, and of the latter, one manifested style 3 and the other style 4. If we changed the sample to include a larger number of obsessive-compulsive personalities, the factors yielded by analysis would very likely change, as Meehl and Rosen (1955) point out. Thus, we cannot say that we have definitively shown that specific personality disorders do not reliably predict given defense styles.

Another limitation of the study is related to the fact that the patients were tested at only one phase of their illness. Although all outpatients were tested at the time of their intake interview, inpatients might have been very decompensated or on the road to recovery when tested. Although we do not have test-retest data from the same time frame, we do plan to carry out an 8-year follow-up to obtain data that will shed some light on the state-or-trait issue.

Even with these limitations, the difference in patients with affective disorders—that is, their resemblance to the control group in their responses to the questionnaire—is interesting. This group of patients and the nonpatients rate themselves as either using defenses that are toward the adaptive end of the hierarchy or behaving in a way that was not tapped by the questionnaire.

It is possible that the defense or coping styles that nonpatients use are different than those used by patients with affective disorders and that both are not measured by the questionnaire. It is also possible that people with affective disorders are different on the basis of a dimension other than defense style—for example, psychodynamic conflicts (Perry and Cooper 1986). A third possibility is that patients with affective disorders do have defense styles similar to those of nonpatients and that their decompensation into patienthood is related to a biochemical factor rather than to the defense style itself.

Our main finding in the follow-up study was that there was not a clear relationship between defense style as measured by the questionnaire and DSM-III diagnosis. However, this finding does not mean that we have proved that defense style and diagnosis are independent dimensions. Our data are consistent, however, with the notion that people with the same diagnosis can use many different defense styles.

This echoes the views of Karasu and Skodol (1980) and those of Strayhorn (1983), who advocate a sixth axis for DSM-III in order to offer more discriminating information about the psychodynamics or resources of patients with the same Axis I or II diagnosis. Along this line, Clarkin et al. (1983) point out the heterogeneity within the diagnostic category of borderline personality disorder and find prototypical typology to be responsible. Defense styles constitute one way of describing those heterogeneous features.

When used in conjunction with clinical data, information about patients' defense styles can help the clinician to plan the subtleties of treatment. The form that a sixth axis should take is properly the task of a work group to revise the DSM-III-R, but our data would suggest that defense mechanisms or styles certainly would not be a redundant addition to the diagnostic schema.

Further Attempts at Validating the Measurement of Defense Mechanisms

A second study involving 156 subjects was carried out in order to compare subjects' responses on the DSQ with their scores on the Defense Mechanism Rating Scales (DMRS) (Perry and Cooper 1986) in which judges rated defense mechanisms from a videotaped clinical assessment interview (Bond et al. 1989). These ratings are assumed to be as valid a measure of defense mechanisms as one can achieve empirically and thus were used as a standard with which to compare the self-report scores.

Subjects

In the period from July 1985 to October 1986, 333 people who came for psychiatric assessments to the department of psychiatry of the Jewish General Hospital, Montreal, were asked to participate in our research project. Of these, 179 agreed to participate and signed informed consent forms. Complete data were collected on 156 subjects, of whom 66 were male and 90 female. Their ages ranged from 16 to 73, with a median of 39, a mode of 24, and a mean of 36 (SD = 14.7).

There were 130 patients from the adult outpatient department and 26 patients from an outpatient youth service for patients ages 16 to 20. Of these patients, 66 were single, 69 married, 9 separated, and 12 divorced.

Methods

The four measures were the DSQ, the DMRS, the Life Events Scale (LES; Pilkonis et al. 1985), and the Health-Sickness Rating Scale (HSRS; Luborsky 1962).

The Defense Style Questionnaire.   All the patients in the study filled out the revised version of the DSQ, which consists of 88 statements (see Appendix 6), at the time of their initial assessment, and 39 subjects filled it out again at 6-month follow-up.

Defense Mechanism Rating Scales.   Three raters who have master's degrees in counseling or a degree in social work, and who graduated from a 2-year psychoanalytic psychotherapy course given by the department of psychiatry, Sir Mortimer B. Davis–Jewish General Hospital, were trained by J. C. Perry in the use of his manual and clinical rating scale. The scale contains 22 defense mechanisms and gives criteria for rating them as absent, probably present, and definitely present. The manual gives operational definitions of each defense and compares them to similar but theoretically different defenses. Eight mature defenses with provisional definitions were also added.

The defenses are grouped into four levels: immature, image-distorting, neurotic, and mature. For our study we moved neurotic denial from the immature level to the neurotic level because we felt that it better belonged in the neurotic group. Neurotic denial involves more of a titration of stressful information and affect than gross avoidance as in the immature defenses.

In addition, Perry and Cooper (1986) created five summary scales: 1) action defenses (acting out, passive aggression, and hypochondriasis), 2) borderline defenses (splitting self-images, splitting other images, and projective identification), 3) narcissistic defenses (omnipotence, devaluation, primitive idealization, and mood-incongruent denial), 4) disavowal defenses (projection, neurotic denial, bland denial, and rationalization), and 5) obsessional defenses (isolation, undoing, and intellectualization). These groups are based on empirical correlations, whereas the four groups based on hierarchy of maturity are arranged according to theory. (For further details, see Chapter 10 of this volume.)

Subjects were interviewed by approximately 20 different interviewers, mostly psychiatric residents, and the interviews were videotaped. These interviewers did nonstandardized psychiatric assessment of patients coming to our outpatient department for help.

Life Events Scale.   A checklist questionnaire about life events as developed by Pilkonis et al. (1985) was given to each of the 39 subjects who had a 6-month follow-up. After completing the checklist, each subject listed his or her 10 most stressful events of the past 6 months. A research assistant then assigned each of these events a rating from 1 to 7 based on the severity of psychosocial stressor guidelines for Axis IV of DSM-III. The total of these ratings comprised each subject's life events score.

Health-Sickness Rating Scale.   The HSRS, as devised by Luborsky (1962), yields a score from 0 to 100 (100 being the healthy end of the scale). The interviewer assigned a score using the scale's guidelines. The 39 subjects who were followed up at 6 months received a score at that point either from their therapist, if in treatment, or as determined by the principal investigator after a brief interview.

Diagnosis.   The interviewer assigned a DSM-III diagnosis after the psychiatric interview. The diagnoses were then grouped into broad categories: psychoses, major affective disorders, personality disorders, anxiety disorders, dysthymic disorders, adjustment disorders, miscellaneous, and no psychiatric disorders.

Results

Defense Style Questionnaire.   Styles 1 (maladaptive), 2 (image-distorting), and 3 (self-sacrificing) were significantly correlated with DMRS immature defenses and negatively correlated with healthy functioning on the HSRS (see Table 7-5). Style 1 was negatively correlated with DMRS mature level defenses. Styles 1 and 2 were positively correlated with a high LES score and negatively correlated with age. Style 2 was correlated with divorced or single status.

The 67 items from the original questionnaire were examined for correlations with ratings on Perry and Cooper's (1986) defense scale. Of the 25 items previously identified as tapping maladaptive action patterns, 23 items correlated with the immature group of DMRS defenses. Of the 12 statements that loaded on the DSQ image-distorting factor in the previous study, only 5 correlated with the DMRS image-distorting group of defenses but also correlated positively with the DMRS immature group of defenses. Only one other statement, tapping suppression, positively correlated with another DMRS group of defenses, the neurotic group.

Table 7–5. Significant ($P < .01$) correlations of defense (using the DSQ) with the DMRS, age, HSRS, and LES

Defense style (DSQ)	DMRS Levels of defense	Summary scales	Age	HSRS	LES
Maladaptive	Immature ($r = .36$)* Mature ($r = -.16$)	Action ($r = .31$)	$r = -.22$	$r = -.23$	$r = .42$
Image-distorting	Immature ($r = .32$)*	Action ($r = .32$)	$r = -.27$	$r = -.23$	$r = .45$
Self-sacrificing	Immature ($r = .23$)*	Action ($r = .21$) Disavowal ($r = .18$)	—	$r = -.20$	—
Adaptive	—	—	—	—	—

Note. DSQ = Defense Style Questionnaire; DMRS = Defense Mechanism Rating Scales; HSRS = Health-Sickness Rating Scale; LES = Life Events Scale.
*Significant at $P < .001$ level. (All other correlations are significant at the $P < .01$ level.)
Source. Reprinted from Bond et al. 1989, with permission of the Guilford Press. Copyright 1989, Guilford Press.

Of the 21 new statements, 4 of the 6 items supposedly measuring the theoretically adaptive mechanisms either correlated with Perry and Cooper's mature subscale or loaded with the adaptive items on the DSQ. The three items designed to tap help-rejecting complaining positively correlated with the immature defenses on both the DSQ and the DMRS. Two items designed to tap undoing positively correlated with the immature DMRS defenses. Two items designed to tap isolation positively correlated with the image-distorting DMRS defenses, and two items designed to tap projection positively correlated with immature DMRS defenses and with the maladaptive DSQ defense style. When individual items on the DSQ were correlated with individual defenses on the DMRS, 20 DSQ items were positively correlated with the specific DMRS defense that they were designed to measure.

In 39 cases, the DSQ was repeated 6 months later. The correlations using a t test for the four defense styles at the two times were highly significant ($P = .001$): for style 1, $r = .73$; for style 2, $r = .71$; for style 3, $r = .68$; and for style 4, $r = .69$. In other words, the style used by an individual did not change in relation to the group of subjects. However, there was a tendency for subjects to report less use of styles 1 and 2 when tested 6 months later ($P < .005$ and .003, respectively), and for them to report more use of style 4 ($P < .01$). Thus, although the defense style profile of an individual remained stable, there was a trend toward more mature defense style reporting 6 months later. This trend might reflect spontaneous improvement, treatment effect, or regression toward the mean.

Two case examples are provided below. (The criterion for the use of a style is a score of 0.5 SD above the mean for that style.)

Case 1

Mrs. N., a 54-year-old married woman, presented to the outpatient department with a 7-month history of early morning wakening and a 3-month history of decreased appetite: weight loss of 18 pounds; withdrawal; loss of interest, energy, and concentration; feelings of worthlessness; sadness; and suicidal thoughts. She worried about losing her job and not having enough money for her old age. She was diagnosed as having a major depression.

On her initial visit, she was shown, according to the DSQ, to be using defense styles 1, 2, 3, and on the DMRS she was shown to be using hypochondriasis, passive aggression, reaction formation, and devaluation. After treatment, 6 months later, she was doing well. Her HSRS score improved by 10 points, and the questionnaire showed her to be using style 4. Thus with improvement, her defense style changed from immature to mature. Her treatment consisted of antidepressants and group and milieu therapy in a day hospital. She was actively encouraged to focus on others, not on herself. In this case the change in defense style was dramatic and in the direction of the therapeutic focus, which encouraged suppression, sublimation, affiliation, and altruism. Defense style behaved like a state phenomenon, changing with improvement.

Case 2

This 23-year-old single female nurse's aide, who lived alone, used the maladaptive and image-distorting defense styles on initial testing and also on testing 6 months later. The HSRS score dropped by 25 points despite 10 sessions of psychotherapy. Her DMRS showed use of immature, neurotic, and image-distorting defenses on initial presentation.

She presented with suicidal ideas, having taken an overdose of over-the-counter sleeping medications while drinking wine 6 months previously. A friend helped her get over this episode, but her suicidal thoughts recurred whenever she felt overwhelmed by stress. She was in recurrent financial crisis and had a relationship with a man whom she perceived as taking advantage of her. She felt unrecognized at her job in spite of her hard work.

She presented as an attractive, friendly, fashionably dressed young woman who smiled a lot, did not seem depressed, and denied suicidal intent. She was seen as having an adjustment disorder and referred for psychotherapy. After 10 sessions of psychotherapy she was "somewhat confused about her life" and appeared depressed and regressed (looking and acting like a teenager). She was not attending school, had difficulty coping at work, and was living with a married man. At this point she was suspected of having borderline personality disorder.

This is an example of how defense style remained as a trait. The maladaptive and image-distorting defense styles are consistent with the behavioral outcomes of acting out, regression, and problematic relationships, and might have been an important warning of problems ahead, despite her superficially healthy presentation that led to a falsely hopeful diagnosis.

Defense Mechanism Rating Scales.   The inter-rater reliabilities were calculated as intraclass reliability coefficients (IRs) ($N = 20$, raters = 3) (see Table 7-6). Coefficients were calculated for individual defenses, and for subscales or groups of defenses, using Perry's scoring method. For the 32 individual defenses, the median IR was .41 (range, .04 to .80). When the summary defense scales were used, the interpolated median reliability was .57, with a range of .30 to .66 (see Table 7-6).

The group of immature-level defenses was correlated with younger age ($P < .003$), low score on the HSRS ($r = -.29$, $P < .001$), and divorced or single marital status. The image-distorting defenses were correlated with

Table 7–6. Inter-rater reliabilities for the DMRS, each expressed as an intraclass correlation coefficient (IR)

	Median IR	Range of IRs
Defense groups by level of maturity		
Immature	.47	.09–.80
Image-distorting	.32	.06–.60
Neurotic	.40	.04–.51
Mature	.52	.04–.65
Summary defense scales		
Action	.62	.51–.80
Disavowal	.63	.04–.40
Borderline	.51	.31–.60
Narcissistic	.51	.06–.42
Obsessional	.30	.05–.51
Mature	.66	.04–.65
Individual defenses (32)	.41	.04–.80

Note. IRs based on $N = 20$; three raters.
Source. Reprinted from Bond et al. 1989, with permission of the Guilford Press. Copyright 1989, Guilford Press.

divorced marital status. The mature defenses were significantly positively correlated with a high score on the HSRS ($P < .02$, $r = .18$).

The immature-level defenses were significantly positively correlated with the first three DSQ defense styles: .36 with the maladaptive group, .32 with the image-distorting style, and .23 with the self-sacrificing group. The DMRS image-distorting defenses were not correlated with any DSQ defense style, nor were the DMRS neurotic defenses. The DMRS mature defenses were significantly negatively correlated with the DSQ maladaptive defense style ($r = -.16$, $P < .04$).

When correlations were done with the DMRS summary defense scales, the action defenses correlated positively with the DSQ maladaptive action defense style ($r = .31$), the image-distorting defense style ($r = .32$), and the self-sacrificing defense style ($r = .21$). The disavowal defenses correlated positively with the DSQ self-sacrificing defense style ($r = .18$). The borderline, narcissistic-obsessive, and mature summary defense scales did not significantly correlate with any DSQ defense style (see Table 7-5).

Health-Sickness Rating Scale. As already mentioned, healthy functioning was negatively correlated with the use of the immature defenses on both the DSQ and the DMRS. When 39 subjects were retested 6 months later, their mean scores went from 62.6 ± 11.6 to 66.1 ± 12.6, a mean difference of 3.5 ($t = 1.94$). The correlation was .53 ($P < .001$). Thus, an individual's score at the time of the initial interview was a significant predictor of his or her score 6 months later.

Life Events Scale.   As previously stated, a high score on the LES was significantly and positively correlated with the use of image-distorting and maladaptive defense styles.

Diagnosis.   The intake diagnoses were distributed as follows: psychoses ($n = 8$), personality disorders ($n = 27$), major affective disorders ($n = 25$), dysthymic disorders ($n = 22$), anxiety disorders ($n = 22$), adjustment disorders ($n = 32$), miscellaneous ($n = 18$), and no psychiatric diagnosis ($n = 2$). No diagnostic group was significantly correlated with any defense style or defense subscale, using one-way ANOVAs. When the personality disorder group was broken down into borderline personality disorder versus others, the only statistically significant differences were that the six borderline patients scored higher on the DMRS immature and image-distorting groups of defenses ($P < .05$ and .01, respectively).

The results of both studies reported in this chapter were combined to look at the particular issue of whether the image-distorting defenses were specifically correlated with borderline personality disorder. This question had different answers depending on whether the defenses were measured by the DSQ or by the DMRS. The results are summarized in Table 7-7.

In both studies, there was no significant difference in the reported use of the DSQ image-distorting defenses between patients with borderline personality disorder and those with other personality disorders and between patients with borderline personality disorder and the patient sample at large.

In the first study, patients with major affective disorders reported using a different defense profile from the other patients (Bond and Sagala Vaillant 1986). The affective disorder patients used less of the first three styles than did the other patients ($X^2 = 28.1$, df = 4, $P < .001$). In the second study, using one way ANOVAs, no diagnostic group (including 27 persons with personality disorders, 8 with psychoses, 25 with major affective disorders, 22 with dysthymic disorders, 22 with anxiety disorders, and 52 others) was significantly correlated with any DSQ defense style or DMRS subscale.

However, in the second study, the 6 patients with borderline personality disorder scored higher on the DMRS immature and image-distorting groups of defenses ($P < .05$ and .01, respectively) compared with other personality-disordered individuals and the sample at large.

As shown in Table 7-7, 12 out of 25 patients with borderline personality disorder and 12 out of 26 patients with other personality disorders reported using DSQ image-distorting defenses. Thus, within the larger category of personality disorders, patients with borderline personality disorder did not stand out in their reported use of these defenses. Whereas when the image-distorting defenses were measured by judges rating clinical interviews, patients with borderline personality disorder were deemed to use these defenses significantly more. Using the DMRS, patients with borderline personality disorder were rated as using immature defenses (mean = 4.00) and image-distorting defenses (mean = 4.83) significantly more than patients with other personality disorders (means = 2.67 and 2.29, respectively) and the sample at large (means = 2.40 and 2.54, respectively).

Table 7–7. Defense styles (based on the DSQ) used by patients with borderline personality disorder and by patients with other diagnoses in two studies

	Number (%) of subjects			
	Maladaptive action	Image-distorting	Self-sacrificing	Adaptive
Study 1				
Borderline personality disorder (*n* = 19)	8 (42)	8 (42)	6 (52)	6 (32)
Other personality disorders (*n* = 5)	3 (60)	3 (60)	2 (40)	1 (20)
Psychoses (*n* = 22)	8 (36)	8 (36)	9 (41)	8 (36)
Major affective disorders (*n* = 16)	3 (19)	2 (13)	4 (25)	5 (31)
Study 2				
Borderline personality disorder (*n* = 6)	2 (33)	4 (66)	2 (33)	0 (0)
Other personality disorders (*n* = 21)	7 (33)	9 (43)	11 (52)	3 (14)
Borderline personality disorder (total) (*n* = 25)	10 (40)	12 (48)	8 (32)	6 (24)
Other personality disorders (total) (*n* = 26)	10 (39)	12 (46)	13 (50)	4 (15)

Source. Reprinted from Bond 1990, with permission from the Guilford Press. Copyright 1990, Guilford Press.

Discussion

This research elucidates both what is possible in the empirical measurement of defense mechanisms and what difficulties continue to exist. The DSQ seems to be most accurate when discriminating between adaptive and maladaptive defense styles. The self-reported use of the maladaptive defense style was significantly positively correlated with the group of immature-level defenses rated by the DMRS and significantly negatively correlated with the DMRS mature-level defenses. Of 25 items previously identified as tapping maladaptive defenses, 23 items positively correlated with Perry and Cooper's group of immature-level defenses. When this finding is added to Vaillant et al.'s (1986) results, there is compelling evidence that the DSQ can identify immature defenses as a group validly and reliably.

Defense mechanisms from other groupings did show significant correlations on an individual basis: neurotic denial, splitting, projection, identification, and omnipotence/devaluation all showed significant correlations between their DMRS and DSQ ratings.

The maladaptive defense style also correlated significantly negatively with both age and healthy functioning on the HSRS, and positively with a high LES score. The use of any given defense style remained stable 6 months later. These data are all consistent with what one would theoretically expect, including the notion that a defense style would be stable over a 6-month period. The fact that there is a trend toward greater maturity and toward a higher HSRS score 6 months after seeking help indicates that as patients are functioning better, they report using more adaptive defenses but still maintain the same basic defensive profile. Thus it would seem that the state-or-trait question cannot be given an all-or-none answer. Defense style appears to be a trait phenomenon, but some change within a given profile seems likely over time. Also, much variation exists among individuals, as shown by our case examples. The fact that high life stress correlated with low HSRS scores and with a maladaptive defense style is logically consistent. The three variables are probably all part of a vicious cycle of stress and poor functioning.

The two case examples illustrate the variety among the many dimensions of functioning of human beings. In the first case, there was a change in the use of defense style as the individual's level of functioning or state of crisis changed. This change may have been a result of therapy's encouraging new ways of dealing with conflicts. In the second case, defense style seemed to be more of a trait. In this case the DSQ elicited evidence of a tendency toward regression that was not apparent in the clinical interview, as is often the case with patients with borderline personality disorder who at first appear to be neurotic. Thus the DSQ can be a useful adjunct to clinical diagnosis but is not predictive on its own. The DSQ may be used to indicate directions to take in therapy. If the use of more adaptive defenses can be fostered by therapy, the patient's clinical state could improve.

Our questionnaire relies on patients' self-reports, which are limited by the patients' motivation at the moment of responding, by their openness, and by their self-awareness. Also, the statements are merely indirect measures of defenses, tapping conscious derivatives of these unconscious intrapsychic processes. These limitations require us to be very cautious about disentangling state-or-trait issues from our results. Although Vaillant (1976) was able to show the predictive power of defenses for large groups, we must be wary of predicting outcome with individuals.

There are several explanations for the areas in which the DSQ and the DMRS did not reinforce each other's concurrent validity. First, the DMRS immature-level defenses had the highest base rates and highest reliabilities in this sample. The DSQ has more items measuring immature defenses, and this is the area in which greatest concurrence was seen. Conversely, lower prevalence for the image-distorting, neurotic, and mature DMRS defenses and fewer DSQ items measuring the corresponding defense styles would lead to a Type II error—that is, failing to detect a relationship that is present. One should note that the lowest reliabilities were found in those defenses that were infrequently rated present and therefore yielded the least stable reliability estimates (Grove et al. 1981).

Second, the fact that the interviewers' priority was doing a psychiatric assessment rather than specifically eliciting defense mechanisms probably lowered the base rates on the DMRS. Higher concurrence might have been elicited if interviewers had been trained specially to stimulate the subject's defenses. The low base of the neurotic defenses rated by the DMRS may have been dependent upon interviewer skill in eliciting adequate evidence for determining their presence. On the other hand, the very low base rates for the mature defenses were anticipated, given that these are theoretically supposed to protect against stress most effectively, and the mature defenses have shown the strongest empirical correlations with mental health, both in other samples (Perry and Cooper 1987) and in this one. In all cases, low rates of defenses, whether due to interview effects or not, constrain this study's estimate of the relationship between the DMRS and the DSQ.

Third, the consensus rating of the judges was not available in most cases, and so the less reliable rating by one judge was used. This could have decreased the concurrence.

Fourth, the DSQ is a self-report instrument, and so the context of its administration is very different from that of a videotaped psychiatric assessment. It might be that the different contexts elicited different defense mechanisms.

Finally, when I was designing the questionnaire items, I had somewhat different operational definitions of some defense mechanisms in mind compared with those that Cooper and Perry propose in their manual (S. H. Cooper, J. C. Perry, personal communication, September 1986). The raters used Perry and Cooper's definitions, and this might have contributed to some divergence.

At this point, it is safest to use the DSQ, modified by adding the items that significantly correlated with the expected defense style, as a means of discriminating between mature and immature defense styles. The methods of Perry and Cooper and of Vaillant, although more costly and time consuming, should be used when a finer discrimination is required to detect the range of individual defense mechanisms.

References

American Psychiatric Association: Diagnostic and Statistical Manual of Mental Disorders, 3rd Edition. Washington, DC, American Psychiatric Association, 1980

Aronoff J: A Test and Scoring Manual for the Measurement of Safety, Love and Belongingness, and Esteem Needs. East Lansing, MI, Department of Psychology, Michigan State University, 1971

Bellak L, Hurvich M, Gediman HK: Ego Functions in Schizophrenics, Neurotics, and Normals. New York, John Wiley, 1973

Blasi A, cited by Loevinger J, Wessler R: Measuring Ego Development, Vol 1: Construction and Use of a Sentence Completion Test. San Francisco, CA, Jossey-Bass, 1970

Blasi A: A developmental approach to responsibility training. Unpublished doctoral dissertation, Washington University, St Louis, MO, 1972; see p 53

Bond M: Are "borderline" defenses specific to borderline personality disorder? Journal of Personality Disorders 4:251–256, 1990

Bond M, Sagala Vaillant J: Empirical study of relationship between diagnosis and defense style. Arch Gen Psychiatry 43:285–288, 1986

Bond M, Gardner ST, Christian J, et al: Empirical study of self-rated defense styles. Arch Gen Psychiatry 40:333–338, 1983

Bond M, Perry JC, Gautier M, et al: Validating the self-report of defense styles. Journal of Personality Disorder 3:101–112, 1989

Chodoff P, Lyons H: Hysteria, the hysterical personality and hysterical conversion. Am J Psychiatry 114:734–740, 1958

Clarkin JF, Widiger TA, Frances A, et al: Prototypic typology and the borderline personality disorder. J Abnorm Psychol 92:263–275, 1983

Cox N: Prior help, ego development, and helping behavior. Child Dev 45:594–603, 1974

Frank S, Quinlan D, quoted by Hauser ST: Loevinger's model and measurement of ego development: a critical review. Psychol Bull 83:928–955, 1976

Freud A: The Ego and the Mechanisms of Defense (1937). New York, International Universities Press, 1966

Freud S: Inhibitions, symptoms and anxiety (1926), in The Standard Edition of the Complete Psychological Works of Sigmund Freud, Vol 20. Translated and edited by Strachey J. London, Hogarth Press, 1959, pp 77–175

Grove W, Andreasen NC, McDonald-Scott P, et al: Reliability studies of psychiatric diagnosis: theory and practice. Arch Gen Psychiatry 38:408–413, 1981

Haan NA: Tripartite model of ego functioning values and clinical research applications. J Nerv Ment Dis 148:14–30, 1969

Haan NA, Stroud J, Holstein J: Moral and ego stages in relationship to ego processes: a study of "hippies." J Pers 41:596–612, 1973

Hauser ST: Loevinger's model and measure of ego development: a critical review. Psychol Bull 83:928–955, 1976

Hoppe C: Ego development and conformity behavior. Unpublished doctoral dissertation, Washington University, St Louis, MO, 1972

Karasu T, Skodol A: Sixth axis for DSM-III: psychodynamic evaluation. Am J Psychiatry 137:607–610, 1980

Kernberg O: Borderline personality organization. J Am Psychoanal Assoc 15:641–685, 1967

Klein M: The Psychoanalysis of Children. London, Hogarth Press, 1973

Laplanche J, Pontalis JB: The Language of Psychoanalysis. London, Hogarth Press, 1973

Loevinger J: The meaning and measurement of ego development. Am Psychol 21:195–206, 1966

Loevinger J: Ego Development. San Francisco, CA, Jossey-Bass, 1976

Loevinger J, Wessler R: Measuring Ego Development, Vol 1: Construction and Use of a Sentence Completion Test. San Francisco, CA, Jossey-Bass, 1970

Luborsky L: Clinician's judgment of mental health. Arch Gen Psychiatry 7:33–45, 1962

Meehl PE, Rosen A: Antecedent probability and the efficiency of psychometric signs, patterns or cutting scores. Psychol Bull 52:194–215, 1955

Mellsop G, Varghese F, Joshua S, et al: The reliability of Axis II of DSM-III. Am J Psychiatry 139:1360–1361, 1982

Nie NH, Hull CH, Jenkins JG, et al: Statistical Package for the Social Sciences, 2nd Edition. New York, McGraw-Hill, 1975

Perry JC, Cooper SH: Preliminary report on defenses and conflicts associated with borderline personality disorder. J Am Psychoanal Assoc 34:863–893, 1986

Perry JC, Cooper SH: Empirical studies of psychological defense mechanisms, in Psychiatry, Vol 1. Edited by Michels R, Cavenar JO. Philadelphia, PA, JB Lippincott, 1987, Chapter 30, pp 1–19

Pilkonis PA, Imber SD, Rubinsky P: Dimensions of life stress in psychiatric patients. Journal of Human Stress 11(1):5–10, 1985

Semrad EV, Grinspoon L, Feinberg SE: Development of an ego profile scale. Arch Gen Psychiatry 28:70–77, 1973

Shapiro D: Neurotic Styles. New York, Basic Books, 1965

Spitzer RL, Cohen J, Fleiss J, et al: Quantification of agreement in psychiatric diagnosis: a new approach. Arch Gen Psychiatry 17:83–87, 1967

Spitzer RL, Forman JBW, Nee J: DSM-III field trials, I: initial interrater diagnostic reliability. Am J Psychiatry 136:815–817, 1979

Strauss JS, Harder DW: The case record rating scale: a method for rating symptom and social function data from case records. Psychiatry Res 4:333–345, 1981

Strayhorn G: A diagnostic axis relevant to psychotherapy and preventive mental health. Am J Orthopsychiatry 53:677–696, 1983

Treece C: DSM-III as a research tool. Am J Psychiatry 139:577–583, 1982

Vaillant GE: Natural history of male psychological health, III: empirical dimensions of mental health. Arch Gen Psychiatry 32:420–426, 1975

Vaillant GE: Natural history of male psychological health, V: the relation of choice of ego mechanisms of defense to adult adjustment. Arch Gen Psychiatry 33:535–545, 1976

Vaillant GE, Bond MP, Vaillant CO: An empirically validated hierarchy of defense mechanisms. Arch Gen Psychiatry 43:786–794, 1986

Chapter 8

A Cross-Validation of Two Methods of Investigating Defenses

George E. Vaillant, M.D.
Caroline O. Vaillant, M.S.S.W.

In Chapter 7, Bond reported on the value of his self-administered questionnaire, the Defense Style Questionnaire (DSQ), that taps possible conscious derivatives of defenses. By using factor analysis, Bond demonstrated that statements selected to reflect relatively mature and immature defenses were significantly correlated with mental health and maturity of ego development, as measured by the Sentence Completion Test (Loevinger 1976). Bond's instrument has the obvious advantages of being free from subjective clinical judgment and free from halo and context effects. However, Bond did not demonstrate the capacity of his questionnaire to identify individual defenses.

In Chapters 3 and 6, we introduced our own efforts to validate a hierarchy of defenses on college men and to carry out a replication study based on a sample of socially disadvantaged "CORE CITY" men (see Chapter 6). In this CORE CITY study, maturity of individual defensive styles correlated highly with independent and objective measures of mental health, and rater reliability for overall maturity of defensive style was .84. However, while the difficulty with pencil-and-paper instruments is that their validity is less easy to prove than their reliability, the difficulty with clinical methods is that reliability is often suspect because of observer bias. In our work, reliable clinical identification of defenses could only be achieved by the rater's knowing as much as possible about the subject's inner and outer reality. The problem, then, becomes how to prove that any observed positive correlations of defensive style with outcome are not the result of halo effects?

A possible solution to the complementary limitations of Bond's and our methods was to combine them. Therefore, we administered Bond's context-free questionnaire to the CORE CITY men whose functioning in the real world had been assessed for four decades. First, if Bond's theoretically derived statements correlated with clinical identification of the same defenses, his use of self-report would be validated. Second, if Bond's statements, created in theory to identify specific defensive styles, correlated in fact with independent clinical assessments of those defensive styles, then evidence would be provided that Vaillant's raters were not making their judgments on the basis of halo effects and Bond's choice of item would be validated. Third, because the DSQ was administered in 1983, 6 to 8 years *after* the interview on which the clinical assessment of defense was based, significant correlations would also provide empirical support for the long-established belief that defenses represent trait-like facets of personality. Recently, this belief has been called into question by Brenner (1981), who asserts without empirical evidence that "[n]o one's repertory of defense is limited or repetitive" (p. 569).

Subjects and Methods

Subjects were drawn from the 456 schoolboys who had been chosen as controls for the Gluecks' (1950) study of delinquency. These men have been followed prospectively for 40 years (Vaillant 1983). The subsample described in this chapter included all of the 131 subjects who at an average age of 54 ± 2 years completed Bond's self-report questionnaire. All subjects were white males, 50% of whom had not graduated from high school, and their mean IQ was 97 ± 12.

Measures

Health-Sickness Rating Scale [Age 47 ± 2]

The Health-Sickness Rating Scale (HSRS; Luborsky 1962) was used to assess global mental health by placing individuals on a continuum from 1 to 100 in which institutional dependency receives a rating of 0–25 and multiple manifestations of positive mental health receive a rating of 90–100. Rater reliability was .89.

Maturity (Health) of Defenses (Adaptive Style)

The definitions of the individual defenses are provided elsewhere (Vaillant 1971; see Appendix 3) as is the empirical rationale for equating "maturity" of defensive style with both developmental maturity and freedom from psychopathology (Vaillant 1976). "Adaptive" may be a more accurate term than "mature," but the latter term captures the fact that as young adults grow older or recover from mental illness, their choice of defenses evolves along the hierarchy outlined below.

Raters of defenses were blind both to childhood records and to independent adult ratings. They were given uniform definitions of 15 defenses and trained on interview protocols that had been rated by many others. The 15 defenses were divided into three clusters determined on the basis of prior empirical study:

1. **Mature**—sublimation, suppression, anticipation, altruism, and humor
2. **Intermediate/neurotic**—displacement, repression, isolation (intellectualization), and reaction formation
3. **Immature**—projection, schizoid fantasy, passive aggression (turning against the self), acting out, hypochondriasis, and dissociation (neurotic denial)

Raters were given a 20- to 30-page summary of the men's 2-hour semi-structured interview at age 47. These interviews had been designed to focus on difficulties in each individual's relationships, physical health, and work. In writing the interview summary, the interviewer was instructed to elucidate, but not label, the behaviors by which the individuals had coped with these difficulties. Interview protocols were prepared by the interviewer from verbatim notes taken during the interview. Direct quotations were included in the interview protocols, but the methodology embodied both the scientific limitations and the advantages of journalism. The purpose was to use the interviewer's summary as the first step in data reduction and to retain interview emphasis often lost in transcripts of tape recordings.

For each of the interview protocols, raters were asked to note *all possible* instances of each of the 15 defensive styles. Attention was paid to concrete past behaviors, style of adaptation, past difficulties, and specific vicissitudes of the interview interaction.

In order to control for variation across subjects in the frequency of identified defensive vignettes, the quantitative strategy described in Chapter 4 was adopted to force clinical judgment of the global maturity (health) of defenses into a 9-point scale.

Individual Defenses

For each interview, 10 to 30 instances of defensive behavior were noted, reflecting three to seven different defenses. Weighing of the salience of each individual defense was achieved through *redundancy* (i.e., through frequency, not certainty, of identification). Each rater scored each defense: 0 if absent, 1 if noted once or twice, 2 if it was the most frequently used defense or noted three times or more. Reliability was only modest. The raters had more difficulty agreeing on individual defense ratings, and, depending on the defense, one rater could score a given defense 2 (major) and the other could score it 0 (absent) in 4%–20% of cases. The two raters' ratings were summed, providing an individual rating for each defense that ranged from 0 (both agreed it was absent) to 4 (both agreed it was major).

Clinical illustrations

The evidence by which two men each received a 4 on suppression (a mature defense) is contrasted with the evidence by which two men each received a 4 on schizoid fantasy (an immature defense). These particular defenses were chosen both because they were highly correlated (suppression positively and schizoid fantasy negatively) with objective evidence of mental health and because they were among the most conceptually difficult of the defenses. The examples, which demonstrate the use of redundancy to make clinical judgments, show both the inferred intrapsychic mechanisms and the objective criteria that the blind raters excerpted from the interview protocols in order to make their judgments. The subjects' social class of origin, their education, and their assessed childhood environment were not significantly associated with maturity of defenses.

Schizoid fantasy was defined as creating a gratifying interpersonal relationship inside one's head that had little counterpart in reality. Suppression was defined as stoicism, minimizing but not denying distress, and postponing gratification without denying or repressing the experienced affect.

Case A: Schizoid fantasy (11 grades of school, good childhood environment, parents in social class V).   This man works as a library clerk. He enjoys a vicarious sense of prestigiousness from the slightest association that he has with professions and doctors. "I just like the academic atmosphere," he says. "I just sort of feel a part of it." When asked about his future, he replies, "I will still be at the library, maybe something on the academic level. I'm still interested in photography. . . . I've had so many cameras." He talks with a tinge of grandiosity as he begins to tell the interviewer about certain cousins in the "old country" who were all "8 feet tall." At age 47 and unmarried, he blames religious prejudice. He says he has had little to do with non-Jewish girls. When asked about relationships with women, he recalled a girl at school 35 years ago, in 1942, on whom he had a crush and of whom he had had thoughts of marrying.

He thought that she had married someone else. There has been no one since. He does not drive or have a driver's license, but he says he might be interested in getting a license in the future. He says he knows "intuitively" how to drive a car and so does not require driving instruction. He does not entertain that much but relaxes in his spare time listening to the radio or to records by himself.

Case B: Schizoid fantasy (9 grades of school, childhood environment only fair, parents in social class IV). This person works as a night security guard. He entered into this line of employment for "no special reason" but because he was "fascinated by it." When asked of any job difficulty, he remarks that alertness is the top priority. He says he gets along with people and illustrates this by a story of striking up a conversation with people on a park bench during vacation in California. Mostly he works alone. If he were to live his life over, he would think of being a physical therapist or a lawyer because he wants to help people. He is interested in journalism, and he has occasionally thought of writing a book. He took an electronics course, but nothing came of it. He said that his family is very close-knit. In actual fact, his parents were divorced 25 years ago; recently they remarried each other but live 2,000 miles away. He said he was not particularly close to any one relative: "They are all the same—cousins, aunts, and everybody." He has had no children. Then he said if he had had children, he imagines that he might have had a son killed in Vietnam or a "daughter to worry me sick." Instead, he and his wife have a dog and a cat. He says of his dog, "You could swear that he was human." He says the cat "has a mind of his own." He and his wife get along, although they should not, he says, because he is a Scorpio and she is a Leo. When troubled or angry, he runs up to the attic to listen to his citizen's band radio that has a police scanner. After 5 to 10 minutes, his anger passes. He never did have a special friend. He says that he is not a loner but that he just does not happen to see anyone. There is no one outside his family to whom he would go for help because he "never needs people." He and his wife mostly "keep to ourselves" and "don't need anyone." His hobbies are CB radio, photography, shooting targets (not animals), and fishing. He also likes war movies.

Case C: Suppression (11 grades of school, childhood environment only fair, parents in social class IV). This man's main job is "keeping the peace between customers and the boss," and he finds he "often has to bite his tongue" in his role as diplomat. He has been married for 26 years and says that "nothing really bothers him" about his wife. "She's my whole life. I get to love her more every day. . . . The family just doesn't disagree about much . . . , nothing major." He and his wife both agree that they have worked hard on their marriage but "after 26 years, it's beautiful." He and his wife remember that they had thought of separating in the first years of their marriage.

When he feels bad, he tries to "think positive" and then he tries to "take care of whatever the problem is." For instance, when he is overwhelmed with bills, he just starts to pay them one at a time. Fearing alcoholism, he stopped drinking 19 years ago and has been abstinent since. He says he has not been sick a day in his life. Hearing this, his wife groaned and said, "He would go to work even if he was bleeding." When he gets a cold, he doesn't believe in staying home, as he always says, "I have to work."

Case D: Suppression (9 grades of school, childhood environment only fair, parents in social class V).   This man denies having had any serious problems with other men in his shop. When he gets troubled, he tries not to show it and to "take things in stride." In this way, he maintains an even temperament "at least on the outside." At work he is known as the man with "no emotions" because he never looks rattled. "I want to make sure I know what I am hollering about before I start hollering. . . . I guess I just don't want to make a fool of myself. If you get mad first and then find out you're wrong, well, then it's too late." He did speculate first that his style might have been the reason for his ulcer problem. When he is especially troubled, he talks things over with his wife and they try to settle it together. When he gets very angry, he becomes quiet. He never raises his voice and tries to avoid blowing his top. Sometimes he will sit and play music on his record player until he cools off. He generally tries to avoid fights. On the other hand, he says that he never backed down from a fight if it got to a point where it could not be avoided without losing face.

There are three points to be made by these vignettes. First, suppression looks so reasonable that it is hard to imagine that it is not voluntary, until one reflects that if conscious coping with stress were that easy, more people would use suppression. Second, the inferred intrapsychic mechanisms are based on behaviors that do not just reflect success at working and loving. They have more to do with cognitive and affective styles than with the instrumental behaviors on which outcome ratings were based. Third, when asked to explain their defensive behavior, all subjects could be said to use rationalization. What determines a rater's identification of a defense is the actual behavior, not the subject's explanation of that behavior.

Bond's Defense Style Questionnaire

The DSQ was administered when the men were 54 ± 2 years and 6 to 8 years after the men's defenses had been assessed by clinical interview. The questionnaire was designed to elicit manifestations of a subject's character-istic style of dealing with conflict, whether conscious or unconscious. It is based on the assumption that persons can accurately comment on their defensive behavior.

Subjects were asked to indicate their degree of agreement or disagree-ment with 67 statements (those statements marked with an asterisk in Ap-pendix 6) on a 5-point scale (from 1 = strongly agree to 5 = strongly disagree).

Because the current project was designed to correlate Vaillant's hierar-chy of defenses with the DSQ, each of 67 Bond statements was relabeled to reflect one of Vaillant's 15 defense mechanisms. Originally, Bond designed his statements to reflect behavior not only of the 15 defenses (see Appendix 1) but also of defensive styles suggestive of pseudoaltruism, "as if" behavior, clinging, regression, somatization, withdrawal, omnipotence-devaluation, inhibition, identification, primitive idealization, and splitting.

Labels reflected the consensus of three raters. In 44 items the labels were the same as Bond's. In 23, statements that were originally selected by Bond to reflect the image-distorting terms favored by Otto Kernberg and Melanie Klein were translated into those terms used by Anna Freud and Vaillant (usually turning against the self, fantasy, or projection). Both groups of investigators agreed that the remaining 10 statements constituted a lie scale.

The final labels for the Bond statements included 42 statements reflect-ing immature defenses—projection (11), passive aggression (turning against the self) (10), fantasy (7), dissociation (5), acting out (4), hypo-chondriasis (2), splitting (1), and unclassified (2). Nine statements reflected neurotic or intermediate defenses—reaction formation (7), displacement (1), and isolation (1)—and six reflected mature mechanisms—suppression (2), humor (2), sublimation (1), and altruism (1). (Bond's Factor I was made up exclusively of statements associated with immature defenses, and Bond's Factor IV was made up exclusively of statements reflecting mature defenses.)

Results

Judgment of defensive style required extensive information regarding the men's lives, including their capacity to work and to love. There was no way of completely blinding the raters of defensive behavior from the behaviors underlying the ratings of the outcome variables. Thus, halo effects could be controlled only by finding an independent means of assessing defenses, which in this case was the DSQ.

Only 307 of the 456 subjects could be reliably rated for defenses at age 47. Of these 307 men, 131 returned the DSQ an average of 7 years later. The 131 men who returned the DSQ were contrasted with 325 subjects who did not return it.

Those who returned the DSQ did not differ from the others in ethnicity, multiproblem family membership, emotional illness, boyhood competence, or social class. Those who returned the DSQ did not differ significantly from those who ignored it in terms of global mental health and maturity of defenses, or in terms of personality disorders per se. However, those who did not return the DSQ did differ dramatically in personality subtype. They were more likely to use projection and passive aggression and less likely to use reaction formation and suppression. Those who did not return the questionnaire spent an average of twice as many years (3) unemployed, were three times as likely (11%) to have been in jail, were twice as likely to have abused alcohol (21%), and were twice as likely to have IQs under 85 (21%).

Our ability to predict in advance which Bond statements would correlate with which clinically assessed defense was not perfect. Nor was it as good as it would have been if Bond's statements had been relabeled with the benefit of hindsight. For example, all four of the items selected by both Vaillant's and Bond's groups to predict acting out instead identified men who, on clinical grounds, were judged to use passive aggression or dissociation. This result made sense—after the fact—because acting out was almost never noted in those men who returned the DSQ and because passive aggression and dissociation were the closest "cousins" of acting out.

In 50% or more of the cases, however, the prelabeled Bond statement correlated significantly with the defensive style clinically identified 7 years earlier. On the one hand, more than half of Bond's statements were statistically positively correlated with the clinically identified style that they were supposed to represent. On the other hand, the defensive labels assigned by Vaillant's raters 7 years earlier to clinical vignettes were not just a function of context and halo effects but correlated subsequently with the men's own self-ratings.

Bond identified five statements that he predicted would identify mature mechanisms. All were correlated with mature mechanisms at $P < .01$. Three correlated significantly and positively with global mental health. Bond identified 42 items intended to reflect immature defenses. If the three statements that my group could not relabel are excluded, 24 of the 39 statements were significantly and negatively correlated with maturity of defenses, and 23 were significantly correlated with clinical assessments of the specific defense that each statement was alleged to reflect. Twenty-nine of the 39 statements were significantly and negatively correlated with global mental health. Only three of the 39 statements correlated positively with maturity of defense, and none significantly.

Table 8-1 illustrates the significance and specificity of agreement between prelabeled defense statements and the clinical assessment of representative defensive styles 7 years previously. Statements identified as *mature* correlated positively with mature mechanisms but did not correlate negatively with immature mechanisms. However, those statements reflecting *immature* defensive styles consistently correlated negatively with suppression, a mature mechanism. (Suppression was the defensive style most consistently correlated with all parameters of positive mental health.)

Statements associated with projection appeared to be nonspecifically correlated with other immature defenses, especially with fantasy and splitting. Perhaps because of the selective attrition of antisocial personalities, statements selected by Bond's group (e.g., no. 7) and by Vaillant's group (e.g., no. 27) to identify acting out in fact correlated more highly with dissociation and neurotic denial.

Bond's 10 lie statements were also validated. Designed to identify factitious disagreement, these lie statements included six of the eight statements with which all respondents most strongly agreed. Also, in sharp contrast to statements designed to assess defenses, no lie statement was significantly correlated with outcome variables.

A crude Bond scale of maturity of defenses was constructed by adding all statements prelabeled as mature and by subtracting statements prelabeled projection and fantasy. This scale correlated with the global mental health score from 7 years earlier ($r = .48$; $P < .001$) and with maturity of defenses ($r = .35$; $P < .001$).

Conclusion

By contrasting two very different modes of assessing defensive style on the same sample of subjects examined 7 years apart, we were able to obtain mutual support for both methods. Valid but subjective clinical judgment was contrasted with a reliable but artificial pencil-and-paper test. The findings suggested that clinical assessments of defensive style based on interview protocols were not just artifacts of context. The assessments correlated significantly and specifically with self-report statements chosen to reflect that style.

Equally important, the findings supported the hypothesis that defenses reflect enduring facets of personality that are relatively stable over several years. Finally, the results validated Bond's hypothesis that individuals have some self-awareness of their dominant defensive style.

Table 8–1. Specificity of individual Bond Defense Style Questionnaire statements

Bond statement (defense label)	Projection	Fantasy	Hypochondriasis	Passive aggression	Dissociation	Repression	Altruism	Suppression	Sublimation	Maturity of ego defenses
								Strength of correlation[a] with clinical assessment of defense 8 years earlier		
#1 I get satisfaction from helping others, and if this were taken away from me, I would get depressed. (Altruism)							.21**			.18*
#3 I'm able to keep a problem out of my mind until I have time to deal with it. (Suppression)						.24**		.26**		
#5 I work out my anxiety through doing something constructive and creative like painting or wood-work. (Sublimation)									.26**	.16*
#18 I often feel superior to people I work with. (Fantasy)	.24**									
#50 I'm shy about sex. (Isolation)	.25**									

Item								
#7 I keep getting into the same type of frustrating situations and I don't know why. (Passive aggression)	.18*	.15*	.20*		-.16*		-.23**	-.25**
#34 My friends see me as a clown. (Passive aggression)[b]	.18*	.31***	.15*			-.22**		-.16*
#27 I often act impulsively when something is bothering me. (Acting out)	.18*	.16*	.26**	.20**	.18*	-.21**		-.26**
#66 I am sure I get a raw deal from life. (Projection)	.20**	.31***	.21**			-.26**	-.21**	-.28**
#25 People tell me I have a persecution complex. (Projection)	.29**	.24**		.16*		-.31***	-.22**	-.24***
#53 As far as I am concerned, people are either good or bad. (Projection/splitting)[c]	.25**	.22**			-.21**	-.25**	-.18**	-.24**

[a]Pearson product moment correlation coefficient.
[b]Correlation with humor is − .12.
[c]Correlation with humor is −.17 (P < .05).
*P < .05. **P < .01. ***P < .001.
Source. Reprinted, with permission, from Vaillant et al. 1986. Copyright 1986, American Medical Association.

References

Brenner C: Defense and defense mechanisms. Psychoanal Q 50:557–569, 1981

Glueck S, Glueck E: Unraveling Juvenile Delinquency. New York, The Common Wealth Fund, 1950

Loevinger J: Ego Development. San Francisco, CA, Jossey-Bass, 1976

Luborsky L: Clinicians' judgments of mental health. Arch Gen Psychiatry 8:407–417, 1962

Vaillant GE: Theoretical hierarchy of adaptive ego mechanisms. Arch Gen Psychiatry 24:107–118, 1971

Vaillant GE: Natural history of male psychological health, V: the relation of choice of ego mechanisms of defense to adult adjustment. Arch Gen Psychiatry. 33:533–545, 1976

Vaillant GE: The Natural History of Alcoholism. Cambridge, MA, Harvard University Press, 1983

Chapter 9

Toward Reliability in Identifying Ego Defenses: Clinical Techniques

Leigh McCullough, Ph.D.

The empirical verification of ego defenses has been impeded by the lack of methods for objective measurement. Although taxonomies of ego defenses have been developed (Freud 1937; Meissner et al. 1975; Vaillant 1971), a reliable methodology for labeling and distinguishing defensive behaviors has been difficult to achieve. The problem with achieving reliable identification of defenses is threefold: 1) ego defenses are intrapsychic constructs; 2) the specific behaviors that identify these mental dispositions are widely heterogeneous, and no single behavior is either necessary or sufficient to identify a defense; and 3) different raters view and code defenses from different perspectives so that what may appear to be defensive behavior to one rater may not to another. Thus, traditional methods of item-by-item identification are not applicable here.

To the untrained observer most deciduous trees look alike. To distinguish the maple from the oak, one must learn the differences in, for example, shape of leaf or type of bark. Likewise, to the untrained eye, the behavioral manifestations of ego defenses might appear as quirks, eccentricities, or just plain personality traits. A reliable classification system would allow the differential distinction of such behavioral manifestations of inferred constructs into discrete defenses. But alas, leaves and trees can be seen, touched, and examined, whereas ego defenses will ever remain hypothetical constructs.

In an impressive discussion of how to make intrapsychic constructs admissible to scientific study, Zuriff (1985) has suggested a possible solution. He reminds us that the Wittgensteinian concept for family resemblance might be a fruitful approach here. Looking at a photograph of a large family, one may note that although not every family member has the same eyes, nose, or mouth, there is a similarity of features. Each family member shares the same resemblance, even though there is no one feature that characterizes each and every member. Thus reliability can be achieved in heterogeneous samples by a consensus of agreement regarding their resemblance to an inferred construct.

In this chapter our goal is to work toward shortening the empirical distance between manifest behavior and hypothesized underlying mechanisms by consensus of agreement across raters. First the concept of ego defenses will be defined. Then the results of a reliability study will be presented with specific examples of defensive behavior found in the case histories of the Grant Study of Adult Development (Vaillant 1977).

Definition of Ego Defenses

Defenses may be defined as intrapsychic coping mechanisms that have the function of keeping anxiety within manageable limits. In contrast to "coping skills," a term used by behaviorists for techniques that are taught to help a patient voluntarily manage anxiety, deployment of defenses is not voluntary. We hypothesize that ego defenses represent certain naturally selected-for cognitive "distortions" of internal and external reality that diminish cognitive dissonance and dysphoria that result from sudden changes in the internal and external milieu. An inherent difficulty in reliably identifying defenses is that what may be a defense in one context may not be defensive in another. For example, the act of forgetting can be a manifestation of active repression of a painful stimulus, or it may indicate the normal decay of a memory trace. Thus, in order to decide that a defense is present, assumptions must be made about the subject's internal state or motivation. Furthermore, the identification of defenses is often influenced by the personality (or defenses) of the viewer. These obstacles to reliability will be discussed in regard to the examples found in the case histories.

Methods

Vaillant's hierarchy of defenses (see Appendix 3) was used as the guiding conceptual model to identify ego defenses in case histories from a longitudinal study of college men. Two independent raters were trained to over .80 reliability criterion ($r = .82$ for specific defenses; $r = .95$ for overall defensive style) on approximately 150 examples of defenses embedded in 10 interview reports. Each rater then read and coded seven extensive case histories spanning the past 40 years that included not only research interviews but also biannual self-report questionnaires. There were roughly 300 pages of data in each case dossier.

Each rater's objective was to find examples of defensive behavior in the verbal statements, quotations, excerpts, or descriptions of behavior in the subject's record. The problem that these raters faced was that vignettes were not preselected. Hundreds of pages of unstructured descriptive information in several forms (e.g., self-report, significant-other report, research interviews) were contained in bulky, aging file folders. The raters had the challenge of reviewing this varied material, trying to select the most salient examples, and then deciding which of 18 defense labels best fit the example. To achieve reliability, not only would the independent raters have to assign the same labels to a given example, but they would also have to select the same example. This is a far more stringent test of rater reliability than exists in most clinical studies.

Results

A total of 517 examples were gleaned from seven cases for an average of 73.8 examples per case (range = 32–87). In 324 instances the two raters both identified the same example. An additional 193 examples were identified by either one or the other of the two raters but not by both. Rater A identified 68 and Rater B identified 125 such examples. Thus, the raters agreed in item selection for 63% of the examples selected (see Table 9-1).

Of the 324 examples listed by both raters, there was agreement across specific defenses (e.g., repression, suppression) on 214, or 66%, of the examples. When the specific defenses were clustered into their hierarchical

Table 9–1. Breakdown of defenses coded by two raters according to both identification of items and agreement on examples

Agreement on identification of items	
Examples identified by both raters:	324 (63%)
Examples identified only by Rater A:	68 (13%)
Examples identified only by Rater B:	125 (24%)
Total different examples	
identified in seven charts:	517 (100%)
Agreement on categories of defense among the sample (324 examples)	
Agreement:	254 examples (78%)
Disagreement:	70 examples (22%)
Agreement on specific defenses among the sample (324 examples)	
Agreement:	214 examples (66%)
Disagreement:	110 examples (34%)

categories—the immature, intermediate, and mature categories (see Appendix 3)—the agreement between raters increased to 254 cases, or 78%.

The level of agreement of the two raters on specific defense mechanisms is presented in Table 9-2. The raters showed greater reliability on mature defenses (only 13% disagreements) than on intermediate or immature defenses (44% and 43%, respectively). In assessing the rate of disagreements, it must be realized that by chance, raters would agree in only 7% of the cases.

Disagreements on defenses provide an opportunity to isolate problems in coding. Taking into consideration only the examples identified by both raters, the four defenses that were most agreed upon (percent agreement

Table 9-2.   Agreement between the two raters in labeling those examples that both raters identified as reflecting defensive behaviors

Defense	Agreements (214 examples)	Disagreements (110 examples)
Suppression	22	4
Altruism	11	2
Anticipation	2	1
Sublimation	3	6
Humor	5	0
Total mature defenses	43 pairs (87%)	13 examples (13%)
Repression	15	7
Reaction formation	1	7 (!)
Intellectualization	17	12
Displacement	4	30 (!)
Total intermediate defenses	37 pairs (57%)	56 examples (44%)
Dissociation	4	16 (!)
Hypochondriasis	0	6 (!)
Schizoid fantasy	6	4
Acting out	3	1
Passive aggression	12	11
Projection	2	2
Mild denial	0	1
Total immature defenses	27 pairs (57%)	41 examples (43%)
Totals	**214 examples**	**110 examples**
	(107 agreement pairs)	

Note.   ! underscores rater disagreement.

of total items coded) were suppression, altruism, acting out, and repression (Table 9-2). The five defenses that were least agreed upon were sublimation, dissociation, reaction formation, displacement, and hypochondriasis.

There seemed to be three major reasons for high disagreement. First, there was a lack of clinical salience (e.g., reaction formation and hypochondriasis). In the seven cases rated by two raters, only nine examples of reaction formation and six of hypochondriasis were noted. Thus, lack of agreement may have simply reflected that these mechanisms were not dominant styles used by the seven individuals selected. Second, in the case of displacement, the defense had several "close relatives." Of 31 instances in which one rater coded an item *displacement,* the other rater coded it as *sublimation* (6 times), *intellectualization* (5 times), *dissociation* (5 times), *hypochondriasis* (4 times), and *some other defense* (11 times). Three of the four alternative defenses are conceptually closely related to displacement. Sublimation is the "mature" defense most closely related to displacement, and hypochondriasis is the closest "immature" defense. In obsessional patients intellectualization (isolation of affect) and displacement are commonly paired. The explanation was not that one rater idiosyncratically favored displacement. Rather, the disagreements appear to be due more to a problem of definition and also because displacement can take so many forms. Thus, the importance of sharpening criteria to achieve mutually exclusive definitions is underscored. This point is emphasized in other chapters in this book. The third cause of rater unreliability was rater idiosyncrasy. Of the 16 disagreements over dissociation, 13 of the 16 were coded as dissociation by Rater A and only three were coded as dissociation by Rater B. Additional clarification of definition, as well as training, is required here.

Case Examples

To illustrate some of the specific issues addressed above, two defenses will be presented with a brief definition and examples of agreements and disagreements from the case records. One example will be drawn from one of the most agreed-upon defenses (i.e., repression) and the other from one of the most disagreed-upon defenses (i.e., displacement).

Repression

Repression is seemingly inexplicable naiveté, memory lapse, or failure to acknowledge input from a selected sense organ. This defense protects the subject from being aware of what he or she is feeling. The emotional elements are clearly experienced, but the cognitive elements remain outside of consciousness. Repression is characterized by, when an individual is asked a question, repeated responses such as "I don't know," "I can't remember," or "My mind goes blank," or by not acknowledging the obvious.

Case examples

The following examples are from a single individual:

1. Said "I don't know" to everything. When asked, "Was your career a poor choice?" he replied, "Yes—but I'm not sure why I said yes."
2. (Later) "I don't know why I drifted into engineering. I might be happy with it—but I'm not at all sure."
3. *Question:* "What are your beliefs over rough spots? *Answer:* "How does anyone answer that question? I'm afraid I don't know."
4. *Question:* "Have you met your expectations 20 years after college? *Answer:* "I haven't the slightest idea what I expected 20 years ago."
5. *Question:* "Is sexual tension a problem?" *Answer:* "Damned if I know—unless it is subconscious."
6. He reported that he loses his temper frequently, but cannot remember even one incident.
7. *Question:* "What do you do in your spare time?" *Answer:* "Questions like this make me wonder what I do. I don't have any idea. I seem to keep busy."
8. *Question:* "What do you do over rough spots?" *Answer:* "I don't know what you mean. I haven't had any." [But he had!]
9. (Shortly after World War II) "I can't say how the danger affected me. I guess I'm still reacting."
10. "I can't remember whether I had sexual thoughts as a boy."
11. "The way I handle problems is to forget them."

Repression, more broadly defined, plays a part in many other defenses. We tried to code repression only when it stood alone. Also, in self-report data, it is often unclear whether the subject was consciously withholding information from us when an "I don't know" or "I'm not sure" answer was given, or whether the information reflected genuine repression. Clearly, redundancy, as in the example above, provided the only assurance. Clinical salience is as important in rating defenses as it is in biography.

Displacement

Displacement is the redirection of feelings toward a relatively less-cared-for object. Displacement refers to the expression of an affect, an impulse, or an action toward a person, bodily part, or object instead of toward the one that aroused the affect feeling in the first place. The affect is fully acknowledged but is redirected to a less conflictual target. Behavioral examples associated with displacement, as presented below, are categorized by the targets to which they are directed and the valence they carry. On these case examples the raters agreed.

Displacement toward objects

1. "I was so mad that I went out and slammed a tennis ball." [But if the subject reported winning tennis tournaments or feeling the thrill of competition, this would be coded *sublimation*.]
2. "When work goes bad I blow off steam in my garden." [If working in the garden were a mindless way of escaping work problems *without acknowledging the anger,* this would be coded *dissociation*. And, as in the tennis example above, if the subject's gardening created something of beauty rather than merely hacking at the ground, this could be coded *sublimation*.]

Bodily ailments under stress

1. "I got a terrific headache after the boss yelled at me."
2. "During that bad year at work, I ended up with chronic indigestion."

Displacement through wit or sarcasm

1. "At one time I was drinking so much I could have put the National Distillers on a second shift!" [The subject is his own target.]
2. When the subject was asked if he ever had psychiatric treatment, he wrote [to the Grant Study psychiatrist], "Anyone who goes to a psychiatrist should have his head examined." [These examples are distinguished from humor, in which no one is attacked.]

Displacement of positive feelings

1. "We treat our dog like the child we don't have. . . . We are even taking Rover to Europe this summer!"

Displacement was one of the defenses for which we initially had difficulty in obtaining reliability. Evident in the varied list of behaviors above is the diversity of the ability of the human mind to direct emotion to multiple targets. As already noted, displacement was one of the most disagreed-upon defenses in this study. There are multiple objects: people, places, body parts, things, and objects. Also, there are multiple ways to displace that run the gamut of emotion: anger (criticism), apparent "humor" (wit or sarcasm), or fears or phobias (anxiety). When is prejudice projection and when is it displacement? When is play displacement and when is it sublimation? These can be fine distinctions. Below are some examples on which the raters *disagreed:*

1. "I am extremely happy doing surgery." [Is this *creative fulfillment* or *displaced aggression?*]
2. As a boy, the subject always mercilessly teased his sister. [This was coded *passive aggression* by one rater and as *displacement* by the other. Could it not be both?]
3. "I am not excited by my life's work, but this doesn't bother me a bit." [One rater coded this *dissociation,* and the other coded it *reaction formation.* Like the preceding example, it has components of both.]

The above examples do not really provide sufficient data to make the necessary distinctions. More data are required so that patterns in defensive style can be determined by consensus rather than by item agreement. This brings us to a second important point. In coding these case histories, what we were seeking was agreement on the overall pattern of behavior. Reliability is generally established on a predetermined set of items, but data in this report were generated from unstructured cases. As with facial recognition or hidden figures, individual raters may not attend to identical families of stimuli on which judgments are based, but they may agree on the family nonetheless. Defensive behaviors reflect fragments of personality as nose and eyes reflect parts of the face. Thus, in Table 9-1, 193 examples of defenses were coded by either Rater A or Rater B but not by both. However, 56% of the individually identified examples by Rater B illustrated defensive styles already identified as a predominant style for a given individual by Rater A. Therefore, in coding defenses one objective may be to arrive at consensus by redundancy, not certainty, for each single item. Reliability on every item can only be achieved by standardized stimuli in the laboratory, and the study of defenses occurs in the wilds, not the laboratory.

Conclusion

The surface event (recorded verbal behavior) will never totally represent a complex, multifaceted intrapsychic state of mind. When we try to squeeze science out of art, some of the beauty and mystery is lost. On the other hand, what is gained are data that we can get our hands on and test by consensual validation. Popper has said that the best we can ever achieve is a "woven web of conjectures." In this chapter we have attempted to weave the conjectural web for ego defenses somewhat tighter.

In our efforts to rate relative maturity of defensive behavior, we intentionally cast a wide net. The trade-off was that false positives occurred frequently. For example, we knew that all cases of "I don't know" in response to personal questions did not represent repression. However, clinical experience suggests that high frequency of "I don't knows" does correlate with repression. The check on our inclusive style of rating was redundancy. Consensus was necessary before a choice received significance.

The scientific study of ego defenses has been impeded by the lack of methods for their objective measurement. We have attempted an orderly classification of defensive behaviors by isolating manifestations of psychological defense mechanisms in written records and systematically arranging this verbal behavior according to specific criteria. Using Vaillant's (1971) hierarchy, two raters coded defensive behavior in case histories from a longitudinal study (spanning 40 years) of men chosen for physical and emotional health. The raters' objective was to identify examples of defensive behavior in the verbal excerpts or in descriptions of behaviors in the subjects' records. Steps toward enhancing the reliability of the coding of defenses involved the examination of inter-rater agreement versus disagreement for each defense, as well as the attempt to minimize the level of inference required in each behavioral example.

References

Freud A: The Ego and the Mechanisms of Defense. London, Hogarth Press, 1937

Meissner WW, Mack JE, Semrad EV: Theories of personality and psychopathology: classical psychoanalysis, in Comprehensive Textbook of Psychiatry, 2nd Edition, Vol 1. Edited by Freedman AM, Kaplan HI, Sadock BJ. Baltimore, MD, Williams & Wilkins, 1975, pp 482–566

Vaillant G: Theoretical hierarchy of adaptive ego mechanisms. Arch Gen Psychiatry 24:107–118, 1971

Vaillant G: Adaptation to Life. Boston, MA, Little, Brown, 1977

Zuriff G: Behaviorism: A Conceptual Reconstruction. New York, Columbia University Press, 1985

Chapter 10

An Approach to Evaluating Adolescent Ego Defense Mechanisms Using Clinical Interviews

Alan M. Jacobson, M.D.
William Beardslee, M.D.
Elizabeth Gelfand, Ed.D.
Stuart T. Hauser, M.D., Ph.D.
Gil G. Noam, Dipl.Psych.
Sally I. Powers, Ed.D.

Call me Ishmael. Some years ago . . . I thought I would sail about a little and see the watery part of the world. It is a way I have of driving off the spleen, and regulating the circulation. Whenever I find myself growing grim about the mouth; whenever it is a damp, drizzly November in my soul; whenever I find myself involuntarily pausing before coffin warehouses, and bringing up the rear of every funeral I meet; and especially whenever my hypos get such an upper hand of me, that it requires a strong moral principle to prevent me from deliberately stepping into the street, and methodically knocking people's hats off—then, I account it high time to get to sea as soon as I can. This is my substitute for pistol and ball.

H. Melville *Moby Dick*

The perspective that underlying issues can motivate thoughts and actions has gained wide acceptance as part of our cultural ideology. Yet the relationships between inner dialogue and overt behavior are often complex and circuitous—novelists and psychiatrists alike strive to unravel them. In their efforts at explicating some of these connections, dynamically oriented psychotherapists regularly utilize the concept of ego mechanisms of defense in their formulations about patients and also in the theoretical and clinical literature (A. Freud 1937; S. Freud 1926). Yet as authors in the previous chapters of this volume have noted, definitions of individual defenses often vary among researchers and clinicians, and relatively few investigators have developed empirical methods for appraising these constructs (Bond et al. 1983; Haan 1977; Vaillant 1977). Reliable and valid methods of assessing defense mechanisms could prove useful in systematic research, in clinical practice, and in the training of clinicians. This potential was recognized, for example, in the consideration given to including a diagnostic axis for defense and coping mechanisms in DSM-III and its revision, DSM-III-R (Klerman et al. 1984). Yet as a result of the lack of consensus among clinicians and researchers about definitions of defenses and means of rating them, this potential has yet to be fully realized.

As a consequence of our research group's interest in assessing developmental processes that are relevant for understanding coping during adolescence, we have devised an objective method of evaluating ego defense mechanisms from clinical interview material.

The work of constructing this coding procedure has been but one facet of two longitudinal studies of family contexts of adolescent development conducted by our group.

The first study, the Adolescent Development Study, has two primary, interrelated aims: 1) to use rigorous empirical methods to investigate specific psychological processes identified by clinical observations as relevant during early and middle adolescence, and 2) to assess the influence of family interaction patterns on adolescent psychosocial development (Hauser et al. 1983). Among the developmental processes we evaluate are adolescent ego defenses, self-images, ego development, and self-esteem (Jacobson et al. 1982, 1984).

In the second study, the Health and Illness Study, the interacting relationships between adolescent development and a chronic medical illness, insulin-dependent diabetes mellitus (IDDM), are examined. The Health and Illness Study has two aims: 1) to assess the impact of IDDM on adolescent psychological processes, and 2) to evaluate early psychosocial predictors of the subsequent course of illness. Family environments and interactions are studied, as are adolescent ego development, self-esteem, adjustment, and use of ego defense mechanisms (Hauser et al. 1982, 1990; Jacobson et al. 1987a, 1987b, 1990).

Assessing ego defenses provides one way of characterizing a discrete and important aspect of adolescent psychosocial maturation—one that may prove particularly relevant in understanding individual adaptations to this complex phase of development. In this chapter we present our approach to evaluating ego defense mechanisms and information regarding the reliability and validity of the rating scales.

Assessment of Defense Mechanisms

Background

Two basic approaches have been taken to assessing defense mechanisms: 1) self-report questionnaires and 2) clinical observer ratings. Self-report questionnaires depend on the conscious description or recognition by the subject of his or her own typical behaviors (Bond et al. 1983; Gleser and Ihilevich 1969). As described in Chapter 7, Bond et al. developed a measure of individual defenses that relies on the individual's responses to statements designed to tap characteristic styles of dealing with conflictual situations. Subjects report their level of agreement or disagreement with each statement. This type of approach has the virtue of minimizing problems of inter-rater reliability, assessment time, and professional participation in the evaluation process. This approach can be used to derive characteristic and consciously recognized behavior patterns for individuals and groups. Its major disadvantage stems from the data source: a limited number of standardized statements that the subject can consciously evaluate and select between. Thus, such measures assess conscious derivatives of defenses but may fail to identify particular areas of individual conflict in which defense style may be more critical and in which the subject remains unaware of defense usage. Indeed, from a theoretical perspective, individuals would be expected to remain unaware of defense mechanisms engaged in response to unconscious conflicts. In addition, subjects may select responses in terms of socially or personally desired behaviors. Finally, this type of measure is used to identify hypothetical rather than actual patterns of defense.

Clinician ratings or judgments of defenses have been utilized by several researchers (Bibring et al. 1961; Grinker et al. 1968; Haan 1977; Prelinger and Zimet 1964; Semrad et al. 1973; Vaillant 1977). The major value of this approach includes the closeness of the data to the kinds of observations made in clinical practice, the richness of data, and the opportunity to detect unconscious processes present in the behaviors of the patient, which can be observed during interactions with staff and in associations during interviews. Ratings of defenses from directly observed behavior, including clinical interviews, may be particularly useful in studies that evaluate psychotherapeutic outcomes. The limitations of these approaches include difficulty in developing reliable ratings, the need for professional input, subject time, and variability in the data base caused by interview style or method of observation.

Within the group of investigators using the clinical rating approach, there have been a variety of differences such as conception of defenses, sources of data, and methods of rating. Investigators often hold strikingly different conceptions of the nature of defense mechanisms. For example, Haan views defenses as pathological and as at one end of an adaptation spectrum, with coping at the opposite end. On the other hand, Vaillant views defenses as being on a hierarchy from more immature or pathological to more adaptive or mature. In addition to defenses, Prelinger and Zimet (1964) assessed ego functioning from the perspective of competencies found in styles of thinking and behaving. Terming this aspect of ego functioning "adaptive strengths," the authors did not view defenses as specifically pathological. Vaillant (1977) and Prelinger and Zimet (1964) utilized defense ratings that derive from traditional psychoanalytic definitions and conceptualizations.

Sources of data vary widely, ranging from interviews (e.g., Prelinger and Zimet 1964) and interviews plus biographical information (Vaillant 1977), to observations in ward settings (e.g., Semrad et al. 1973). However variable, the data that form the basis of evaluations consistently derive, at least in part, from direct observations of subjects.

Approaches to coding defenses also vary. Haan (1977) used trained coders to rate defense and coping using a Q-sort method. Prelinger and Zimet (1964) used defense and adaptive strength codes with definitions having scaled levels of intensity and examples from interviews that exemplify scale points. Vaillant (1977) reviewed interview material and biographical information to draw vignettes that demonstrate defenses in action. Coders then rated these vignettes in terms of specific defenses.

The complexity involved in developing a systematic, reliable coding system for assessing clinical material has limited the number of investigations that use clinical rating approaches and thwarted the construction of a single method that is widely accepted by multiple researchers. In forming our coding method, we have built on these prior efforts to rate ego defenses clinically. In addition to using defense assessments for understanding adolescent development and coping, this work may stimulate the further evolution of a more widely applicable coding method for assessing defense mechanisms from clinical material.

To broaden our perspective on the assessment of coping, we have also been engaged in constructing an additional coding method for assessing adaptive ego processes, based on a psychoanalytic ego psychological framework (Prelinger and Zimet 1964) and on work in the assessment of competence in children, as reported elsewhere (Beardslee et al. 1985, 1990; Hauser et al. 1982). By using two distinct approaches to the evaluation of coping, like Prelinger and Zimet, we assume that defenses can serve adaptive functions and do not simply represent a pathological end of the spectrum of individual coping. This conception is quite consistent with that of Vaillant (1977), but differs distinctly from that of Haan (1977).

Samples

Adolescent Development Study. To identify a wide range of adolescent developmental patterns, we have followed clinically defined samples of adolescent subjects who are likely to be developmentally impaired or at risk for future impairment. A nonpatient sample not at apparent risk for developmental impairment has also been followed. The three groups of early adolescent subjects in this study, described below, were recruited between the ages of 12 and 16:

1. Diabetic adolescents were drawn from consecutive registrants at a camp for patients with diabetes or from consecutive admissions to the teaching and treatment unit of the Joslin Diabetes Center. Patients hospitalized in this setting were not acutely ill but had been admitted to refine their understanding or control of their diabetes.
2. Psychiatric patients were drawn from consecutive admissions to the adolescent inpatient unit of a large private teaching hospital. We excluded patients for whom admission evaluation suggested a diagnosis of psychosis or organic brain syndrome.
3. Adolescents without known chronic illness were drawn from freshman volunteers who were attending a suburban high school.

Detailed descriptions of the samples and procedures used for their assessment can be found elsewhere (Hauser et al. 1983; Jacobson et al. 1984).

Health and Illness Study. Two samples of patients, ages 9 to 16, were studied:

1. The diabetic sample consisted of patients presenting at the Joslin Diabetes Center's Pediatric Unit who had been diagnosed as having IDDM in the prior year.
2. The other group of patients consisted of children with a recent acute medical problem that necessitated at least some change in their daily activities. These children were recruited from a local health maintenance organization. The diagnostic breakdown of the sample was as follows: fractures (48%), infections (15%), appendicitis (13%), and lacerations and other injuries (24%). Change in daily activities was defined as two or more visits to a physician, or hospitalization and loss of at least one day in school or, during vacation periods, one missed day of extracurricular activities. Subjects who presented for treatment of the same acute medical problem within the preceding 6 months were excluded from the study.

A more detailed description of the samples is found elsewhere (Jacobson et al. 1987b).

The Interviews

In both studies, children and adolescents were interviewed yearly by trained mental health professionals (psychiatrists, psychologists, or psychiatric social workers). The interview style was exploratory, using open-ended questions. Several topics were covered, including school and home life, peer relationships, illness experiences, and hopes for the future. One related topic cut across all others: the ways in which conflicts, affects, and external crises were perceived and handled by the subject. This interview, therefore, covered a broad range of concerns relevant to the adolescent subject in a manner similar to an initial, open-ended clinical interview. The interviewers explored various aspects of the adolescents' life experiences. However, individual interviews differed in the extent to which topics were covered. The coverage variations stemmed from the adolescents' own areas of special interest or concern, which were explored in more depth as determined by the capacity of the subject. For example, the presence of parental conflicts or divorce often led to prolonged discussions of the family and of the subject's own concerns and coping patterns in response to this problem area.

The interviews were audiotaped and transcribed. The transcripts served as the material from which ego defenses were rated. This approach was used in both studies.

The Defense Codes

In order to generate an inclusive set of ego defenses with usable definitions, we reviewed relevant literature, most especially the work of A. Freud (1937), Prelinger and Zimet (1964), and Vaillant (1977). However, Valenstein's work (as reported in Bibring et al. 1961), in particular, provided us with conceptually oriented definitions of defense mechanisms. From the above sources, we selected defenses that were both widely recognized and pertinent for a population of adolescents. Currently, we assess subjects by means of rating 12 defenses. In addition, we have established a separate code for overall defensive success (see Table 10-1). Some other defenses included in earlier versions of our coding manual were excluded subsequently for various reasons. For example, identification with the aggressor and identification with the lost object were initially included. The definitions of these defenses required the coder to determine the object with whom the subject was identifying, which proved extremely difficult from a single interview. We also excluded defenses such as those used by

Table 10–1. Reliabilities for defense codes

Defense	Intraclass correlation
Acting out	.69
Altruism	.54
Asceticism	.76
Avoidance	.67
Denial	.37
Displacement	.74
Intellectualization	.56
Projection	.32
Rationalization	.38
Repression	.46
Suppression	.62
Turning against self	.67
Overall	**.60**

patients with borderline character disorders. This decision stemmed more from our focus on adolescent development than from any particular view of the overall merits of these particular defenses. We believe that our approach could be used to develop other defense codes, such as those for rating defenses used by patients with severe character disorders.

While definitions used by the Valenstein and Bibring group and others provided a major starting point for our codes, we have refined them in three ways:

1. Where definitions were confusing, changes were made in the definitions themselves.
2. Based on Prelinger and Zimet's (1964) approach, we developed a 5-point scale of intensity from minimally to maximally present. Brief descriptions were provided for each point on the scale.
3. From a subset of our interviews we then generated case examples for each scale point. Our manual for scoring ego defense mechanisms is presented in Appendix 5 of this book. For each of the defenses, the manual provides a conceptual definition, descriptive scale points, and clinical examples for each scale point.

Using the combination of a definition, specified scale points, and examples, raters judge each subject on all defenses. They can withhold ratings on specific defenses if sufficient information is lacking, but in practice this has occurred very infrequently. Raters are instructed to use the entire interview to make each rating. The coder uses both the frequency of episodes found in the entire interview and the strength of particular vignettes to judge the subject. For example, in the manual presented in Appendix 5, the subject who was rated as using a moderate level of asceticism presented different instances of relatively subtle ascetic responses. If she had shown only one, stronger instance of ascetic attitudes, such as strong disgust over sexual activity, this could also have been rated as demonstrating a moderate level of asceticism. The subject examples rated as showing higher levels of asceticism demonstrated more frequent and/or stronger instances of ascetic attitudes.

In each rating, information derives from both the interview behavior and the self-reports of the subject. For example, altruism may be shown both through charitable actions to friends and by specific attempts at being helpful in providing information to the interviewer. Acting out may be identified through reports by the subject as well as by impulsivity motivated by anxiety during the interview.

Reliability of the Defense Codes

On a subset of 18 transcripts, inter-rater reliability was assessed (three raters were compared) for all codes using the intraclass correlation statistic (Bartko and Carpenter 1976). The sample size for the three-way reliability study was selected with statistical consultation (J. Bartko, personal communication, 1982). Table 10-1 shows the defenses and the intraclass correlation reliabilities. Based on previously developed guidelines for evaluating intraclass correlations (Cichetti and Sparrow 1982), 3 of the 13 codes showed fair levels of agreement ($r = 0.40$–0.59), 6 showed good levels of agreement ($r = 0.60$–0.74), and 1 showed an excellent level of agreement ($r = 0.75$–1.00). These findings suggest that on the whole these codes can be reliably used by trained coders.

We have now also trained two additional sets of raters to use these codes. Although these raters range widely in clinical experience and training, their levels of reliability are quite similar to those presented here. This suggests that these defense codes can be taught and used by other groups interested in evaluating defense profiles from clinical interviews.

However, our own experience with these codes indicates that certain problems interfere with their reliable use. These stem in part from the theory of defenses and its application to clinical material. A major problem is that raters have widely different expectations about the amount of inference that should be used. The trained clinician often looks for subtle cues from which to hypothesize the presence of certain conflicts and defensive processes.

This serves the clinician well in actual practice but can create problems in coding reliably, because a turn of phrase can be interpreted in many distinct ways. By providing brief descriptions of how subjects have been rated, the case examples are particularly useful in moderating the amount of inference used in evaluating defenses. Thus, after reading a transcript, the coder reviews each code definition and scale points and rates the subject on that scale. Then, using the examples, the rater reviews the decision. This approach parallels the method of scoring used by Loevinger and Wessler (1970) in developing a sentence completion test of ego development, which has led to acceptable levels of inter-rater reliability for the use of their instrument by many different groups of investigators.

Validity of the Defense Codes

Empirical studies by our group have demonstrated the validity—external, convergent, and predictive—of these defense scales. In the Adolescent Development Study, patterns of ego defense use distinguished a sample of psychiatric patients from age-matched peers (see Table 10-2). The psychiatric sample employed significantly more "immature" defenses (acting out, avoidance, displacement, projection, and turning against the self) than did

Table 10–2. Ego defenses (by subject group)

Defense	Diabetic	Psychiatric	Nonpatient	F
Acting out	1.26	2.59[a]	1.58	28.47**
Altruism	2.03	1.56[a]	2.00	7.74*
Asceticism	2.10	1.74[a]	1.97	5.83*
Avoidance	1.35	2.52[a]	1.55	31.42**
Denial	2.00	2.41	2.18	2.61
Displacement	1.16	2.26[a]	1.06	27.70**
Intellectualization	1.90[b]	1.56[a]	2.27	10.62*
Projection	1.26	1.96[a]	1.52	8.57**
Rationalization	2.13	1.93	2.06	0.73
Repression	1.71	1.78	1.58	1.01
Suppression	2.42[b]	1.44[a]	2.03	24.60**
Turning against self	1.19	1.85[a]	1.00	19.79**
Overall	**3.00**	**2.11**[a]	**3.15**	**52.25**

*$P < .004$. **$P < .0001$.
[a]Significantly different from diabetic and nonpatient groups using Fischer's test of least significant differences.
[b]Significantly different from the nonpatient group using Fischer's test of least significant differences.

the other two groups and also utilized significantly fewer "mature" defenses (altruism, asceticism, intellectualization, and suppression) than did the others (Jacobson et al. 1986). These results support our predictions from theory and demonstrate the external validity of this measure. Additionally, in this study, subjects' scores on the ego defense measures correlated in the expected directions with their scores on a well-established measure of ego development, the Sentence Completion Test (Loevinger and Wessler 1970) (see Table 10-3). These findings confirm theoretical predictions and provide evidence of convergent validity for this measure.

The Health and Illness Study tested the effectiveness of employing defense usage as a predictor of relevant patient coping behaviors (i.e., self-care activities by young patients with IDDM). We anticipated, based on prior research on psychosocial factors associated with adjustment to illness, that use of mature defenses would be positively associated with adherence to the diabetes treatment regimen and that use of less mature defenses would be negatively related to adherence.

Based on the results of the Adolescent Development Study, we organized the 12 defense mechanisms into three clusters that we labeled immature, midrange, and mature. The immature grouping was comprised of acting out, avoidance, displacement, projection, and turning against the self; the mature cluster included altruism, asceticism, intellectualization, and suppression; the midrange defenses were denial, rationalization, and repression. The cohesive patterning of the mature and immature defense cluster was borne out by statistical analysis: Cronbach's alpha was .76 for the

Table 10–3. Pearson correlations between ego development scores and defenses

Altruism	.39****
Intellectualization	.34****
Suppression	.30***
Overall	.38****
Acting out	−.26**
Avoidance	−.44****
Denial	−.30***
Displacement	−.19*
Projection	−.26**
Repression	−.30***
Turning against self	.11
Asceticism	.05
Rationalization	−.05

Note. Item sum scores were used in these correlational analyses.
*$P < .04$. **$P < .007$. ***$P < .002$. ****$P < .001$.

immature cluster, indicating that this cluster was strongly intercorrelated. Cronbach's alpha for the mature cluster was .43, suggesting a moderate interrelationship among these defenses. The midrange defenses are commonly utilized and can, at high levels of use, be considered neurotic or maladaptive. These defenses do not seem to describe as cohesive a pattern of coping in that the Cronbach's alpha for this cluster was only .29. It should be noted that midrange defenses are the least reliable to rate, so conclusions regarding this cluster must be drawn with caution.

Diabetic patients were interviewed shortly after study entry, and these clinical interviews were rated in terms of defense usage. Patterns of patient adherence evaluated by the patient's health care provider were recorded at subsequent medical visits. The relationship of defense usage to adherence was examined.

The results of analyses over the first 18 months of follow-up largely confirmed our expectations. We found that higher levels of mature defense use were somewhat positively correlated with greater adherence, whereas higher levels of immature and midrange defense use were clearly associated with poor adherence (Jacobson et al. 1987a) (see Table 10-4). More recently, we have examined patterns of defense use in relationship to adherence over a 4-year period of follow-up (Jacobson et al. 1990). In this instance, we constructed a single defense strength index that included all 12 defenses. To create this index, mature defenses were reverse scored and added to the immature and midrange defenses. This total, or summary, scale had a Cronbach's alpha of .75. A higher score on the defense strength index reflects less use of mature defenses and greater use of immature defenses. A higher defense score was associated with lower average adherence over the 4-year follow-up ($r = -.52$, $P \leq .0007$). These findings confirm theoretical formulations about defense use and also support the predictive validity of these defense codes.

Table 10–4. Pearson correlations of defense clusters with adherence over 18-month follow-up

Defense clusters	Adherence	
	0–9 months	10–18 months
Immature	−.48***	−.33**
Midrange	−.33**	−.33**
Mature	.25*	.18

*$P \leq .05$. **$P \leq .01$. ***$P \leq .0001$.

Discussion

We have described our method of assessing ego defense mechanisms from clinical interview material and the studies that we have done to determine the validity and reliability of these scales. The codes were able to distinguish a sample of psychiatrically hospitalized adolescents from their age peers without psychiatric diagnosis: the psychiatric group used more maladaptive defenses (i.e., acting out, avoidance, displacement, projection, and turning against the self) and fewer adaptive defenses (i.e., altruism, asceticism, suppression, and intellectualization) than did healthy subjects or those with diabetes. We also found that subjects' scores on the defense codes correlated in theoretically expected ways with their ego development as measured by Loevinger's Sentence Completion Test. Subjects who scored high on ego development utilized "mature" defenses such as altruism, asceticism, intellectualization, and suppression, whereas those with low ego development scores tended to use more "immature" defenses like acting out, avoidance, displacement, projection, and turning against the self. Additionally, we have evidence for the predictive validity of these measures in that defense use was associated with adherence to a diabetes self-care regimen over 4 years of follow-up. Again, use of mature defenses seemed to correlate positively with better adherence, whereas use of immature and midrange or neurotic defenses corresponded with poor adherence. In sum, the defense rating codes have strong evidence of validity. Some caution needs to be exercised, however, when drawing inferences from some of the scales (the midrange defenses in particular) because of lower reliability.

In conclusion, we have presented a method for systematically assessing ego defense mechanisms from in-depth exploratory interviews. This approach to coding defense use may be applicable in several areas of psychiatry, including the study of development during adolescence and the evaluation of change in psychotherapy. Additionally, codifying and quantifying definitions of ego defenses may be useful in training therapists.

References

Bartko J, Carpenter W: On the methods of theory of reliability. J Nerv Ment Dis 16:307–317, 1976

Beardslee W, Jacobson AM, Hauser ST, et al: An approach to evaluating adolescent adaptive processes: scale development and reliability. Journal of the American Academy of Child Psychiatry 24:637–642, 1985

Beardslee W, Powers S, Hauser S, et al: Adaptation in adolescence: the influence of time and severe psychiatric disorder. J Am Acad Child Adolesc Psychiatry 29:429–439, 1990

Bibring G, Dwyer T, Huntington D, et al: A study of the psychological processes in pregnancy and of the earliest mother-child relationship, II. Psychoanal Study Child 16:25–72, 1961

Bond M, Gardner ST, Christian J, et al: Empirical study of self-rated defense styles. Arch Gen Psychiatry 40:333–338, 1983

Cichetti D, Sparrow S: The Behavioral Inventory for Rating Development (BIRD). Proceedings of the Social Statistics Section, American Statistical Association, 1982, pp 218–223

Freud A: The Ego and the Mechanisms of Defense (1937). New York, International Universities Press, 1966

Freud S: Inhibitions, symptoms and anxiety (1926), in The Standard Edition of the Complete Psychological Works of Sigmund Freud, Vol 20. Translated by Strachey J. London, Hogarth Press, 1953, pp 77–175

Gleser GD, Ihilevich D: An objective instrument for measuring defense mechanisms. J Consult Clin Psychol 33:51–60, 1969

Grinker RR, Weble B, Drye R: The Borderline Syndrome. New York, Basic Books, 1968

Haan N: Coping and Defending: Processes of Self-Environment Organization. New York, Academic, 1977

Hauser ST, Powers S, Jacobson AM, et al: Family interactions and ego development in diabetic adolescents. Pediatric and Adolescent Endocrinology 10:69–76, 1982

Hauser ST, Jacobson AM, Noam G, et al: Ego development and self-image complexity in early adolescence: longitudinal studies of psychiatric and diabetic patients. Arch Gen Psychiatry 40:32–33, 1983

Hauser ST, Jacobson AM, Lavori P, et al: Adherence among children and adolescents with IDDM over a four-year longitudinal follow up, II: immediate and long-term linkages with the family milieu. J Pediatr Psychol 15:527–542, 1990

Jacobson AM, Hauser ST, Powers S, et al: Ego development in diabetics: a longitudinal study. Pediatric and Adolescent Endocrinology 10:1–8, 1982

Jacobson AM, Hauser ST, Powers S, et al: The influences of chronic illness and ego development level on self-esteem in diabetic and psychiatric patients. Journal of Youth and Adolescence 13:489–507, 1984

Jacobson AM, Beardslee W, Hauser S, et al: Evaluating ego defense mechanisms using clinical interviews: an empirical study of adolescent diabetic and psychiatric patients. J Adolesc 9:303–319, 1986

Jacobson AM, Gelfand E, Hauser ST, et al: Ego mechanisms of defense and compliance in diabetes, in New Research Abstracts, American Psychiatric Association Annual Meeting, Chicago, May 1987a, p 136

Jacobson AM, Hauser S, Wolfsdorf J, et al: Psychologic predictors of compliance in children with recent onset of diabetes mellitus. J Pediatr 110:805–811, 1987b

Jacobson AM, Hauser S, Lavori P, et al: Adherence among children and adolescents with IDDM over a four-year longitudinal follow up, I: the influence of patient coping and adjustment. Journal of Pediatric Psychology 15:5–11, 1990

Klerman GL, Vaillant GE, Spitzer RL, et al: A debate on DSM-III. Am J Psychiatry 141:539–553, 1984

Loevinger J, Wessler R: Measuring Ego Development, Vol 1: Construction and Use of a Sentence Completion Test. San Francisco, CA, Jossey-Bass, 1970

Prelinger E, Zimet C: An Ego Psychological Approach to Character Assessment. Glencoe, IL, Free Press, 1964

Semrad EV, Grinspoon L, Feinberg SE: Development of an ego profile scale. Arch Gen Psychiatry 28:70–77, 1973

Vaillant GE: Adaptation to Life. Boston, MA, Little, Brown, 1977

Chapter 11

What Do Cross-Sectional Measures of Defense Mechanisms Predict?

J. Christopher Perry, M.D., M.P.H.
Steven Cooper, Ph.D.

I n this chapter we report on the development, reliability, and some aspects of validity of the Defense Mechanism Rating Scales (DMRS), which can be applied to clinical interview and life vignette data. The findings presented in this chapter comprise one of a series of empirical studies of the psychodynamic and descriptive psychopathology of individuals with personality and affective disorders. Validity of the DMRS is examined in relation to prospective data on symptoms and on both psychosocial and defensive functioning.

Research methods for measuring defenses have employed projective tests, self-report instruments, or clinically based rating procedures. Projective test methods have been reviewed elsewhere (Cooper et al. 1988; Perry and Cooper 1987). Self-report measures have the advantage of not requiring an observer's clinical judgment; however, they are restricted to conscious derivatives of defenses, the clinical meaning of which is difficult to specify in the absence of external validation. There are currently two such instruments: the Defense Mechanism Inventory (Gleser and Ihilevich 1969; Ihilevich and Gleser 1986) and the Bond Defense Style Questionnaire (Bond et al. 1983). Most research on defenses has applied definitions of defenses to a specified clinical data base, generally interview data. The applicability of these methods to both clinical work and research, along with

This chapter was originally published as "An Empirical Study of Defense Mechanisms, I: Clinical Interviews and Life Vignette Ratings" in *Archives of General Psychiatry* 46:444–452, 1989. Reprinted with permission of the American Medical Association. Copyright 1989, AMA.

their clinical findings, is reviewed elsewhere (see Perry and Cooper 1987; Chapter 5, this volume).

We designed the DMRS with the following features in mind:

1. Definitions of the defenses should include a description of how each defense functions and how to discriminate it from related defenses.
2. Each definition should have an accompanying rating scale anchored with concrete examples to facilitate reliable scoring.
3. The scales should measure defensive functioning directly with minimal use of inference and should not rely solely on self-report derivatives of defenses.
4. The scales should be applicable to data from clinical interviews or ongoing psychotherapy as well as life vignette data.

These points should ensure that the scales in fact measure the same phenomena that concern clinicians, rather than some derivative.

Subjects

The subjects for the present study were drawn from an ongoing naturalistic study of borderline personality disorder (BPD) in comparison with two relatively established diagnoses: antisocial personality disorder and bipolar type II affective disorder. The sample and diagnostic methods have been described elsewhere (Perry 1985; Perry and Cooper 1985). The sample of adults aged 18–39 was originally recruited in 1980–1981 from clinical settings at the Cambridge Hospital (49%), advertisements in a local newspaper (45%), and the local probation department (7%). Severity of psychopathology did not differ across source of recruitment on the major diagnostic variables.

Definite BPD was diagnosed if the subject met DSM-III criteria and scored above 150 on the Borderline Personality Scale, Second Version (BPS-II), an earlier version of the Borderline Personality Disorder Scale (Perry and Cooper 1985). Borderline traits were diagnosed if the subject met four DSM-III criteria and scored above 130 on the BPS-II, but did not meet all criteria for BPD.

Antisocial personality disorder was diagnosed according to DSM-III, whereas bipolar type II was diagnosed according to the Research Diagnostic Criteria (Spitzer et al. 1978). Subjects with neurotic character problems who did not meet criteria for personality disorders were drawn from a clinic setting for inclusion in the reliability study only. All other assessments were made blind to initial diagnostic assessment.

Methods

Instrument Construction

The DMRS consist of 30 defense mechanisms representing four defensive levels posited by others: immature[1] (Vaillant 1971), borderline (Kernberg 1967) or image-distorting (Bond et al. 1983), neurotic (Kernberg 1967), and mature (Vaillant 1971). We selected specific defenses relevant to the study of personality pathology, omitting both psychotic and mature-level defenses in the cross-sectional studies presented here. The mature-level defenses were subsequently added after the follow-up data on life vignette data became available.

The manual provides a formal definition of each defense, an explanation of the function of the defense, and a discussion of how to discriminate it from other defenses.[2] Each defense has a three-point rating scale (not present, probably present, definitely present) anchored with examples. The scales are applicable to dynamically oriented interview data such as might be obtained in an initial psychotherapy interview.

One of the defense scales, hypochondriasis, is given in Table 11-1. To help use the scale, hypochondriasis is described as follows:

Definition: Hypochondriasis involves the repetitious use of a complaint or series of complaints in which the subject ostensibly asks for help. However, covert feelings of hostility or resentment toward others are expressed simultaneously by the subject's rejection of the suggestions, advice, or whatever others offer. The complaints may consist of either somatic concerns or life problems. Either type of complaint is followed by a "help-rejecting complainer" response to whatever help is offered.

Function: Hypochondriasis is a defense against the anger the subject experiences whenever he or she feels the need for emotional reliance on others. The anger rises from the conviction that nobody will really satisfy the subject's perceived needs. The subject expresses the anger as an indirect reproach by rejecting help as "not good enough" while continuing to ask for more of it.

---

[1]No assumptions are made about the developmental aspects of defenses that may appear to be implied in categorizing defenses by levels such as immature or mature. These terms are employed because of convention. Whether they have developmental significance is an empirical question.

[2]A glossary containing the definitions of the 30 defenses is available in Appendix 4 and in the DMRS manual obtainable from the authors.

Table 11–1. Scoring method for hypochondriasis characteristics

Score

0: No examples present.

1: Probable use of hypochondriasis. At least one of the following is present:

    a. The subject mentions several complaints but doesn't appear to protest or to act helpless when others fail to attempt to help with the complaints.

    b. The subject mentions the same complaint several times asking what should be done.

    c. When others offer advice or commentary on a particular problem that the subject introduced, the subject tends to say "Yes, but . . . ," that is, he or she seems to find a reason to reject the advice as not useful.

    d. The subject acts as if unconsolable about some problem(s) that doesn't strike one as being so hard to deal with or live with. It isn't obvious why the subject should be inconsolable.

    e. The subject mentions feeling like giving up without offering a clear sense of what is so burdensome.

2: Definite use of hypochondriasis. Examples stand out and tend to be somewhat vexing for the interviewer or observer. At least one of the following is present:

    a. The subject is the classic medical "crock" who gives an "organ recital" of physical complaints, skipping from one symptom to the other, eluding attempts to inquire fully into one complaint and effectively deal with or understand it, while nonetheless complaining about the lack of help.

    b. The subject complains spontaneously about how others (e.g., doctors, therapists, relatives, etc.) don't really care, or haven't actually tried to help, even when there is clear evidence to the contrary based on the subject's own account.

    c. The subject presents a seemingly insoluble dilemma about an important problem in life (e.g., threatened job loss, health, marriage) and systematically rejects all suggestions that others offer to a degree that prevents any progress toward a solution.

    d. The subject mentions problem after problem and describes how helpless he or she is to deal with any of them. It is not evident why the subject should feel so helpless.

Instead of driving the other person away by the expresssion of the anger, the use of hypochondriasis binds the person to the subject by the overt request for help. The subject's expression of helplessness over the problem at hand reflects the subject's sense that he or she is powerless to get the comfort and attention desired while discharging his or her resentment for the expected disappointment that help will not be forthcoming.

Differentiation: With passive aggression, the subject's needs (e.g., dependency) are unclear, and there is usually no direct request that the subject makes of the other. Rather, there is the indirect expression of hostility toward the other for real or imagined demands on the subject, or for failure to meet some need of the subject. Passive aggression does not bind the other person to the subject, because it invites retaliation. In fact, it is usually not used except when there is some preexisting relationship that already binds the subject and object, such as an authority hierarchy or work relationship in which neither party can escape one another easily. In contrast, with hypochondriasis both an overt or implied request and a veiled reproach occur.

Dissociation and hypochondriasis frequently present together when the complaint refers to a functional symptom such as headaches or vague aches and pains. Dissociation represents the affect or impulse that is diverted from consciousness and displaced into a physical complaint. Hypochondriasis, then, is present if and only if the subject is also requesting help for a physical symptom and yet rejecting attempts to help. When the person is unconcerned with the symptom and does not hinder the object from helping, then dissociation is in use without hypochondriasis.

In undoing, the subject is not requesting help. It is undoing, not hypochondriasis, when a subject responds to an interviewer by stating the opposite of the interviewer's comment or by qualifying his or her own previous statement. It becomes hypochondriasis only when the interviewer's comment was a clear attempt to offer help on a particular problem.

Hypochondriasis differs from devaluation in that the subject is very bound to the helpgiver. In devaluation, the subject makes negative comments in a way to dismiss someone's importance, power, prestige, and so on, not to bind himself or herself further to getting help from that person. Devaluation serves to dismiss the object before the subject experiences disappointment of his or her wishes for something from the object.

To facilitate data analysis, we combined conceptually related defenses that intercorrelated into five summary defense scales. Each summary defense scale is defined by the shared features of the constituent defenses; their descriptive titles differ from the above-mentioned "levels" of defenses.

Action defenses. Acting out, passive aggression, and hypochondriasis were combined because each defense releases feelings and impulses through action, often toward others.

Borderline defenses. Splitting of self and others' images, and projective identification were combined because they distort self and object images to conform with a particular meaning or emotional state. The distinction between borderline and narcissistic defenses was supported by previous factor analysis (Perry and Cooper 1986).

Disavowal defenses.   Projection, neurotic (minor) denial, bland denial, and rationalization were combined because they all disavow experiences, affects, or impulses.

Narcissistic defenses.   Omnipotence, primitive idealization, and devaluation were combined because each serves to regulate self-esteem and mood. Based on a factor analysis of the eight borderline level defenses as defined by Kernberg (1967), which we have reported elsewhere (Perry and Cooper 1986), we added mood-incongruent denial (manic or depressive denial).

Obsessional defenses.   Isolation, intellectualization, and undoing, which neutralize affects without distorting external reality, were combined.

The low intercorrelation of repression and other conceptually related neurotic defenses in this data set did not support construction of a hysterical summary defense scale. When the follow-up life vignette data became available, we constructed a sixth summary defense scale consisting of all eight mature-level defenses (Table 11-2).

Cross-Sectional Procedures

Each subject received a psychodynamically oriented interview that was videotaped, usually within 6 weeks of joining the study. The interviews were not a part of any psychotherapy, which some subjects were undergoing. Interviewing clinicians were dynamically oriented and blind to any information about the subjects. The videotaped interviews served as the data base from which ratings were made.

The reliability of rating the DMRS from the videotaped interviews was assessed in two phases. The first phase consisted of subjects ($n = 22$) with personality disorders or bipolar type II affective disorder, while the second phase ($n = 24$) contained equal proportions of subjects with personality disorders, bipolar type II affective disorder, and neurotic character problems.

Six research assistants served as raters, half of whom were in graduate school; only one had had no previous clinical experience. Raters were divided into two groups of three each. After observing a videotape, the individuals independently rated the subject on 22 defenses. (Mature-level

Table 11–2. Intraclass reliabilities of defenses assessed by videotaped interview and life vignette

Individual defenses	Videotaped interview inter-rater consensus (raters = 6)	(groups = 2)	Life vignette inter-rater consensus (raters = 2)
Immature			
Neurotic (minor) denial	.42	.57	.71
Nondelusional projection	.34	.42	.61
Hypochondriasis	.53	.68	.40[a]
Passive aggression	.34	.52	.18
Acting out	.59	.60	.88
Schizoid fantasy	.55	.79	.77
Image-distorting (borderline and narcissistic)			
Splitting—self	.34	.67	—[a]
Splitting—others	.44	.62	.80
Mood-incongruent denial	.21	.62	—[a]
Bland denial	.38	.54	—[a]
Projective identification	.44	.51	.03[a]
Primitive idealization	.43	.75	.46
Omnipotence	.56	.70	.12[a]
Devaluation	.37	.61	.59[a]
Neurotic			
Repression	.43	.70	.23
Dissociation	.31	.40	.41
Displacement	.33	.47	.35
Reaction formation	.27	.53	.19
Isolation	.26	.54	.40
Intellectualization	.26	.35	.68
Rationalization	.11	.41	.56
Undoing	.31	.56	.02[a]
Mature			
Affiliation			.57
Anticipatory problem solving			.24
Suppression			.73
Self-observation			.56
Self-assertion			.40
Humor			.99[a]
Altruism			.98[a]
Sublimation			.49
Summary defense scales			
Action	.65	.74	.67
Borderline	.54	.76	.80
Disavowal	.43	.70	.72
Narcissistic	.53	.78	.72
Obsessional	.39	.57	.65
Mature	—	—	.65
Overall maturity of defenses	—	—	**.61**

Note . For videotaped interviews, *n* = 46; for life vignette method, *n* = 130 life vignettes from 34 subjects. — indicates no variance.
[a]Defense rated as present in only 5% or less of reliability sample.

defenses were not included in this procedure.) Each group then discussed each defense and settled on a consensus rating. For the reliability subsamples (combined $n = 46$) there were six individual ratings and two group consensus ratings, whereas the remaining 38 subjects were rated by one group only. Altogether, initial defense ratings were available on 76 subjects with personality disorders or bipolar type II affective disorder, and on 8 subjects with neurotic character problems.

Follow-up Procedures

Phase 1.   After the videotaped interview, the subjects with BPD and antisocial personality disorder or bipolar type II affective disorder entered a follow-up phase lasting 1–2 years, during which they were interviewed every 3–6 months (median 20.5 weeks) by research assistants. At each interview, four types of observer-rated symptom measures were obtained. These included the Hamilton Rating Scales for Depression (Hamilton 1960) and Anxiety (Hamilton 1959) and the Modified Manic Rating Scale (Blackburn et al. 1977), each rated for the past week; and the Alcohol, Drug Abuse and Antisocial Symptom scales from the Psychiatric Status Schedule (Spitzer et al. 1970), obtained for the previous month. The self-report Profile of Mood States (POMS) (McNair et al. 1971) was also administered at each follow-up. The general level of symptoms for each subject over the entire first-phase follow-up period was summarized by the median score on each scale.

Phase 2.   Beginning in the second or third year of follow-up, a new interview format was introduced. Each subject was assessed in seven areas of psychosocial functioning on 5-point scales on a month-by-month basis. Based on a previous factor analysis, these seven roles were collapsed into two dimensions for presentation. Factor 1 included occupation, relatives, and general satisfaction, and factor 2 consisted of spouse/lover, friends, general socializing, and recreation. Global functioning was rated using the Global Assessment Scale (GAS) (Endicott et al. 1976) (intraclass coefficient of reliability $I_R = .82$) on a month-by-month basis. Each subject's mean score over the Phase 2 follow-up period was used in data analyses.

   The Phase 2 follow-up interview also contained a systematic inquiry about significant life events that had occurred over each subject's follow-up. Research assistants used a semistructured interview format, adapted from Brown and Harris (1978), to obtain descriptive information about each event, the subject's role in bringing it about, resources for dealing with the event, and the subject's emotional response and efforts to cope with the event. This information about the life event is collectively known as a *life vignette.* The life vignettes from each Phase 2 follow-up interview served as the data base for rating subjects' prospective use of defenses, including mature-level defenses.

Defense ratings were made as follows. A pair of clinician raters read the life vignettes obtained from a single follow-up interview and independently rated the use of anywhere from zero to five defenses per vignette. The same DMRS manual was used, including the eight mature defenses. Only absence or presence of a particular defense was scored. In addition to the 30 defenses, an additional overall rating of splitting was made for each subject's follow-up, after considering the self and object representations across all the vignettes within the follow-up. After discussion, raters made consensus ratings for the defenses employed in each vignette. Only consensus ratings were used in data analyses.

The subject's score for each defense was calculated as the proportion of defensive responses attributible to each defense (0 to 100%) within each life vignette. Defense scores for the follow-up were then obtained by taking the mean of the individual scores for all of the life vignettes within the follow-up. An overall maturity-of-defenses scale was calculated by weighting each instance of a defense from least to most adaptive as follows: 1, action; 2, borderline; 3, disavowal or fantasy; 4, narcissistic; 5, other neurotic; 6, obsessional; 7, mature. The maturity score was calculated as the average maturity weight for all the defenses rated for the follow-up. When multiple follow-ups were available on a given subject, the mean score across the follow-ups was used for each defense and for overall maturity of defenses.

Ninety-one subjects entered the study, 76 of whom were videotaped and rated on the first 22 defenses. These 76 subjects included the following diagnostic groups: definite BPD (n = 22, 86% female); concurrent BPD (definite or traits) and antisocial personality disorder (n = 12, 50% female); borderline traits only (n = 13, 38% female); antisocial personality disorder (n = 12, 50% female); and bipolar type II affective disorder (n = 17, 47% female). The mean age was 28 (range = 18 to 38) and did not differ significantly by diagnostic group.

Of the above subjects, 67 had at least two administrations of the symptom scales (range = 2–7) during follow-up in Phase 1 (during the first 2 years of the study), and 53 had a 1 year of follow-up interviews in Phase 2.

Data Analysis

Inter-rater reliability was assessed by the intraclass correlation coefficient calculated by the method of Shrout and Fleiss (1979). Reliability coefficients are presented in the results section for both individual (r = 6) and group consensus ($r = 2$). The reliability for each defense was first calculated separately for subsamples 1 and 2. Because the results were similar, the subsamples were combined. The reliability coefficients presented are from the combined ($n = 46$) group. Reliability was calculated for the 27 defenses actually rated from the follow-up life vignettes using individual raters only ($r = 2$) rating 130 follow-ups with an average of three life vignettes per follow-up. Subsequent data analyses used the two raters' consensus ratings, although consensus reliability was not obtained.

Because the intraclass correlation is unstable under the condition of very high or low base rates of the phenomenon being measured (Grove et al. 1981), it is noted when the scores for each defense have a distribution with less than 5% in any category. In the life vignette rating procedure, some defenses were never rated, and reliability was therefore not calculated, although there was 100% agreement on their absence. Reliability figures were separately calculated for the five summary defense scales.

Each follow-up variable from Phases 1 and 2 was summarized by calculating each subject's mean value. Because many variables were not normally distributed, Spearman correlations were used to measure associations between defenses and these variables.

Results

Reliability

The reliability of the defense ratings for both the videotaped interview and the life vignette methods is presented in Table 11-2. For the individual nonprofessional raters, the median I_R was .36, with a range from .11 to .59. The reliability of the group consensus ratings was generally higher (median I_R = .57, range = .35 to .79). Seventeen (77%) of these coefficients were above .50.

The inter-rater reliabilities for the life vignette scoring method were available only for professional raters. The median I_R was calculable for 27 defenses yielding a median of .46. If defenses with a low base rate (rated in less than 5% of the subjects) are excluded, the median I_R was .53 (range = .19 to .87) among the remaining 20 defenses.

The reliabilities of the summary defense scales also are given in Table 11-2. For the videotaped interview method, the median I_R was .53 (range = .39 to .65). However, for the consensus ratings the median I_R value was .74 (range = .57 to .78). For the life vignette method, the interpolated median I_R for the summary defense scales was .69 (range = .65 to .80). Reliability of the consensus ratings was not obtained.

Phase 1 Follow-up: Prospective Symptoms

The correlations between defensive functioning at intake and median symptom scale scores measured prospectively across all interviews over Phase 1 follow-up are presented in Table 11-3.

The Action Defense Summary Scale correlated significantly with general levels of symptoms for all scales except one. The correlations of greatest magnitude were with observer-rated affective symptom scales, followed by the POMS scales for anger-hostility, fatigue-inertia, and depression-dejection. The action defenses also correlated higher than other defense summary scales with drug abuse and equally high with the disavowal defenses for alcohol abuse and antisocial symptoms.

Table 11–3. Spearman correlations between defense scores (videotaped interview method) and median symptom scale scores over Phase 1 follow-up (*n = 67*)

	Summary defense scale[a]				
	Action	**Borderline**	**Disavowal**	**Narcissistic**	**Obsessional**
Observer rated					
HRS depression	.51	.29	.25	.07	−.32
HRS anxiety	.44	.26	.26	.11	−.39
Modified manic RS	.48	.25	.54	.18	−.17
PSS drug	.33	.16	.17	.18	.10
PSS alcohol	.29	−.03	.32	.14	−.03
PSS antisocial	.30	.06	.33	.25	.07
Self-report POMS					
Tension-anxiety	.26	.35	.06	−.04	−.29
Depression-dejection	.35	.40	.03	−.01	−.39
Anger-hostility	.38	.39	.26	.09	−.31
Vigor-activity	−.27	−.17	−.07	−.11	.19
Fatigue-inertia	.37	.33	.23	.10	−.41
Confusion-bewilderment	.23	.25	.02	−.02	−.25
Total POMS score	**.37**	**.41**	**.11**	**.02**	**−.41**

Note. HRS = Hamilton Rating Scale, for depression (Hamilton 1960), and for anxiety (Hamilton 1959); RS = Rating Scale; PSS = Psychiatric Status Schedule (Spitzer et al. 1970); POMS = Profile of Mood States (McNair et al. 1971).
[a]$r > .24$ ($P < .05$); $r > .31$ ($P < .01$); $r > .38$ ($P < .001$); $r > .45$ ($P < .0001$).

The Borderline Defense Summary Scale was associated with observer-rated depressive, anxiety, and manic symptoms, but not substance abuse or antisocial behaviors. However, the Borderline Defense Summary Scale correlated significantly with six of the POMS scales, especially the total score, and the scales for depression-dejection and anger-hostility.

The Disavowal Summary Defense Scale was associated with five of the six observer-rated scales, especially manic symptoms, alcohol abuse, and antisocial behaviors, and, to a lesser extent, with Hamilton Rating Scale anxiety and depressive symptoms. However, there was only one significant correlation with the self-report POMS scales, the anger-hostility scale, suggesting a lack of subjective awareness of symptoms.

The Narcissistic Defense Summary Scale was associated with antisocial behaviors only.

Finally, the Obsessional Defense Summary Scale demonstrated negative associations with observer-rated anxiety and depressive symptoms. In line with the minimization of affects that these defenses accomplish, the correlations with six of the self-report POMS scales were significant and negative in direction. Unlike the other defense summary scales, the obsessional scale correlated with fewer observed or reported symptoms.

Phase 2 Follow-up: Prospective Psychosocial Role Impairment

The relationship between the individual defenses at intake and GAS (both at intake and over follow-up) and psychosocial role impairment assessed during Phase 2 of the follow-up period is shown in Table 11-4. A negative correlation with subjects' median GAS score reflects an association with poorer global functioning, whereas a positive correlation with psychosocial role factors reflects an association with poorer functioning on that variable.

All of the immature defenses except fantasy had negative correlations with global functioning at intake and over Phase 2 follow-up. Except for neurotic (minor) denial, the immature defenses correlated significantly with poorer psychosocial role functioning. This correlation was generally more significant for factor 1 roles (occupation, relatives, satisfaction) than for factor 2 roles (spouse/lover, friends, socializing, recreation). The converse was true for fantasy, in which poorer functioning in relationships was observed. Three defenses stand out as most consistently and significantly associated with poorer functioning and impairment: hypochondriasis, passive aggression, and acting out. Among the image-distorting defenses, the borderline defenses correlated with poorer global functioning. Of these, splitting of self-images and others' images correlated with poorer functioning on factor 1 social roles, with nonsignificant trends evident on factor 2

Table 11–4. Spearman correlations between individual defenses and Global Assessment Scale and psychosocial role functioning over 1 year of follow-up

	GAS		Mean score over 1 year	
	Intake	Follow-up mean	Factor 1[a]	Factor 2[b]
	(*n* = 76)	(*n* = 53)		
Individual defenses				
Immature				
Neurotic denial	−.27*	−.04	.08	−.10
Projection	−.24*	−.21	.29*	.24
Hypochondriasis	−.21	−.37**	.33*	.18
Passive aggression	−.18	−.29*	.31*	.14
Acting out	−.37***	−.42**	.34**	.18
Fantasy	−.01	.00	.10	.30*
Image-distorting				
Splitting—self	−.31**	−.36**	.39**	.13
Splitting—other	−.42***	−.34**	.38**	.14
Projective identification	−.02	−.11	.21	.27*
Bland denial	−.15	−.03	.08	.01
Manic denial	−.13	−.09	.17	.04
Primitive idealization	.01	−.10	.11	−.09
Omnipotence	−.09	−.19	.17	.15
Devaluation	−.24	−.18	.21	.26
Neurotic				
Repression	.09	.05	−.04	.05
Dissociation	−.15	−.12	.21	.22
Displacement	−.15	−.18	.24	.18
Reaction formation	.15	−.04	.06	−.18
Isolation	.17	.10	−.21	−.07
Intellectualization	.22	.21	−.21	−.32*
Rationalization	.13	−.04	.17	.00
Undoing	.08	.11	−.06	−.11
Summary defense scales				
Action	−.38***	−.49***	.41**	.29*
Borderline	−.30*	−.34**	.40**	.22
Disavowal	−.19	−.12	.27*	.06
Narcissistic	−.14	−.22	.23	.13
Obsessional	.21	.20	−.24	−.25
Overall defense maturity scale	**.38***	**.37**	**−.39**	**−.28***

Note.   GAS = Global Assessment Scale (Endicott et al. 1976).
*P < .05. **P < .01. ***P < .001.
[a]Factor 1 involves occupation, relatives, and satisfaction.
[b]Factor 2 involves spouse/lover, friends, socializing, and recreation.

roles as well. Projective identification demonstrated a reverse pattern, show-ing significantly poor functioning on factor 2 (relationships). Among the four narcissistic defenses, the only finding was that devaluation correlated negatively with GAS at intake and correlated positively with poor factor 2 social roles during Phase 2 follow-up.

The neurotic level defenses generally demonstrated no significant correlations with GAS at intake or follow-up, or with either psychosocial role factor. There were, however, two exceptions. Displacement correlated (trend) with poor functioning on factor 1 social roles. Intellectualization correlated with higher GAS at intake (trend) and with better functioning on factor 2 social roles during Phase 2 follow-up.

The relationships between the five summary defense scales and the same outcome variables also are shown in Table 11-4. The strongest relationships with poor global functioning and poor psychosocial role functioning were demonstrated by action and borderline defenses for all variables. The dis-avowal defenses showed a similar pattern of correlations, but with fewer sig-nificant findings. The narcissistic defenses also displayed a pattern that was consistently toward poorer functioning, although only factor 1 role func-tioning reached a statistical trend. The obsessional defenses correlated with higher GAS and better social role functioning, though only at trend levels.

Defensive Functioning on Follow-up

The proportion of defenses used in dealing with life events over the follow-up was calculated for each summary defense scale and expressed as percent-ages of total defensive functioning: action, 11.4%; borderline, 6.4%; dis-avowal, 38.3%; narcissistic, 11.7%; obsessional, 5.4%; mature, 22.6%. The defenses not included in the summary scales (e.g., fantasy, reaction forma-tion) filled out the remaining percentages of defensive functioning. The mean ($\pm$ SD) overall maturity-of-defenses score for the sample was $4.1 \pm .92$ (range = 2.2 to 6.3), putting the mean functioning at the level of the narcissistic defenses.

We examined the stability of the defense summary scales across meth-ods and across time (video interview at intake vs. life vignettes 3 years later) (see Table 11-5). In descending order of magnitude, the borderline and ac-tion summary defense scales at intake were significantly correlated with their respective scales on follow-up, whereas nonsignificant trends were evident for the obsessional, disavowal, and narcissistic scales. These correlations represent the stability of the summary defense scales across methods and time (approximately 3 years later). Considering these stability estimates as a group, they have a mean of $.26 \pm .12$, so no estimate is less than a standard deviation from the group mean.

Table 11–5. Spearman correlation matrix of summary defense scales: videotaped interview method (at intake) by life vignette method (2–3 years later) (*n* = 53)

Life vignette method	Videotaped interview method				
	Action	Borderline	Disavowal	Narcissistic	Obsessional
Action	.32*	.06	.25	.15	−.30*
Borderline	.01	.45***	.19	.14	−.17
Disavowal	.09	−.11	.17	.03	.26
Narcissistic	.12	.06	.29*	.17	.06
Obsessional	−.21	−.24	.08	.10	.20
Mature	−.34**	−.07	−.26	−.12	.14
Overall defense maturity scale	**−.42****	**−.14**	**−.37****	**−.14**	**.26**

*P < .05. **P < .01. ***P < .001.

The defenses as measured at intake generally correlated with the defenses rated from the life vignettes in the predicted directions. Action defenses (video) correlated most positively with action and most negatively with obsessional and mature defenses on follow-up. Borderline defenses (video) correlated most positively with borderline defenses and most negatively with obsessional defenses on follow-up. (The negligible correlation with mature defenses is discussed below.) Disavowal defenses (video) correlated most positively with action and narcissistic defenses and most negatively with mature defenses on follow-up. Narcissistic defenses (video) had only nonsignificant correlations with other defenses, although the correlation with mature defenses was negative, as anticipated. Obsessional defenses (video) correlated most positively with disavowal, narcissistic, and obsessional defenses and most negatively with action defenses.

Finally, the overall maturity-of-defenses score was calculated for all of the follow-up defense ratings. As predicted, four defense summary scales rated at intake (video) correlated negatively with the overall maturity-of-defenses scale assessed by the life vignette method, whereas obsessional defenses correlated positively.

Discussion

We have examined the reliability and some aspects of the validity of defense mechanisms assessed by our DMRS on two sources of data. The reliability of the individual defenses rated from the videotaped interviews is higher when rated by group consensus than when rated by individual raters alone. This finding undoubtedly reflects the difficulty of scanning a whole interview for evidence of a large number of defenses, each of which is an open, textured concept. The process of comparing different observations, discussing the evidence, and referring to the manual to answer disputes yields reliability coefficients that are nearly 60% higher on average than those from individual raters alone. This might have been less often true if transcripts of the videotaped interviews were available to individual raters, but the cost of the process would have increased considerably. The individual defenses have comparable reliability when rated from life vignette data, although professional raters were used and only individual inter-rater reliabilities were assessed. Our findings compare favorably to the reliability of blind raters reported by Vaillant (1976) using preselected life vignettes (median Pearson's $r = .59$, range $= -.01$ to .95). Nevertheless, we recommend that consensus ratings be used whenever possible to ensure higher reliabilities.

When conceptually and empirically related defenses were aggregated into summary scales, reliabilities increased across the board. Median I_R values were 47% higher for the inter-rater video method (.53 vs. .36), 30% higher for the group consensus video method (.74 vs. .57), and 50% higher for the inter-rater life vignette method (.69 vs. .46). Given higher reliabilities, the summary scales detected more associations with the follow-up data.

This study did not attempt to determine whether nonprofessional raters are as reliable as professional raters. We originally chose nonprofessional raters because they were less costly and less likely to have had previous training about defenses that would interfere with learning and with following the DMRS manual. We did conduct a preliminary trial (not reported here) using four professional raters and found both reasons borne out. Researchers and educators should note that learning to assess defenses reliably is easier in the absence of previous idiosyncratic learning.

The present sample is restricted to individuals who were predominantly personality disordered, highly symptomatic, and psychosocially impaired. We previously reported that the major study diagnostic groups did not differ in their general levels of global functioning during Phase 2 follow-up, as measured by the GAS. Because too few subjects were symptomatically well and high functioning, optimal explorations of the comparative effects of the neurotic and mature defenses were not obtained. This may mean that some positive adaptive aspects of these defenses might have been overwhelmed by the more prevalent but less adaptive defenses. Conversely, however, the sample was excellent for exploring the relationship between defenses and symptoms and impairment.

It is hard to disentangle causal relationships in naturalistic follow-up studies. In a follow-up of 307 men from the Gluecks' study, Vaillant et al. (1986) attempted to tease out the effect of maturity of defenses in adulthood on other indexes of positive functioning. They found that the correlations between defense maturity and psychological health were highest among the subjects who had the bleakest childhood backgrounds. The authors thus suggested that mature defenses exert some causal role in healthy functioning and are not simply epiphenomena of healthy functioning. When the authors controlled for social class of origin, upward social mobility correlated with use of more mature defenses (Snarey and Vaillant 1985). The most impaired individuals used the highest proportion of projection, fantasy, hypochondriasis, passive aggression, and dissociation (this includes neurotic denial under our definition). Furthermore, these defenses plus acting out correlated most highly with the presence of a personality disorder (Vaillant and Drake 1985).

We found that the immature- and image-distorting–level defenses were associated overall with higher general levels of symptoms, and impairment in psychosocial functioning. In addition, they correlated with the use of the same defenses over the Phase 2 follow-up period. We do not believe that a simple causal model will explain these relationships (e.g., defenses at time 1 are necessary and sufficient for symptoms, psychosocial impairment, and defensive functioning at time 2). Instead, a more complicated model will be needed that examines stressful life events, social supports, defensive functioning, symptoms, and Axis I episodes, as well as psychosocial functioning. In addition, it is important to elucidate whether diagnosis predisposes to particular responses.

The DMRS were designed to assess defenses used in clinically significant ways. When these scales are applied to a single videotaped psychodynamic interview, it is difficult to separate out state-vs.-trait aspects of defenses. However, as a rule, the DMRS require multiple examples of subject responses to qualify a defense as definitely present. Taken together with the longitudinal findings, there is reason to conclude that to a large degree the DMRS measure characteristic defenses—that is, defenses as traits.

What Defenses Foretell

One should keep the makeup of the sample in mind when interpreting the meaning of the associations between defenses assessed in cross-section and the longitudinal data. Each of the action defenses hypochondriasis, passive aggression, and acting out allows the individual to direct impulses, feelings, and actions toward others, as if others were the source of all problems and remedies. Awareness of internal conflict over wishes and feelings is largely bypassed. However, this does not protect against symptoms, as evidenced by the moderately high correlations between the Action Defense Summary Scale score and the observer-rated and—to a slightly lesser extent—the self-reported symptom scales. By this standard, individuals who use these defenses count themselves as suffering greatly. Rather than help the individual in solving his or her internal and external problems, these defenses ensnarl others in ways that often turn potential allies into adversaries. The effects of this are evident in the correlations with increased levels of impairment in most psychosocial roles. Individuals rated on these defenses from the videotape also used them in coping with life events over the follow-up.

The defense of hypochondriasis demonstrated some of the strongest relationships to symptoms and psychosocial impairment. It is important to clarify that this defense was not rated simply on the basis of the individual reporting symptoms. Rather, as the defense of the "help-rejecting complainer," it was rated present when this particular type of exchange occurred between subject and interviewer. In the videotaped interviews most of these exchanges centered on dilemmas around solving life problems rather than on reporting physical or emotional symptoms. Thus the "active ingredient" in hypochondriasis is a way of engaging others to help with problems while simultaneously rejecting what is offered. This conclusion is supported by the consistency that hypochondriasis and the other action defenses showed in their associations with the longitudinal data.

The borderline defenses of splitting of self and others' images and projective identification protect one from the awareness of conflict about the good and bad aspects of oneself and others. Confusing or contradictory aspects of oneself or others are temporarily simplified because all aspects are distorted to fit a particular emotional meaning. However, these defenses do not protect their user from the distress associated with ambivalent or contradictory feelings. Borderline defenses were moderately associated with anxiety and affective symptoms as rated prospectively by the interviewer. They demonstrated the highest association of all summary defense scales with self-reported depression, anger, and anxiety. This finding suggests that given objectively high levels of affective symptoms, borderline defenses were associated with increased levels of subjective distress compared with other defenses. Borderline defenses also were associated with lower global functioning at both intake and on follow-up and with greater impairment over follow-up with relatives, general socializing, and satisfaction.

The borderline defenses demonstrated moderate stability from the initial videotaped interview to the life vignettes on follow-up. Methodologically, we noted that the best way to capture splitting was not by rating it within a given life vignette, but by contrasting the description of self and others across vignettes. Splitting was rated infrequently within individual vignettes but was rated with high reliability and moderate frequency across the vignettes within a given follow-up. It may be that splitting would be rated more frequently within vignettes if we used audio recordings rather than summaries of the life vignette interviews.

The disavowal defenses of denial, projection, bland denial, and rationalization allow the individual to deny or disavow something about himself or herself. However, as vividly demonstrated in Table 11-4, these defenses are more effective at hiding things from the person who uses them than from an observer. The disavowal defenses correlated signficantly with symptoms rated by the interviewer (manic, antisocial, alcohol use, anxiety, and depression), but not with self-report measures of some of the same symptoms. This demonstrates that disavowal defenses protect the individual from *awareness* of how symptomatic he or she really is, without dispelling the symptoms. The disavowal defenses also were associated with lower global functioning at intake and greater impairment in functioning with occupation and relatives and in general satisfaction. These defenses demonstrated a nonsignificant trend toward stability over time in coping with life events. Overall, although minimizing awareness of one's emotional problems, these defenses do not vanquish negative consequences.

The narcissistic defenses of omnipotence, primitive idealization, devaluation, and mood-incongruent denial (manic-depressive denial) primarily help the individual with difficulty in regulating self-esteem by focusing on overvalued or undervalued aspects of experience, oneself, and others. These defenses were associated with increased prospective report of antisocial, but not other, symptoms. We previously reported a positive association between these defenses and the diagnosis of antisocial personality disorder (Perry and Cooper 1986). Vaillant and Drake (1985) also noted that narcissistic and antisocial personality disorders shared similar immature defenses (acting out, dissociation, projection, and passive aggression). Together, these data suggest that narcissistic and antisocial personality disorders may share some common problems in self-esteem regulation.

Overall, the narcissistic defenses were only weakly associated with impairment in factor 1 psychosocial functioning. However, devaluation, which occurred frequently in the sample, demonstrated trend associations with lower global functioning (as measured by the GAS) at intake and with greater impairment with factor 2 social roles: spouse/lover, friends, general socializing, and recreation.

As a group, the neurotic defenses demonstrated few associations with symptoms or psychosocial impairment. This finding corroborates Vaillant's observation in his male college sample that neurotic defenses did not correlate with psychological adjustment on follow-up (Vaillant 1976). Neurotic defenses are found in individuals at all levels of psychological functioning and therefore do not individually demonstrate strong relationships to symptoms or psychosocial functioning.

There is one exception to this. In our sample, the obsessional defenses, especially intellectualization, had positive associations to global functioning at intake, negative associations with observer-rated and self-report symptoms on follow-up, and less impairment on factor 1 and 2 social roles. Isolation, intellectualization, and undoing serve to distance their user from feelings but leave awareness of events and ideas intact. In a sample of personality and affective disorders, this defense has some virtues. Battista (1982) also found an association between intellectualization and higher global functioning ($r = .29$) in a sample of psychiatric outpatients. However, in samples that extend into a healthier range of functioning, such as Vaillant's (1976) college sample, this association does not appear to be true, as the mature defenses overshadow the adaptive value of obsessional ones. Though in their follow-up of a largely lower socioeconomic class sample of inner city men, Vaillant et al. (1986) found no association between intellectualization and global functioning ($r = .06$); of all the defenses, intellectualization was most highly associated with upward social mobility, with mature defenses following (Snarey and Vaillant 1985). Thus, in some samples the obsessional defenses demonstrate some adaptiveness not shared by other neurotic defenses.

Our assessment of obsessional defenses by videotaped interview correlated positively, but short of statistical significance, with obsessional defenses on follow-up. In addition, obsessional defenses at intake correlated negatively with life vignette ratings of action and borderline defenses.

We cannot in this report disentangle the reasons for the lack of stronger correlations between the intake and life vignette methods for rating disavowal, narcissistic, and obsessional defenses. Whereas the intake method was qualitative, the follow-up method was quantitative, and the median time interval between the assessments was 2.5 years. It will take comparison of successive years of follow-up data to determine how much of the unexplained variance in Table 11-5 is due to methods, time elapsed, or error.

Our approach in this report has had the least to say about the mature defenses because they were not initially included when the videotaped interviews were rated. In the life vignette ratings, the individual mature defenses were by and large highly reliable. The Mature Defense Summary Scale has only moderately high reliability, however, which suggests that it measures more than one dimension of mature functioning. Finally, the Mature Defense Summary Scale did correlate negatively with all other defense summary scales, except the scale for obsessional defenses. This finding is consistent with the higher adaptive value that others (Battista 1982; Bond and Vaillant 1986; Bond et al. 1983; Snarey and Vaillant 1985; Vaillant 1976; Vaillant and Drake 1985; Vaillant et al. 1986) have found associated with the mature defenses.

Psychodynamic clinicians have long stressed the role of defense mechanisms in normal and pathological personality functioning. Recent years have brought some advancement in methodology that allows more precise study of the defenses. Although different researchers utilize different definitions, scales, and sources of data, the similarity of findings across different samples suggests that defenses have a robust relationship to adult personality functioning and psychopathology. As measurement issues, such as instrument reliability, stability, and predictive validity, continue to resolve, it is worthwhile to explore the relationship of psychodynamic variables (such as defense mechanisms) to the onset, maintenance, and resolution of psychopathology. Finally, studying the interrelationship of life stress, biology, psychodynamics, social learning, and social supports may yield a more complete, if complicated, understanding of the movement between clinical psychopathology and psychological health.

References

Battista JR: Empirical test of Vaillant's hierarchy of ego functions. Am J Psychiatry 139:356–357, 1982

Blackburn IM, Loudon JB, Ashworth CM: A new scale for measuring mania. Psychol Med 7:453–458, 1977

Bond MP, Vaillant JS: An empirical study of the relationship between diagnosis and defense style. Arch Gen Psychiatry 43:285–288, 1986

Bond MP, Gardner ST, Christian J, et al: Empirical study of self-rated defense styles. Arch Gen Psychiatry 40:333–338, 1983

Brown GW, Harris T: Social Origins of Depression: A Study of Psychiatric Disorder in Women. New York, Free Press, 1978

Cooper SH, Perry JC, Arnow D: An empirical approach to the study of defense mechanisms, I: reliability and preliminary validity of the Rorschach defense scales. J Pers Asses 52:187–203, 1988

Endicott J, Spitzer RL, Fleiss JL: The Global Assessment Scale. Arch Gen Psychiatry 33:766–771, 1976

Gleser GC, Ihilevich D: An objective instrument for measuring defense mechanisms. J Consult Clin Psychol 33:51–60, 1969

Grove W, Andreasen NC, McDonald-Scott P, et al: Reliability studies of psychiatric diagnosis: theory and practice. Arch Gen Psychiatry 38:408–413, 1981

Hamilton M: The rating of clinical anxiety. Br J Med Psychol 32:30–55, 1959

Hamilton M: A rating scale for depression. J Neurol Neurosurg Psychiatry 23:56–62, 1960

Ihilevich D, Gleser GC: Defense Mechanisms: Their Classification, Correlates, and Measurement With the Defense Mechanisms Inventory. Owosso, MI, DMI Associates, 1986

Kernberg O: Borderline personality organization. J Am Psychoanal Assoc 15:641–685, 1967

McNair DM, Lorr M, Droppleman LF: Profile of Mood States. San Diego, CA, Educational and Industrial Testing Service, 1971

Perry JC: Depression in borderline personality disorder: lifetime prevalence at interview and longitudinal course of symptoms. Am J Psychiatry 142:15–21, 1985

Perry JC, Cooper SH: Psychodynamics, symptoms, and outcome in borderline and antisocial personality disorders and bipolar type II affective disorder, in The Borderline: Current Empirical Research. Edited by McGlashan TH. Washington, DC, American Psychiatric Press, 1985, pp 19–41

Perry JC, Cooper SH: Preliminary report on conflicts and defenses associated with borderline personality disorder. J Am Psychoanal Assoc 34:863–893, 1986

Perry JC, Cooper SH: Empirical studies of psychological defenses, in Psychiatry, Vol 1. Edited by Cavenar JO, Michels R. Philadelphia, PA, JB Lippincott, Basic Books, 1987, Chapter 30, pp 1–19

Shrout PE, Fleiss JL: Intraclass correlation: uses in assessing rater reliability. Psychol Bull 86:420–428, 1979

Snarey JR, Vaillant GE: How lower- and working-class youth become middle-class adults: the association between ego defense mechanisms and upward social mobility. Child Dev 56:899–910, 1985

Spitzer RL, Endicott J, Fleiss J: The Psychiatric Status Schedule: a technique of evaluating psychopathology and impairment in role functioning. Arch Gen Psychiatry 23:41–55, 1970

Spitzer RL, Endicott J, Robins E: Research Diagnostic Criteria: rationale and reliability. Arch Gen Psychiatry 35:773–782, 1978

Vaillant GE: Theoretical hierarchy of adaptive ego mechanisms. Arch Gen Psychiatry 24:107–118, 1971

Vaillant G: Natural history of male psychological health: the relation of choice of ego mechanisms of defense to adult adjustment. Arch Gen Psychiatry 33:535–545, 1976

Vaillant GE, Drake RE: Maturity of ego defenses in relation to DSM-III Axis II personality disorder. Arch Gen Psychiatry 42:597–601, 1985

Vaillant GE, Bond M, Vaillant CO: An empirically validated hierarchy of defense mechanisms. Arch Gen Psychiatry 43:786–794, 1986

Chapter 12

A Q-sort Approach to Identifying Defenses

Diane Roston, M.D.
Kimberly A. Lee, A.B.
George E. Vaillant, M.D.

E ver since Freud first proposed the existence of ego defense mechanisms, many researchers have worked to develop a systematic, empirical method for studying these unconscious processes. This search has been called "either a field filled with mines, or with challenges and opportunities" (Hauser 1986). The "land mines" center around three major difficulties: 1) there is as yet no universally accepted set of defense mechanisms; 2) recognition of defenses is generally left to clinical judgment, which may not lend itself to objective study; and 3) there is as yet no consensus regarding the best data source. In this book, sources have included videotaped interviews, written transcripts, autobiographical statements, self-reports, psychological tests, and combinations thereof. The Q-methodology (Mowrer 1953) described in the present chapter offers another tool for systematizing the study of defense mechanisms. In our discussion of this work in progress, we will address several questions:

1. Is the Q-method useful in evaluating ego defenses?
2. How well do primary defense mechanisms and maturity of ego defenses determined by the Q-method correlate with both standard clinical assessment (discussed in Chapter 11) and the Bond Defense Style Questionnaire (DSQ)?
3. How well do Q-sort and clinical assessment of maturity of defense style correlate with measures of general psychological well-being as reflected by the Health-Sickness Rating Scale (HSRS; Luborsky 1962) and the Global Assessment of Functioning (GAF) scale?

Those readers who are unfamiliar with Q-methods may be surprised to learn that this approach was first described by Stephenson over 50 years ago (Stephenson 1935, 1953). The literature using Q-methodology now numbers over 1,500 bibliographic entries and includes many applications to behavioral and psychological research (McKeown and Thomas 1988). Stephenson originally devised the Q-methodology as a departure from statistical factor analysis that was based on correlations between tests or variables. He performed correlations between persons, rather than between tests, and termed this new approach Q to distinguish it from standard R factor analysis. Although Stephenson originally devised the Q-methodology to provide data suitable for these studies in Q (or "inverse" factor analysis), the technique is not bound by one particular statistical orientation. The prefix letter "Q" has remained from its original historical roots and otherwise has no special significance (Block 1978).

The Q-method is based on a system of rank ordering a set of statements that describe aspects of the domain of study. This set of descriptive statements or words is carefully constructed to represent aspects of the area to be investigated. For example, to assess ego defenses, the Q-statements used in this study include "Gets pleasure out of giving to and caring for others" (representing altruism) and "Forgets aspects of trying circumstances" (representing repression). Each Q-statement is printed on a separate index card so that the deck may be easily arranged and rearranged. The statements are then sorted according to a given criterion, such as, in this study, nine categories ranging from "most characteristic" to "least characteristic." The number of cards placed in each category is predetermined. This "forced choice" aspect of the Q-sort methodology provides a quasi-normal distribution curve and indicates that an identical set of criteria is applied to each individual. In some cases, the person who rank orders the Q-statements (the "Q-sorter") is the subject himself or herself, but more often the Q-sorter is an outside evaluator. (See Block 1978 for a discussion of the rationale and validity of these technical restraints and other methodological issues.)

Three aspects of Q-methodology deserve particular attention. These aspects serve to differentiate this research method from both subjective clinical assessment and many empirical study designs. First, the Q-method is a person-centered, or *ipsative*, method that compares an individual to himself or herself. This is in contradistinction to normative studies that compare subjects to each other and to sample norms. Thus, like a fingerprint, a Q-sort preserves the unique and subtle qualities of each individual. When one wants to understand as complex an intrapsychic system as defenses, this is a distinct advantage. An added benefit is that because sample norms do not enter into the scoring, data from individuals in different samples, as well as data from within the same sample, can be compared.

Second, personality traits or defensive styles cannot be measured in discrete units as can, for example, blood pressure (e.g., in millimeters of mercury) or temperature (e.g., in degrees Fahrenheit). Instead, the Q-sort method highlights the significance, the rank order, and the salience of a variable, rather than its specific value. Because Q-sort data are based on ordinal ranking, they are more accessible to scientific and statistical study than are purely qualitative descriptions. Thus, the Q-methodology can translate nonlinear, clinically gleaned interview data into a precise rank-ordered list that can then be empirically studied. Admittedly, if Q-statements representing the defense mechanism repression are ranked as "most characteristic" for two subjects, the researcher cannot know which individual employs repression more frequently. All that could be said is that repression was felt to be a characteristic defense for both subjects.

A third advantage of the Q-methodology is that a relatively untrained person can perform a Q-sort. Other methods may require that the evaluator have a working knowledge of clinical practice or terminology, such as the definitions of defense mechanisms. But as should be clear from Appendix 7, Q-statements avoid the difficulties of conflicting nomenclatures that were outlined in Chapter 3. Of course, Q-methods are vulnerable to the same advantages and disadvantages as other study designs that employ human raters rather than scientific instruments. Because ego defenses are like metaphors, the Q-method is still susceptible to the subjective biases of the rater. However, the Q-sort is less dependent on the idiosyncratic nature of the evaluator because he or she works with a predetermined set of statements within an externally imposed distribution curve, and inter-rater reliability can be determined with precision.

Norma Haan (1965) was the first investigator to develop a set of Q-statements for assessing ego mechanisms of defense. She selected three statements to represent each of 10 coping and 10 defending ego mechanisms, for a set total of 60 statements (Haan 1977). Evaluators based their ratings on material available in clinical interview transcripts and clinical observation of the subjects of the Institute of Human Development (IHD) at the University of California at Berkeley.

Haan also developed a self-report technique for assessing ego defenses involving the use of scales from the item pools of the Minnesota Multiphasic Personality Inventory (MMPI) and the California Psychological Inventory (CPI) (Haan 1965). Although some studies were encouraging regarding the validity of these scales, neither the Q-sort design nor the test-based self-report was cross-validated in the more than 30 studies that have applied these methods (Morrissey 1977) until Joffe and Naditch (1977) improved the ego process scales by selecting only those items from the MMPI and CPI scales that predicted clinicians' ratings of the Q-sort items.

Methods

Subjects

The TERMAN sample.   Some 672 women, who averaged 11 years of age when Lewis Terman began his study of gifted children, have been followed by means of a written questionnaire every 5 years until age 76 (Terman and Oden 1959; Oden 1968; Sears 1984). From the surviving active participants, 53 women who met the criteria of birth date between 1909 and 1913 and residence within a selected metropolitan area were selected for interview (refer to Chapter 6 for methods). Of these 53 women, 40 consented to an interview that lasted for approximately 2 hours. These 40 women were generally indistinguishable from those who were not included, except for physical health after age 70, since the most common reason for refusal to participate was poor health.

Each interview was conducted by a clinician who was blind to the subject's past record. The interview was built around a series of questions that covered topics ranging from work and social activities to reflections on what makes for successful aging. Also present was a second researcher, who, having reviewed all past data, would ask clarifying questions in the absence of the interviewer and who recorded and dictated the interview.

The transcriptions of these interviews were as a journalist might record them rather than as a tape recorder. Direct quotations were retained, as well as the observer's description of significant facial expressions, movements, and circumstances of the interview. The advantages of this approach include a potential for data reduction and more succinct and accented reporting of conversation, as well as the opportunity to note inconsistencies between what the subject remembers or chooses to discuss, and what actually happened. On the other hand, the method is vulnerable to observer bias.

The CORE CITY sample.   The CORE CITY subjects were a group of 456 schoolboys selected over 40 years ago as a control group for the Gluecks' study of delinquency (Glueck and Glueck 1950). All subjects were white males, and half had not completed high school. A large group of these subjects (n = 376) have been followed by biennial questionnaire since the mid-1970s and were reinterviewed in person between 1974 and 1978, when the men were between the ages of 45 and 50. These interviews covered topics ranging from work, family, and general health to ways the men dealt with problems. The interviewer included in each transcript his or her overall subjective impressions of the individual (see Chapter 6). Prior to this study, clinical assessments of ego defenses had been completed based on these interview transcripts.

A subsample of 30 CORE CITY subjects who represented the full range of maturity of defensive styles were chosen for this investigation of Q-methods. Of the 30 men in this subsample, 18 had previously completed the DSQ (see Chapters 7 and 8).

Measures

Global Assessment of Functioning Scale.   GAF ratings were done on all TERMAN subjects by an independent rater prior to the start of this study. This scale, which is part of a comprehensive psychological assessment according to the DSM-III-R (American Psychiatric Association 1987), asks the rater to assess a subject's psychological health on a scale from 1 to 90.

Health-Sickness Rating Scale.   HSRS ratings of mental health had been made on all CORE CITY subjects by an independent rater not involved in this study or familiar with the ratings of defenses. Like the GAF, the HSRS rates global mental health on a continuum from 1, representing total inability to function independently, to 100, reflecting various qualities of mental health (Luborsky 1962). Thus, as in the TERMAN sample, the correlations of defensive style with other measures of mental health can be studied.

Q-sort statements.   We began with Haan's 60 "Q-sort of ego processes" statements (Haan 1977). Nineteen additional statements representing Vaillant's defenses of hypochondriasis, acting out, fantasy, passive aggression, reaction formation, and anticipation were added. This initial deck was pretested by five clinicians. Twenty-eight unclear items from Haan's 60 statements were eliminated, leaving a total of 51 Q-statements (see Appendix 7).

With two exceptions, each of Vaillant's 15 defenses (see Appendix 3) was represented by a set of three Q-statements. Six, rather than three, of Haan's statements were retained to represent suppression, and six of Haan's statements were retained to represent isolation. The purpose of these exceptions was to alter Haan's instrument as little as possible. To preserve equal statistical representation for each of the 15 defenses, each of the six Q-statements representing suppression and isolation, respectively, received only half weighting.

The Bond Defense Style Questionnaire.   The DSQ (Bond et al. 1983) is described in detail in Chapter 7.

Procedure

Two clinicians and two independent Q-sorters each read 18 of the TER-MAN women's interviews. The two clinicians identified the subject's prominent defenses by using clinical judgment to assess the number of times each defense mechanism appeared in a transcript in the fashion described in Chapter 9. These numbers were totaled to obtain the clinicians' consensus score.

The second pair of raters applied the Q-methodology, as described. One rater was a psychiatrist and the other a research assistant with a baccalaureate degree in psychology. Each rater sorted the Q-statements along a continuum according to which statements the rater felt most closely represented each subject's defensive style.

The cards were distributed in a 9-point sort, quasi-normal distribution, as shown in Figure 12-1. The same procedure was followed for 30 CORE CITY men except that only one Q-sorter was employed.

The defense mechanism deemed to be represented by each Q-statement was written on the back of its index card. To determine which defense mechanisms were ranked as most characteristic for a subject, the cards were turned over; each defense mechanism that was represented by a card in row 1, the "Most Characteristic" ranking, received 4 points, each in row 2, 3 points, and each in rows 3 and 4, 2 points and 1 point, respectively. The scores from these top four rows were totaled, and the raw scores for each subject's defenses were ranked based on these scores.

In addition, these scores for individual defenses were then used to calculate a score for maturity of defensive style. The scores for defenses represented in the top four rows were distributed into *mature, intermediate* (neurotic), and *immature* groups (see Appendix 3). A total of 8 points was divided among these three groupings to reflect the relative proportion of each group, with a minimum of 1 point and a maximum of 5 points allowed per group (see Chapter 8). The score for maturity of defensive style was calculated by subtracting the adjusted score for mature defenses (1–5) from the adjusted score for immature defenses (1–5), and then adding 5 points, to bring the final score into a range from 1 (i.e., most mature) to 9 (i.e., least mature).

Data Analysis

All correlations were calculated using Pearson's product-moment correlation coefficient, or Spearman's r, which was felt to be most appropriate for those data in which relative ranks, rather than specific values, were being compared.

Ranking		Most characteristic = 1		Least characteristic = 9		Case #: 26	Date: 9//90	Rater: A

Rank Weighting

Rank	(wt)								
1	(4)	10 Isolation	59 Repression	60 Repression					
2	(3)	11 Isolation	46 Displacement	58 Repression	71 Fantasy				
3	(2)	12 Isolation	28 Projection	29 Projection	30 Projection	47 Displacement	72 Fantasy		
4	(1)	2 Isolation	8 Isolation	19 Anticipation	48 Displacement	51 Suppression	57 Suppression	63 Humor	70 Fantasy
5		1	3	21	41	42	45	49	56	68
6		17	20	25	31	36	54	61	67	
7		16	27	32	53	55	62			
8		4	5	18	69					
9		64	65	66						

Maturity scores of defensive style:

	Raw scores	8 points distributed
I = Immature	12	2
N = Neurotic	23	5
M = Mature	3	1

2 − 1 + 5 = 6

Distribution of characteristic cards x weighting for defense rank

1. Repression (N)	$4 + 4 + 3 = 11$		6. Isolation (N)	$1 + 1 = 2$
2. Isolation (N)	$4 + 3 + 2 = 9$		7. Anticipation (M)	1
3. Fantasy (I)	$3 + 2 + 1 = 6$		8. Humor (M)	1
4. Displacement (N)	$3 + 2 + 1 = 6$		9. Suppression (M)	1
5. Projection (I)	$2 + 2 + 2 = 6$			

Figure 12–1. An example of Q-sort of ego defenses for an individual

Results

A case example (see Figure 12-1) clarifies how the Q-sort method was applied. A TERMAN woman had suffered four major depressive episodes in her life but had made no mention of her mental illness throughout her interview at age 78. Her son had also experienced significant psychiatric difficulties throughout much of his life, and she "forgot" to mention anything about this even when asked explicitly about her children. Instead, she focused on her dreams of being a famous writer and lamented the fact that she had written nothing in the past 10 years because she could not decide between writing her autobiography or a book about sewing. At times, she blamed her family for her writer's block. Her main attention was upon issues of fabric and dress design. She described feeling no enjoyment from her life with her elderly but active husband; she simply explained that it was "stressful choosing clothing for him" because of the difference in their tastes. She summed herself up by saying, "I don't think broadly."

Each Q-sorter ranked the set of Q-statements based on which statements best reflected this woman's defensive style. One of the Q-sort worksheets for this subject is shown in Figure 12-1. The Q-sorter selected the following three statements as "most characteristic":

> Q-statement 10: "Produces intellectualizations rather than cogent solutions. Talks on a level of abstraction not quite appropriate to the situation." (Isolation)
> Q-statement 59: "Forgets aspects of trying circumstances." (Repression)
> Q-statement 60: "Unable to recall painful experiences." (Repression)

Each of the defense mechanisms represented by these statements received 4 points. The defense mechanisms represented by the Q-statements sorted into the next row, Q-statements 11 (isolation), 46 (displacement), 58 (repression), and 71 (fantasy), were given 3 points. The next two rows were scored with 2 points and 1 point, respectively.

The method for calculating this subject's maturity of defensive style is illustrated in the lower left corner of Figure 12-1. The raw scores for immature, neurotic, and mature defenses were 12, 23, and 3, respectively. Transformed into an 8-point scale, these scores became 2, 5, and 1, respectively. Subtracting the adjusted score for mature defenses (1) from the adjusted score for immature defenses (2) and adding 5 points results in a global maturity of defense score of 6. The other blind Q-sorter gave the subject an overall score of 7, as one can calculate from Table 12-1.

The total raw scores for this subject's defenses based on the top four rows of rankings of each Q-sorter are shown in Table 12-1. The clinicians'

Table 12–1. Inter-rater reliability between Q-sorters and clinicians for one subject

	Q-sorter A	Q-sorter B	Average of 2 Q-sorters	Clinicians' consensus
Humor (M)	1	0	0.5	0
Anticipation (M)	1	0	0.5	0
Sublimation (M)	0	0	0	1
Altruism (M)	0	0	0	0
Suppression (M)	1	1	1	0
Repression (N)	11	9	10	0
Displacement (N)	6	5	5.5	1
Isolation (N)	5.5	5	5.25	0.5
Reaction formation (N)	0	0	0	0
Dissociation (I)	0	5	2.5	6
Projection (I)	6	0	3	0
Hypochondriasis (I)	0	2	1	0
Passive aggression (I)	0	2	1	1
Fantasy (I)	6	9	7.5	12
Acting out (I)	0	0	0	0

Note. Pearson *r* based on 15 defenses for Q-sorters A vs. B is .73. The correlation is statistically significant at *P* < .001. Pearson *r* based on 15 defenses for the average of the Q-sorters vs. the average of the clinicians is .41. M = mature; N = neurotic; I = immature.

consensus scores are also listed. The reader can see that the dominant defenses for this subject, as assessed by the Q-method, are repression, displacement, isolation, and fantasy. The raw scores of the two Q-sorters on their ratings of 15 defense mechanisms correlated with a Pearson's *r* of .73. The distribution of scores illustrates how recovery from a schizoaffective psychosis, from which this subject had suffered, resulted in a shift toward neurotic defenses, but both sets of raters saw schizoid fantasy still a prominent defense.

Table 12-2 presents the level of agreement in the TERMAN sample of three comparisons: 1) between the Q-sorters on the ranking of all 51 Q-statements; 2) between the Q-sorters for rankings of the 15 defenses, as calculated from the Q-statement ranking raw scores; and 3) between the Q-sorters' average raw scores and the clinicians' consensus scores for the 15 defenses. When comparing all 51 Q-statements, the results of the Pearson correlations indicate that the two Q-sorters reached statistical significance for all 18 cases. Two-thirds of these correlations reflect very strong agreement between Q-sorter A and B (*P* < .001). When we collapse the Q-statements into the 15 defenses they represent, there appears to be

Table 12–2. Inter-rater reliability of the ego mechanisms of defense for the TERMAN sample ($n = 18$)

Subject #	Correlations for Q-sorter A vs. B		Clinicians' consensus vs. average of the Q-sorters
	51 Cards[a]	15 Triads[b]	15 Triads[b]
1	.66***	.25	.41
2	.65***	.67**	.67**
3	.65***	.22	.68**
5	.31*	.07	.48*
7	.35**	.70**	.34
10	.38**	.14	.77***
26	.63***	.73***	.41
28	.28*	.27	.48*
29	.49***	.48*	−.06
31	.80***	.93***	.96***
32	.39**	.09	.70**
33	.73***	.70**	−.06
34	.75***	.73***	.67**
35	.24*	.37	.62**
36	.48***	.31	.69**
38	.77***	.59**	.73***
39	.78***	.84***	.65**
40	.46***	.52*	.11
Average of 18 cases:	.54	.48	.51

[a]The correlations are based on the whole Q-sort deck for all nine ranks.
[b]The correlations are based on the 15 sets of defenses for the top four ranks only.
*$P < .05$. **$P < .01$. ***$P < .001$.

slightly weaker agreement. In comparing the average of the Q-sorters' scores with the clinicians' consensus scores, there was statistical significance in two-thirds of the 18 cases. What is most striking is the wide range of agreement between raters, from .07 for subject no. 5 to .93 for subject no. 31 for Q-sort comparisons. This confirms the findings of past investigators that assessing metaphorical constructs with reliability is not easy.

Rater reliability may be examined defense by defense instead of case by case. As shown in Table 12-3, there was greater agreement for the mature and immature defenses than for the neurotic defenses. When comparing the Q-sorters' scores to the clinicians', the same pattern held. There was good agreement on the mature and immature defenses (except for dissociation) and unacceptable agreement on the neurotic defenses (except for isolation).

Table 12–3. Inter-rater reliability of the Q-sort and clinical assessments for 15 defenses in the TERMAN sample (*n* = 18)

	Q-sort A vs. B	Q-sort vs. clinicians' consensus
Humor (M)	.73***	.54**
Anticipation (M)	.42*	.76***
Sublimation (M)	.69***	.80***
Altruism (M)	.71***	.82***
Suppression(M)	.60**	.64**
Repression (N)	.44*	.11
Displacement (N)	.51*	.05
Isolation (N)	.37	.51*
Reaction formation (N)	.10	.13
Dissociation (I)	.59**	.24
Projection (I)	.31	.60**
Hypochondriasis (I)	.63**	.44*
Passive aggression (I)	.68***	.67**
Fantasy (I)	.45*	.61**
Acting out (I)[a]	NA	NA
Average of 14 Defenses:	.52	.49

Note. NA = not applicable. M = mature; N = neurotic; I = immature.
[a]Correlations for this defense could not be calculated because of the almost perfect agreement of its absence.
*P < .05. **P < .01. ***P < .001.

We examined inter-rater reliability for the assessment of maturity of defensive style for the TERMAN women and CORE CITY men, respectively (see Tables 12-4 and 12-5). When the 15 defenses are grouped into three categories of mature, neurotic, and immature types, inter-rater reliability improves dramatically. The results indicated that regardless of the comparison, inter-rater reliability for the maturity of defensive style was statistically significant. The lowest agreement for the TERMAN women was Q-sorter A vs. B (Pearson's r = .64, P < .01) (Table 12-6). The highest agreement was between the clinicians (Pearson's r = .83, P < .001). Similarly high inter-rater reliabilities were observed for the CORE CITY sample. The more labor-intensive clinical ratings appeared to be more reliable than the Q-sort ratings.

For the CORE CITY sample, the measures of maturity of defensive style derived by Q-sort and by clinical assessment were also highly correlated. We compared the results of the Q-sort with maturity ego defenses obtained by self-report as reflected by the DSQ (see Table 12-6). The greatest consensual validation was when the Q-sort and the labor-intensive assess-

Table 12–4. Maturity scores of defensive style for the TERMAN sample
($n = 18$)

Subject #	Q-sorter A	Q-sorter B	Average of 2 Q-sorters	Blind clinician	Not blind clinician	Average of 2 clinicians
1	1	6	3.5	6	8	7.0
2	6	7	6.5	7	8	7.5
3	1	3	2.0	3	2	2.5
5	1	8	4.5	5	3	4.0
7	4	7	5.5	9	8	8.5
10	1	4	2.5	2	1	1.5
26	6	7	6.5	9	9	9.0
28	7	6	6.5	8	9	8.5
29	4	7	5.5	6	6	6.0
31	1	1	1.0	1	1	1.0
32	3	8	5.5	4	4	4.0
33	1	1	1.0	5	4	4.5
34	1	1	1.0	2	1	1.5
35	5	8	6.5	7	6	6.5
36	1	3	2.0	4	4	4.0
38	1	2	1.5	1	1	1.0
39	1	1	1.0	4	2	3.0
40	3	8	5.5	8	6	7.0
Average of 18 cases:	2.67	4.89	3.78	5.06	4.61	4.83

Note. Maturity scores range from 1 to 9, with 1 the most mature and 9 the most immature.

ment by clinicians on the summaries of the same interview were compared, rather than when either of these was compared with the DSQ self-report.

Finally, we sought construct validity for the Q-sort. The assessment of maturity of defenses by the Q-sort correlated with the global mental health (as measured by the GAF) of the TERMAN women ($r = .56$; $P < .01$) and with the global mental health of the CORE CITY men (as measured by the HSRS) ($r = .65$; $P < .001$). Assessment of maturity of defensive style by the two clinicians correlated with the mental health of the TERMAN women ($r = .82$) and with the CORE CITY men ($r = .78$).

Discussion

These results support the mutual applicability of both the Q-sort methodology and clinical assessment for studying defensive style. This pilot study

Table 12–5. Maturity scores of defensive style for the CORE CITY sample
($n = 30$)

Subject #	Q-sorter	Blind clinician	Not blind clinician	Average of 2 clinicians
728	3	3	5	4
741	8	3	7	5
812	2	6	5	5.5
836	6	6	5	5.5
885	3	5	2	3.5
889	1	1	1	1
892	4	3	2	2.5
914	9	8	8	8
919	1	3	2	2.5
930	9	7	4	5.5
933	9	7	6	6.5
937	4	4	4	4
938	3	4	5	4.5
951	7	6	6	6
954	8	8	9	8.5
959	7	7	8	7.5
960	7	8	8	8
962	3	3	3	3
969	3	3	3	3
971	5	4	5	4.5
973	6	7	7	7
975	1	2	1	1.5
976	9	7	7	7
984	4	4	3	3.5
985	9	9	9	9
991	1	4	3	3.5
994	1	2	4	3
995	9	9	9	9
997	6	6	6	6
999	7	4	4	4
Average of 30 cases:	5.17	5.10	5.03	5.07

Note. Maturity scores range from 1 to 9, with 1 the most mature and 9 the most immature.

Table 12–6. Correlations of maturity of defensive style as assessed by clinical, Q-sort, and Bond Defense Style Questionnaire (DSQ) measures for the CORE CITY and TERMAN samples

| | Pearson's correlations | |
	CORE CITY men (*n* = 30)	TERMAN women (*n* = 18)
Q-sorters vs. clincians	.83***	.83***
Q-sorters vs. blind clinician	.80***	.82***
Clinician: blind vs. not blind	.83***	.93***
Q-sorter A vs. B		.64**
***n* = 18[a]**		
Q-sorter vs. self-report (Bond DSQ)	.13	
Q-sort vs. average of 2 clinicians	.86***	
Average of 2 clinicians vs. self-report (Bond DSQ)	.46*	
Q-sorter A vs. average of 2 clinicians		.80***
Q-sorter B vs. average of 2 clinicians		.72***

[a]Of the original 30 CORE CITY men who were Q-sorted, only 18 of them had self-report data.
*$P < .05$. **$P < .01$. ***$P < .001$.

also reveals that further work needs to be done and that the tool of the Q-sort method may be honed more sharply if we consider several aspects of these results that were problematic. First, looking over inter-rater reliabilities for both defense mechanisms and maturity-of-defensive style scores in the TERMAN sample, we see that there are striking discrepancies between Q-sorter A and Q-sorter B. Although their overall correlations with the clinicians are comparable (.80 for Q-sorter A, .72 for Q-sorter B; $P < .001$; Table 12-6.), Q-sorter A tended to perceive the subjects' defensive style as more mature than did Q-sorter B. For maturity of defensive style, Q-sorter A averaged a score of 2.67 for all 18 subjects, whereas Q-sorter B averaged a score of 4.89 (indicating a less mature style) for the 18 subjects (Table 12-4). The clinicians' consensus average score was 4.83, much closer to the average score of Q-sorter B than to that of Q-sorter A. In all cases in Table 12-4 in which the raw scores between Q-sorter A and Q-sorter B differed by 3 or more points (subjects nos. 1, 5, 32, 40), Q-sorter A's score was always the lower number (indicating more mature style).

Q-sorter A was a psychiatrist who did not work closely with the clinicians outside of this study. Q-sorter B had earned a baccalaureate in psychology and worked closely with the clinicians as a research assistant on several studies. One wonders whether Q-sort variability would decrease if all Q-sorters had the same level of training and clinical experience, as well as the same exposure to the clinical philosophy of ego defenses espoused by the clinicians in this study.

Two subjects (nos. 29 and 33) (Table 12-2) produced negative correlations between the average Q-sort scores and the clinicians' consensus. In both cases, the clinicians' consensus was that reaction formation was a dominant defense (raw scores of 12 and 5, respectively), whereas the averaged Q-sort scores showed reaction formation as being insignificant in these cases (0 and 1.5, respectively). In both women, the Q-sorters distributed points for the prominent defenses among at least four defenses. The clinicians' consensus, however, was that for subject no. 29 reaction formation dominated, and that for subject no. 33 reaction formation and displacement (raw score of 6) surpassed all other defenses. On review this discrepancy reflects the difficulty in interpreting the meaning of reaction formation, and Haan's specific Q-statements representing this defense (nos. 53 and 54) were inadequate or unclear. As a result, these two items (see Appendix 7) have been replaced with statements that encompass reaction formation more clearly. In addition, the fact that the clinicians' consensus for both women pointed to only one or two defenses instead of several may also explain why their clinical assessments correlate so poorly with the Q-sort data, which by convention fits into a quasi-normal distribution. In women for whom clinical assessments correlated more highly with Q-sort data (e.g., subject nos. 31, 34, 36, and 38), the clinicians' consensus scores were more broadly distributed among several defenses. One might speculate that imposing some distribution requirements on the clinical assessments would improve their correlation with Q-method data. Broader distribution may reflect a potential advantage of Q-sorting subjective clinical data.

Also of interest is the relative difficulty of both Q-sorters and clinicians in rating not only reaction formation, but all neurotic defenses, as compared with mature or immature ones (Table 12-3). This finding is consistent with similar findings in other studies (Perry et al. 1987). Were the Q-statements that reflected neurotic defenses more ambiguous than other Q-statements? Could these statements be examined more closely and revised so that the Q-methodology could be an improvement over other methods in defining this territory? Further work is needed.

On the positive side are the highly significant correlations between the global measures of mental health and the Q-sort assessment of maturity of defensive style (.56 and .65 for the TERMAN and CORE CITY samples, respectively). Because the Q-sort method of assessing defenses offers advantages over clinical methods in computational clarity, labor costs, and reproducibility, the Q-sort method has clear advantages over clinical assessment, even though the latter methods correlated more highly than did

Q-sort data with global measures of mental health. Certainly, the Q-sort method lends itself to measuring ipsative changes in ego function in clinical situations, especially psychotherapy research, better than the quantitatively less tightly controlled clinical methods.

Conclusion

In this chapter we contrast three methods for assessing ego defenses: the DSQ, clinical assessment, and our modification of Haan's Q-sort methodology. The DSQ offers the most direct and convenient approach but sacrifices validity when compared with other methods. Conscientious clinical assessment is a reliable method, given well-trained clinicians and adequate time; however, this design produces data that are susceptible to human bias, that may be difficult to interpret in a statistically sound fashion, and that are less reproducible across studies.

In this pilot study, as in Haan's earlier studies, it seems clear that the Q-methodology offers a promising third method for the empirical study of defense mechanisms. This method provides more statistically accessible data with less need for advanced clinical expertise on the part of the raters. By comparing this technique with clinical assessment methods, both methods were validated. Further, both Q-sorting and clinical judgment correlated significantly with broader measures of mental health, namely, the GAF scale and the HSRS. The significant agreement between Q-sort and clinical methods of assessing defense mechanisms provides further evidence and encouragement that the field of ego defenses is as solid a terrain to map and explore as it is a powerful, poetic metaphor for describing qualitative clinical assessment.

References

American Psychiatric Association: Diagnostic and Statistical Manual of Mental Disorders, 3rd Edition, Revised. Washington, DC, American Psychiatric Association, 1987

Block J: The Q-Sort Method in Personality Assessment and Psychiatric Research. Palo Alto, CA, Consulting Psychologists Press, 1978

Bond M, Gardner ST, Christian J, et al: Empirical study of self-rated defense styles. Arch Gen Psychiatry 40:333–338, 1983

Glueck S, Glueck E: Unraveling Juvenile Delinquency. New York, The Common Wealth Fund, 1950

Haan N: Coping and defense mechanisms related to personality inventories. Journal of Consulting Psychology 29:373–387, 1965

Haan N: Coping and Defending: Processes of Self-Environment Organization. New York, Academic, 1977

Hauser ST: Conceptual and empirical dilemmas in the assessment of defenses, in Empirical Studies of Ego Mechanisms of Defense. Edited by Vaillant GE. Washington, DC, American Psychiatric Press, 1986, pp 89–99

Joffe P, Naditch MP: Paper and pencil measures of coping and defense processes, in Haan N: Coping and Defending: Processes of Self-Environment Organization. New York, Academic, 1977, pp 280–297

Luborsky L: Clinicians' judgments of mental health. Arch Gen Psychiatry 7:407–417, 1962

McKeown B, Thomas D: Q Methodology (Quantitative Applications in the Social Sciences Series). Newbury Park, CA, Sage, 1988

Morrissey RF: The Haan model of ego functioning: an assessment of empirical research, in Haan N: Coping and Defending: Processes of Self-Environment Organization. New York, Academic, 1977, pp 250–279

Mowrer OH: Q-technique—description, history, and critique, in Psychotherapy Theory and Research. Edited by Mowrer OH. New York, Ronald Press, 1953, pp 140–157

Oden MH: The fulfillment of promise: 40-year follow-up of the Terman gifted group. Genet Psychol Monographs 77:3–93, 1968

Perry JC, Cooper SH: Empirical studies of psychological defenses, in Psychiatry, Vol 1. Edited by Cavenar JO, Michels R. Philadelphia, PA, JB Lippincott, Basic Books, 1987, Chapter 30, pp 1–19

Sears RR: The Terman Gifted Children Study, in Handbook of Longitudinal Research, 9th Edition. Edited by Mednick SA, Herway M, Finello KM. New York, Praeger, 1984, pp 398–414

Stephenson W: Technique of factor analysis. Nature 136:297, 1935

Stephenson W: The Study of Behavior: Q-Technique and Its Methodology. Chicago, IL, University of Chicago Press, 1953

Terman L, Oden MH: Genetic Studies of Genius, Vol 5: The Gifted Group at Midlife. Stanford, CA, Stanford University Press, 1959

Appendixes

Seven Assessment Schemes for
Defense Mechanisms

Appendix 1

DSM-III-R Glossary of Defense Mechanisms

Defense Mechanisms

Patterns of feelings, thoughts, or behaviors that are relatively involuntary and arise in response to perceptions of psychic danger. They are designed to hide or to alleviate the conflicts or stressors that give rise to anxiety. Some defense mechanisms, such as projection, splitting, and acting out, are almost invariably maladaptive. Others, such as suppression and denial, may be either maladaptive or adaptive, depending on their severity, their inflexibility, and the context in which they occur. Defense mechanisms that are usually adaptive, such as sublimation and humor, are not included here.

Acting out   A mechanism in which the person acts without reflection or apparent regard for negative consequences.

Autistic fantasy   A mechanism in which the person substitutes excessive daydreaming for the pursuit of human relationships, more direct and effective action, or problem solving.

Denial   A mechanism in which the person fails to acknowledge some aspect of external reality that would be apparent to others.

Devaluation   A mechanism in which the person attributes exaggeratedly negative qualities to self or others.

Displacement   A mechanism in which the person generalizes or redirects a feeling about an object or a response to an object onto another, usually less threatening, object.

This glossary is reprinted, with permission, from the *Diagnostic and Statistical Manual of Mental Disorders*, 3rd Edition, Revised (DSM-III-R). Washington, DC, American Psychiatric Association, 1987, pp. 393–395. Copyright 1987, American Psychiatric Association.

This glossary is the result of the work of the Advisory Committee on Defense Mechanisms: Drs. David Barlow, Michael Bond, Allen Frances, William Frosch, J. Christopher Perry, George Vaillant, Jeff Young, and Robert Spitzer (Chairman, Work Group to Revise DSM-III).

Dissociation   A mechanism in which the person sustains a temporary alteration in the integrative functions of consciousness or identity.

Idealization   A mechanism in which the person attributes exaggeratedly positive qualities to self or others.

Intellectualization   A mechanism in which the person engages in excessive abstract thinking to avoid experiencing disturbing feelings.

Isolation   A mechanism in which the person is unable to experience simultaneously the cognitive and affective components of an experience because the affect is kept from consciousness.

Passive aggression   A mechanism in which the person indirectly and unassertively expresses aggression toward others.

Projection   A mechanism in which the person falsely attributes his or her own unacknowledged feelings, impulses, or thoughts to others.

Rationalization   A mechanism in which the person devises reassuring or self-serving, but incorrect, explanations for his or her own or others' behavior.

Reaction formation   A mechanism in which the person substitutes behavior, thoughts, or feelings that are diametrically opposed to his or her own unacceptable ones.

Repression   A mechanism in which the person is unable to remember or to be cognitively aware of disturbing wishes, feelings, thoughts, or experiences.

Somatization   A mechanism in which the person becomes preoccupied with physical symptoms disproportionate to any actual physical disturbance.

Splitting   A mechanism in which the person views himself or herself or others as all good or all bad, failing to integrate the positive and the negative qualities of self and others into cohesive images; often the person alternately idealizes and devalues the same person.

Suppression   A mechanism in which the person intentionally avoids thinking about disturbing problems, desires, feelings, or experiences.

Undoing   A mechanism in which the person engages in behavior designed to symbolically make amends for or negate previous thoughts, feelings, or actions.

Appendix 2

Meissner's Glossary of Defenses

A. Narcissistic Defenses

Denial   Psychotic denial of external reality. Unlike repression, it affects the perception of external reality. Seeing but refusing to acknowledge what one sees and hearing but negating what is actually heard are examples of denial and exemplify the close relationship of denial to sensory experience. However, not all denial is necessarily psychotic. Like projection, denial may function in the service of neurotic or even adaptive objectives.

Distortion   Grossly reshaping external reality to suit inner needs—including unrealistic megalomanic beliefs, hallucinations, wish-fulfilling delusions—and using sustained feelings of delusional superiority or entitlement.

Projection   Frank delusions about external reality, usually persecutory; it includes both perception of one's own feelings in another and subsequent acting on the perception (psychotic paranoid delusions).

B. Immature Defenses

Acting out   Direct expression of an unconscious wish or impulse to avoid being conscious of the accompanying affect. The unconscious fantasy, involving objects, is lived out impulsively in behavior, thus gratifying the impulse more than the prohibition against it. On a chronic level, acting out involves giving in to impulses to avoid the tension that would result from postponement of expression.

Blocking   Inhibition, usually temporary in nature, of affects (usually), thinking, or impulses.

This glossary is reprinted, with permission, from Kaplan HI, Sadock BJ: *Modern Synopsis of Comprehensive Textbook of Psychiatry,* 3rd Edition. Baltimore, MD, Williams & Wilkins, 1981, pp. 137–138.

Hypochondriasis   Transformation of reproach toward others—arising from bereavement, loneliness, or unacceptable aggressive impulses—into self-reproach and complaints of pain, somatic illness, and neurasthenia. Existent illness may also be overemphasized or exaggerated for its evasive and regressive possibilities. Thus, responsibility may be avoided, guilt may be circumvented, and instinctual impulses may be warded off.

Introjection   With a loved object, introjection involves the internalization of characteristics of the object with the goal of establishing closeness to and constant presence of the object. Anxiety consequent to separation or tension arising out of ambivalence toward the object is thus diminished. Introjection of a feared object serves to avoid anxiety by internalizing the aggressive characteristics of the object, thereby putting the aggression under one's control. The aggression is no longer felt as coming from outside but is taken within and used defensively, turning the person's weak, passive position into an active, strong one. Introjection can also rise out of a sense of guilt, in which the self-punishing introject is attributable to the hostile-destructive component of an ambivalent tie to an object. The self-punitive qualities of the object are taken over and established within one's self as a symptom or character trait, which effectively represents both the destruction and the preservation of the object. This is also called identification with the victim.

Passive-aggressive behavior   Aggression toward an object expressed indirectly and ineffectively through passivity, masochism, and turning against the self.

Projection   Attributing one's own unacknowledged feelings to others; it includes severe prejudice, rejection of intimacy through suspiciousness, hypervigilance to external danger, and injustice collecting. Projection operates correlatively to introjection; the material of the projection is derived from the internalized configuration of the introjects.

Regression   Return to a previous state of development or functioning to avoid the anxieties or hostilities involved in later stages; return to earlier points of fixation, embodying modes of behavior previously given up. This defense mechanism is often the result of a disruption of equilibrium at a later phase of development.

Schizoid fantasy   Tendency to use fantasy and to indulge in autistic retreat for the purpose of conflict resolution and gratification.

Somatization   Defensive conversion of psychic derivatives into bodily symptoms.

C. Neurotic Defenses

Controlling   Excessive attempt to manage or regulate events or objects in the environment in the interest of minimizing anxiety and solving internal conflicts.

Displacement   Purposeful, unconscious shifting from one object to another in the interest of solving a conflict. Although the object is changed, the instinctual nature of the impulse and its aim remain unchanged.

Dissociation   Temporary but drastic modification of character or sense of personal identity to avoid emotional distress; it involves fugue states and hysterical conversion reactions.

Externalization   Tendency to perceive in the external world and in external objects components of one's own personality, including instinctual impulses, conflicts, moods, attitudes, and styles of thinking. It is a more general term than projection, which is defined by its derivation from and correlation with specific introjects.

Inhibition   Unconsciously determined limitation or renunciation of specific ego functions, singly or in combination, to avoid anxiety arising out of conflict with instinctual impulses, the superego, or environmental forces or figures.

Intellectualization   Control of affects and impulses by thinking about them instead of experiencing them. It is a systematic excess of thinking, deprived of its affect, to defend against anxiety due to unacceptable impulses.

Isolation   Intrapsychic splitting or separation of affect from content, resulting in repression of either idea or affect or the displacement of affect to a different or substitute content.

Rationalization   Justification of attitudes, beliefs, or behavior that may otherwise be unacceptable by an incorrect application of justifying reasons or the invention of a convincing fallacy.

Reaction formation   Management of unacceptable impulses by permitting expression of the impulse in antithetical form.

Repression   Expelling and withholding from conscious awareness of an idea or feeling. It may operate by excluding from awareness what was once experienced on a conscious level (secondary repression), or it may curb ideas and feelings before they have reached consciousness (primary repression). The "forgetting" of repression is unique in that it is often accompanied by highly symbolic behavior, which suggests that the repressed is not really forgotten.

Sexualization   Endowing of an object or function with sexual significance that it did not previously have or that it possesses to a lesser degree
to ward off anxieties connected with prohibited impulses.

Somatization   Defensive conversion of psychic derivatives into bodily
symptoms.

D. Mature Defenses

Altruism   Vicarious but constructive and instinctually gratifying service
to others. This defense mechanism must be distinguished from altruistic
surrender, which involves a surrender of direct gratification or of instinctual
needs in favor of fulfilling the needs of others to the detriment of the self,
with vicarious satisfaction being gained only through introjection.

Anticipation   Realistic anticipation of or planning for future inner discomfort.

Asceticism   Elimination of directly pleasurable affects attributable to an
experience. The moral element is implicit in setting values on specific
pleasures. Asceticism is directed against all base pleasures perceived consciously; gratification is derived from the renunciation.

Humor   Overt expression of feelings without personal discomfort or
immobilization and without unpleasant effect on others. Humor allows one
to bear and yet focus on what is too terrible to be borne; in contrast, wit
involves distraction or displacement away from the affective issue.

Sublimation   Gratification of an impulse whose goal is retained but
whose aim or object is changed from a socially objectionable one to a
socially valued one. Libidinal sublimation involves a desexualization of drive
impulses and the placing of a value judgment that substitutes what is valued
by the superego or society. Sublimation of aggressive impulses takes place
through pleasurable games and sports. Unlike neurotic defenses, sublimation allows instincts to be channeled, rather than dammed or diverted. In
sublimation, feelings are acknowledged, modified, and directed toward a
relatively significant person or goal, so that modest instinctual satisfaction
results.

Suppression   Conscious or semiconscious decision to postpone attention to a conscious impulse or conflict.

Appendix 3

Vaillant's Glossary of Defenses

A. "Psychotic" Defenses

> These mechanisms are common in "healthy" individuals before age 5, and common in adult dreams and fantasy. For the user, these mechanisms alter reality. To the beholder, they appear "crazy." They tend to be immune to change by conventional psychotherapeutic interpretation; but they are altered by change in reality (e.g., chlorpromazine, removal of stressful situation, developmental maturation). In therapy they can be given up temporarily by offering the user strong interpersonal support in conjunction with direct confrontation with the ignored reality.

1. Delusional projection   Frank delusions about external reality, usually of a persecutory type.

Delusional projection includes both the perception of one's own feelings in another person and then acting on the perception (e.g., florid paranoid delusions), and the perception of other people or their feelings literally inside one's self (e.g., the agitated depressed patient's claim that "the devil is devouring my heart.") This mechanism can be distinguished from projection by the fact that in the former, reality testing is virtually abandoned. It is distinguished from distortion by the absence of wish fulfillment and from introjection in that the responsibility for acknowledged internal feelings is still projected. In toxic psychosis, delusional projection can adaptively organize otherwise chaotic perceptions.

2. Denial (psychotic)   Denial of external reality.

Unlike repression, denial, as here defined, affects perception of external reality more than perception of internal reality (e.g., "girls do so got penises.") It includes the use of fantasy as a major substitute for other people—especially absent other people (e.g., "I will make a new him in my own mind").

3. Distortion   Grossly reshaping external reality to suit inner needs.

Distortion includes unrealistic megalomaniacal beliefs, hallucinations, wish-fulfilling delusions, and employing sustained feelings of delusional superiority or entitlement. It can encompass persistent denial of personal responsibility for one's own behavior. It also includes acting upon, as well as thinking about, unrealistic obsessions or compulsions. In distortion, there may be a pleasant merging or fusion with another person (e.g., "Jesus lives inside me and answers all my prayers"); but in contrast to delusional projection, in which distress is alleviated by assigning responsibility for offensive feelings elsewhere, in distortion unpleasant feelings are replaced with their opposites. As manifested in religious belief, distortion can be highly adaptive.

B. "Immature" Defenses

These mechanisms are common in "healthy" individuals, age 3–15, in persons with character disorder, and in adults in psychotherapy. For the user these mechanisms most often alter distress engendered either by the threat of interpersonal intimacy or by the threat of experiencing its loss. To the beholder these defenses appear socially undesirable. Although refractory to change, they change with improved interpersonal relationships (e.g., personal maturation, a more mature spouse, a more intuitive physician, or a fairer parole officer) or with repeated and forceful interpretation during prolonged psychotherapy.

4. Projection   Attributing one's own unacknowledged feelings to others.

Projection includes severe prejudice, rejections of intimacy through unwarranted suspicion, marked hypervigilance to external danger, and injustice collecting. The behavior of someone using this defense may be eccentric and abrasive but within the "letter of the law." It includes much "devaluation."

5. Schizoid fantasy   Tendency to use fantasy and to indulge in autistic retreat for the purpose of conflict resolution and gratification.

Schizoid fantasy is associated with global avoidance of interpersonal intimacy and the use of eccentricity to repel others. In contrast to psychotic denial, the individual does not fully believe in or insist upon acting out his fantasies. Nevertheless, unlike mere wishes, schizoid fantasies serve to gratify unmet needs for personal relationships and to obliterate the overt expression of aggressive or sexual impulses toward others. It includes much "primitive idealization."

6. Hypochondriasis   The transformation of reproach towards others arising from bereavement, loneliness, or unacceptable aggressive impulses into, first, self-reproach and, then, complaints of pain, somatic illness, and neurasthenia.

Hypochondriasis includes those aspects of introjection that permit traits of an ambivalently regarded person to be perceived within oneself and causing plausible disease. Unlike identification, hypochondriacal introjects are "ego alien." The mechanism may permit the individual to belabor others with his or her own pain or discomfort in lieu of making direct demands upon them or in lieu of complaining that others have ignored his or her wishes (often unexpressed) to be dependent. It does not include illnesses like asthma, ulcer, or hypertension, which may be neither adaptive nor defensive. Unlike hysterical conversion symptoms, hypochondriasis is accomplished by the very opposite of *la belle indifference.*

7. Passive-aggressive behavior   Aggression toward others expressed indirectly and ineffectively through passivity.

This behavior includes failures, procrastinations, or illnesses that (initially at least) affect others more than self. It includes silly or provocative behavior in order to receive attention and clowning in order to avoid assuming a competitive role. People who form sadomasochistic relationships often manifest both passive-aggressive and hypochondriacal defenses.

8. Acting Out   Direct expression of an unconscious wish or impulse in order to avoid being conscious of the affect that accompanies it.

Acting out includes the use of motor behavior, delinquent or impulsive acts, and "tempers" to avoid being aware of one's feelings. It also includes the chronic use of drugs, failure perversion, or self-inflicted injury to relieve tension (i.e., subjective anxiety or depression). Acting out involves chronically giving in to impulses in order to avoid the tension that would result were there any postponement of expression.

9. Dissociation   Temporary but drastic modification of one's character or of one's sense of personal identity to avoid emotional distress.

Dissociation can include fugues, most hysterical conversion reactions, a sudden unwarranted sense of superiority or devil-may-care attitude, and short-term refusal to perceive responsibility for one's acts or feelings. Includes overactivity and counterphobic behavior to blot out anxiety or distressing emotion, "safe" expression of instinctual wishes by acting on stage, and the acute use of religious "joy" or of pharmacological intoxication to numb unhappiness. Dissociation is more comprehensive to others than distortion, more considerate of others, and less prolonged than acting out. It is synonymous with neurotic denial and perhaps with "omnipotence."

C. "Neurotic" Defenses

These mechanisms are common in "healthy" individuals, age 3–90, in persons with neurotic disorder, and in persons as they master acute adult stress. For the user these mechanisms alter private feelings or instinctual expression. To the beholder they appear as individual quirks or neurotic hang-ups. They often can be dramatically changed by conventional, brief psychotherapeutic interpretation.

10. Repression   Seemingly inexplicable naivete, memory lapse, or failure to acknowledge input from a selected sense organ. In isolation, the idea is kept in mind and the affect forgotten; in repression, the idea is repressed and the affect often remains. The "forgetting" of repression is unique in that it is often accompanied by highly symbolic behavior which suggests that the repressed is not really forgotten. The mechanism differs from suppression by effecting unconscious inhibition of impulse to the point of losing, not just postponing, cherished goals. Unlike denial, it prevents the expression and perception of instincts and feelings rather than affecting recognition of and response to external events. If a man were weeping but forgot for whom he wept, this would be repression; if he denied the existence of his tears or insisted that the mourned one was still alive, this would represent denial; if he denied that he felt sad, that would be dissociation.

11. Displacement   The redirection of feelings toward a relatively less cared for (less cathected) object than the person or situation arousing the feeling.

Displacement includes facile "transference" and the substitution of things or strangers for emotionally important people. Practical jokes, with hidden hostile intent, and caricature involve displacement. Most phobias, a few hysterical conversion reactions, and some prejudice involve displacement.

12. Reaction formation   Conscious affect and/or behavior that is diametrically opposed to an unacceptable instinctual (id) impulse.

This mechanism includes overtly caring for someone else when one wishes to be cared for oneself, "hating" someone or something one really likes, or "loving" a hated rival or unpleasant duty. The term can encompass both "identification with the aggressor" and "altruism" as defined by Anna Freud.

13. Intellectualization   Thinking about instinctual wishes in formal, bland terms that leaves the associated affect unconscious.

The term encompasses the mechanisms of isolation, rationalization, ritual, undoing, restitution, magical thinking, and "busy work." While these mechanisms differ from each other, they usually occur as a cluster. Intellectualization includes paying undue attention to the inanimate in order to avoid intimacy with people, or paying attention to external reality to avoid recognition of inner feelings, or paying attention to irrelevant detail to avoid perceiving the whole. Obsessions and compulsions not acted upon are included here, although they can also be thought of as a form of intrapsychic displacement.

D. "Mature" Defenses

These mechanisms are common in "healthy" individuals, age 12–90. For the user these mechanisms integrate reality, interpersonal relationships, and private feelings. To the beholder, they appear as convenient virtues. Under increased stress, they may change to less mature mechanisms.

14. Altruism   Vicarious but constructive and instinctually gratifying service to others.

Altruism can include benign and constructive reaction formation, empathy, philanthropy, and well-repaid service to others. Altruism differs from projection in that it responds to needs of others that are real and not projected; it differs from reaction formation in that it leaves the person doing for others as he or she wishes to be done by at least partly gratified.

15. Humor   Overt expression of feelings without individual discomfort or immobilization and without unpleasant effect on others.

Some games and playful regression come under this heading. Unlike wit, which is a form of displacement, humor lets you call a spade a spade; and humor can never be applied without some element of an "observing ego." Like hope, humor permits one to bear and yet focus upon what is too terrible to be borne; in contrast, wit always involves distraction or displacement away from the affective issue at hand. Unlike schizoid fantasy, humor never excludes other people.

16. Suppression   The capacity to hold all components of a conflict in mind and then postpone action, affective response, or ideational worrying.

Suppression appears as a semiconscious decision to defer paying attention to a conscious impulse or conflict. The mechanism includes looking for silver linings, stoicism, minimizing acknowledged discomfort, employing a stiff upper lip, and "counting to 10" before acting. With suppression, one says, "I will think about it tomorrow," and the next day one remembers to think about it. With repression, one forgets to remember.

17. Anticipation　　Realistic anticipation of or planning for future inner discomfort.

This mechanism includes goal-directed but overly careful affective planning or worrying, anticipatory mourning and anxiety, and the conscious utilization of "insight" gained from psychotherapy.

18. Sublimation　　Indirect or attenuated expression of instincts without adverse consequences or marked loss of pleasure.

Sublimation includes both expression of aggression through pleasurable games, sports, and hobbies, and romantic attenuation of instinctual expression during a real courtship. Unlike humor, with sublimation, "regression in the service of the ego" has real consequences. Unlike the case with "neurotic defenses," in sublimation instincts are channeled rather than dammed or diverted. In projection one's feelings (e.g., anger) are attributed to another person. In displacement one's feelings are acknowledged as one's own, but are redirected toward a relatively insignificant object, often without satisfaction. In sublimation, feelings are acknowledged, modified, and directed toward a relatively significant person or goal so that modest instinctual satisfaction results.

Case Illustration

A woman, married at age 30, after one miscarriage tried for 7 years to have children. Then, following a cervical biopsy that showed early cancer, at age 38 she underwent a total hysterectomy. She had always felt inadequate to her younger sister, who already had four children and had been the one in the family who won praise as "being good with kids." The woman's husband desperately wanted children. (Note the conflict involves instinctual wishes, parental expectations, reality, and the needs of those she loved.) Below are a number of possible responses to her surgery.

A.　The woman, a month after surgery, organized a group of other women who had had breast and uterine surgery to counsel and visit patients undergoing gynecological surgery. They tried to give information, to give advice and comfort, and from their experience to provide answers to questions and fears that such new patients might have. (**Altruism**)

B. Following a slight postoperative wound infection, she wrote long, angry letters to the papers blaming the hospital for unsanitary conditions. Blaming her doctor for not doing a Pap smear earlier, she threatened to institute malpractice proceedings. (**Projection**)

C. She renewed her old college interest in planned parenthood and passionately argued with her younger friends to limit their families. She suddenly "remembered" that she had always been afraid of the pain of childbirth and remarked to her husband how lucky she was to be spared the burden. (**Reaction formation**)

D. She read a lot about uterine cancer and asked the doctor a great many questions about the nature of the operation. She concerned herself with minute details of preventing postoperative infection and caring for her operative wound. She made a hobby in the hospital of learning medical words. (**Isolation**)

E. Emerging from anesthesia she felt no regret but instead enjoyed what she felt was a religious experience. Postoperatively, she told all her friends that her pain gave her a sense of joyous communion with sufferers everywhere. She felt an intense inward sense of good fortune that she had been favored by God to have had her cancer discovered so soon and to have come through surgery so well. (**Dissociation**)

F. She read Marcus Aurelius and Ecclesiastes in the hospital. She took great care to hide her tear-stained tissues from her husband and made no complaint (even though the process was painful) while her sutures were removed. Knowing that baby pictures upset her, she deliberately gave away an unread copy of her favorite magazine, which featured an article on child care. (**Suppression**)

G. She found herself unable to remember the name of the operation, except that it was for "a little nubbin in my tumtum." She "forgot" her first follow-up visit to the physician. On coming home she broke into tears when she broke an inexpensive, amphora-shaped flower vase; she had no idea why. (**Repression**)

H. She started ordering the nurses to move her upstairs to the maternity ward. She wandered about the hospital looking for her baby. By phone she ordered an expensive bassinet and baby clothes to be delivered to her house. She experienced no postoperative pain. (**Denial**)

I. She got great pleasure from "get well" cards from her sister's children, agreed to teach a Sunday School class of preschoolers, and got a poem published in her hometown weekly on the bittersweet joys of the maiden aunt. (**Sublimation**)

J. She became very interested in growing tulips and daffodils in her hospital window. Although she never asked the doctor questions about her own hospital course, she worried about a funny mold on the bulbs she was growing. Knowing his hobby was gardening, she repeatedly asked her surgeon's advice about the growth on her bulbs. (**Displacement**)

K. On the third postoperative day she announced that she was a Christian Scientist and was signing out immediately. Besides, she had to go home because she and her husband were planning a trip to Bermuda that weekend. (In reality, their total income was $200 a week and their Blue Cross had lapsed.) She added with a naughty laugh that they needed a vacation to do a little "spring planting." (**Distortion**)

L. Her doctor was surprised to find out how relaxed and practical she was about her postoperative course and the calm frankness with which she could express her regret at being cheated of children. His surprise was due to the fact that she had spent her preoperative visit anxiously worrying about possible surgical complications and weeping over the fact that she would never be able to bear children. (**Anticipation**)

M. She felt that the hospital was being run by racists who were trying to sterilize her. She tried to telephone the FBI to report the hospital for genocide. She refused her pain medication, claiming it was an experimental drug for thought control. (**Delusional projection**)

N. She asked the nurse not to permit visitors because they made her "sad." She threw out all her flowers and instead read and reread a copy of *Parent's Magazine* and looked repeatedly at *The Family of Man*. She would go down the corridor to the newborn nursery daydreaming about what she would call each child if it were hers, and once a floor nurse had to ask her not to whistle "Lullabye" so loudly. (**Fantasy**)

O. She became worried that the cancer might have spread to her lymph nodes and belabored her visitors with accounts of the tiny lumps in her groin and neck. When her sister came to visit, the patient angrily accused her of caring so much for her own children that she did not care if her own sister died of cancer. (**Hypochondriasis**)

P. When the intern, while inserting an IV, missed her vein, she smiled at him, told him not to worry, and said, "When you're just a medical student, it must be hard to get things right." Unable to sleep, she watched her IV run dry. Later, at 4 A.M., the night nurse had to call the intern to restart the IV. She cheerfully told him that she had not rung for the nurse because she knew how busy everyone in the hospital was. (**Passive aggression**)

Q. Shortly after leaving the hospital she was unfaithful to her husband with four different men in a month, twice picking up men in cocktail lounges and once seducing an 18-year-old delivery boy. Prior to that time she had had no sexual interest in any man but her husband. **(Acting out)**

R. She laughed so hard tears came to her eyes and her ribs ached when she read the *Playboy* definition of a hysterectomy: "throwing out the baby carriage but keeping the playpen." She explained her private mirth to a startled and curious nurse with, "The whole thing is just so damned ironic." **(Humor)**

Appendix 4

Perry's Defense Mechanism Rating Scale
(March 1990)

This glossary contains definitions of those defense mechanisms that are included in the author's *Defense Mechanism Rating Scales*, Fifth Edition (DMRS). The definitions are grouped together in styles or levels, based on similarities in the function of defenses from the same style or level.

Asterisk denotes defense mechanism is not listed in DSM-III-R glossary.

Action Defenses

Acting out   The individual deals with emotional conflicts, or internal or external stressors, by acting without reflection or apparent regard for negative consequences.

Acting out involves the expression of feelings, wishes, or impulses in uncontrolled behavior with apparent disregard for personal or social consequences. It usually occurs in response to interpersonal events with significant people in the subject's life, such as parents, authority figures, friends, or lovers, but the actual victims of the behavior are often relative strangers.

This definition is broader than the original concept of acting out transference feelings or wishes during psychotherapy. It includes behavior arising both within and outside of the transference relationship. It is not synonymous with "bad behavior," or with any symptom per se, although acting out often involves socially disruptive or self-destructive behavior. So-called acting-out behaviors, such as physical fighting or compulsive drug use, must show some relationship to affects or impulses that the person cannot tolerate in order to serve as evidence for the defense of acting out.

A complete rating manual with examples may be obtained from J. Christopher Perry, M.D., M.P.H. (for address see contributors' list).

Passive-aggression (turning against the self)   The individual deals with emotional conflicts, or internal or external stressors, by indirectly, un-assertively, and often self-detrimentally expressing aggression toward others. There is a facade of overt compliance masking covert resistance toward others.

Passive aggression is characterized by venting hostile or resentful feelings in an indirect, veiled, and unassertive manner toward others. Passive aggression often occurs in response to demands for independent action or performance by the subject or when someone has disappointed the subject's wish or sense of entitlement to be taken care of, regardless of whether the subject has made this wish known. Includes "turning against the self."

Hypochondriasis (help-rejecting complaining)*   Hypochondriasis involves the repetitious use of a complaint or series of complaints in which the subject ostensibly asks for help. However, covert feelings of hostility or reproach toward others are expressed simultaneously by the subject's rejection of the suggestions, advice, or help that others offer. The complaints may consist of either life problems or somatic concerns. Either type of complaint is followed by a "help-rejecting complainer" response to whatever help is offered.

Major Image-Distorting Defenses

Splitting   The individual deals with emotional conflicts, or internal or external stressors, by viewing himself or herself or others as all good or all bad, failing to integrate the positive and negative qualities of the self and others into cohesive images. Often the same individual will be alternately idealized and devalued.

In splitting of other's images (object images), the subject demonstrates that his views, expectations and feelings about others are contradictory and that he cannot reconcile ambivalent affects to form realistic and coherent views of others. Others' images are divided into polar opposites, such that the subject can see only one emotional aspect or side of the object at a time. At one time an object will seem only to have such traits as being loving, powerful, worthy, nurturant, and kind, but no attributes of opposite emotional significance. At another time that same object may be seen as bad, hateful, angry, destructive, rejecting, or worthless, and the subject is incapable of seeing any positive attributes. The switch from experiencing an object as good or bad to its opposite is unpredictable.

When the subject uses splitting of object images, he or she cannot integrate anything that does not match his or her immediate experience of and feeling about a given object. All of the attributes with the same feeling tone are highlighted, and contradictory views, expectations, or feelings about the object are excluded from emotional awareness, although not necessarily from cognitive awareness.

Splitting of self-images often occurs alongside splitting of others' images, since both these processes were learned in response to the unpredictability of one's early significant others. In splitting of self-images, the subject demonstrates that he or she has contradictory views, expectations, and feelings about himself or herself that cannot be reconciled into one coherent whole.

The self-images are divided into polar opposites: at a given time the subject's awareness is limited to those aspects of the self having the same emotional feeling tone. He or she sees himself or herself in "black or white" terms. At one point in time the subject believes he himself has good attributes, such as being loving, powerful, worthy, or correct and having good feelings; or he believes the opposite—that he is bad, hateful, angry, destructive, weak, powerless, worthless, or always wrong and has only negative feelings about himself. Moreover, the switch from experiencing the self exclusively in one polar feeling tone to the opposite feeling tone is unpredictable.

Projective identification*   In projective identification the subject has an affect or impulse that he or she finds unacceptable and projects onto someone else, as if it was really that other person who originated the affect or impulse. However, the subject does not disavow what is projected—unlike in simple projection—but remains fully aware of the affects or impulses, and simply misattributes them as justifiable reactions to the other person! Hence, the subject eventually admits his or her affect or impulse, but believes it to be a reaction to those same feelings and impulses in others. The subject confuses the fact that it was he himself who originated the projected material, and, unlike simple projection, believes himself to be the just rather than the unjust victim.

This defense is seen most clearly in a lengthy interchange in which the subject initially projects his or her feelings but later experiences his or her original feelings as reactions to the other. Paradoxically, the subject often arouses the very feelings in others he or she at first mistakenly believed to be there. It is then difficult to clarify who did what to whom first. This process is more extensive than simple projection, which involves the denial and subsequent external attribution of an impulse. Projective identification involves attribution of an image so that the whole object is seen and reacted to in a distorted light.

Autistic fantasy   The individual deals with emotional conflicts, or internal or external stressors, by excessive daydreaming as a substitute for human relationships, more direct and effective action, or problem solving.

Fantasy denotes the use of daydreaming as either a substitute for relationships, dealing with or solving external problems, or as a way of expressing and satisfying one's wishes. While the subject may be aware of the "I'm just pretending" quality of the fantasy, nonetheless, it may be the closest that he or she ever comes to expressing or gratifying the need for satisfying interpersonal relationships.

Disavowal Defenses

Denial (neurotic denial)   The individual deals with emotional conflicts, or internal or external stressors, by refusing to acknowledge some aspect of external reality or of his or her experience that would be apparent to others.

The subject actively denies that a feeling, behaviorial response, or intention was or is not present, even though its presence is considered more than likely by the observer. The subject is blinded to both the ideational and emotional content of what is denied. [This excludes "psychotic denial" in which the subject refuses to acknowledge a physical object or event within the subject's field in the present time.]

Projection   The individual deals with emotional conflicts, or internal or external stressors, by falsely attributing his or her own unacknowledged feelings, impulses, or thought to others. The subject disavows his or her own feelings, intentions, or experience by means of attributing them to others, usually others by whom the subject feels threatened and to whom the subject feels some affinity.

Rationalization   The individual deals with emotional conflicts, or internal or external stressors, by devising reassuring or self-serving but incorrect explanations for his or her own or others' behavior.

Narcissistic or Minor Image-Distorting Defenses

Devaluation   The individual deals with emotional conflicts or internal or external stressors by attributing exaggeratedly negative qualities to oneself or others. Unlike reaction formation, devaluation may conceal admiration or positive feelings toward others.

Omnipotence* Omnipotence is a defense in which the subject responds to emotional conflict or internal and external stressors by acting superior to others, as if one possessed special powers or abilities.

Idealization The individual deals with emotional conflicts, or internal or external stressors, by attributing exaggerated positive qualities to self or others.

Other Neurotic Defenses

Repression The individual deals with emotional conflicts, or internal or external stressors, by being unable to remember or unable to be cognitively aware of disturbing wishes, thoughts, or experiences. In contrast to isolation, the affective component often remains in consciousness.

Dissociation The individual deals with emotional conflicts, or internal or external stressors, by a temporary alteration in the integrative functions of consciousness or identity. In the defense of dissociation, a particular affect or impulse of which the subject is unaware may operate in the subject's life out of normal awareness. Both the idea and associated affect or impulse remain out of awareness but are expressed by an alteration in consciousness. While the subject may be dimly aware that something unusual takes place at such times, full acknowledgement that his or her own affect or impulses are being expressed is not made. Dissociation may result in a loss of function or in counterphobic or uncharacteristic behavior.

Reaction formation The individual deals with emotional conflicts, or internal or external stressors, by substituting behavior, thoughts, or feelings that are diametrically opposed to his or her unacceptable thoughts or feelings.

Displacement The individual deals with emotional conflicts, or internal or external stressors, by generalizing or redirectioning a feeling about or a response to an object onto another, usually less-threatening, object. The person using displacement may or may not be aware that the affect or impulse expressed toward the displaced object was meant for someone else.

Obsessional Defenses

Isolation The individual deals with emotional conflicts, or internal or external stressors, by being unable to experience simultaneously the cognitive and affective components of an experience, because the affect is kept from consciousness. In the defense of isolation, the subject loses touch with the feelings associated with a given idea (e.g., a traumatic event) while remaining aware of its cognitive elements (e.g., descriptive details). Only the affect is lost or detached, while the idea is conscious. It is the converse of repression, where the affect is retained but the the idea is detached and unrecognized.

Intellectualization   The individual deals with emotional conflicts, or internal or external stressors, by the excessive use of abstract thinking or generalizing to avoid experiencing disturbing feelings.

Undoing   The individual deals with emotional conflicts, or internal or external stressors, by words or behavior designed to symbolically make amends for or negate previous thoughts, feelings, or actions.

High Adaptive–Level Defenses

Affiliation*   The individual deals with emotional conflicts, or internal or external stressors, by turning to others for help or support. By affiliating with others, the individual can express himself or herself, confide problems, and feel less alone or isolated with a conflict or problem. This may also result in receiving advice or concrete help. It does not imply trying to make someone else responsible for dealing with one's own problems, coercing someone to help, or covertly reproaching others, as in hypochondriasis. Affiliation is characterized by a give and take around conflicts and problems that occurs in the context of belonging to an organization, or by confiding in someone.

Altruism   The individual deals with emotional conflicts over his or her own needs, or internal or external stressors, by dedication to fulfilling the needs of others. This is only to be rated as present when there is a demonstrable, strong functional relationship between the feelings and the response pattern. Unlike the self-sacrifice sometimes characteristic of reaction formation, the individual using altruism receives some partial gratification either vicariously or as a response from others. The subject is usually aware to some extent that his or her own needs or feelings underlie altruistic actions. There may also be a direct reward or overt self-interested component in the subject's altruistic actions.

Anticipation (affective rehearsal)*   The individual deals with emotional conflicts or internal or external stressors by experiencing modest emotional reactions to possible events ahead of time and then considering realistic, alternative responses or solutions (anticipatory problem solving).

The individual trades off experiencing some distress ahead of time in order to plan for an optimal response later when the stressful situation arises.

Humor* The individual deals with emotional conflict and internal or external stressors by emphasizing the amusing or ironic aspects of the conflict or stressor. Humor tends to relieve the tension around conflict in a way that allows everyone to share in it, rather than being at one person's expense, as in derisive or cutting remarks. An element of self-observation or truth is often involved.

Self-assertion* The individual deals with emotional conflict, or internal or external stressors, by expressing one's feelings and thoughts directly in order to achieve goals. Self-assertion is not coercive or indirect and manipulative. The goal or purpose of the self-assertive behavior is usually made clear to all parties affected by it.

Self-observation* The individual deals with emotional conflicts, or internal or external stressors, by reflecting on his or her own thoughts, feelings, motivation, and behavior. The insight gained by self-observation allows the individual to grow and adapt better as he or she deals with stress. The person is able to "see himself as others see him" in interpersonal situations, and as a result is better able to understand other people's reactions to him or her. The defense is not synonymous with simply making comments or observations about oneself.

Sublimation* The individual deals with emotional conflicts, or internal or external stressors, by channeling potentially maladaptive feelings or impulses into socially acceptable behavior. This defense is to be rated present only when a strong functional relationship can be demonstrated between the feelings and the response pattern. Classic examples of the use of sublimation are sports and games used to channel angry impulses, or artistic creation that expresses conflicted feelings.

Suppression The individual deals with emotional conflicts, or internal or external stressors, by voluntarily avoiding thinking about disturbing problems, wishes, feelings or experiences temporarily. This may entail putting things out of one's mind until the right time to deal with them: it is postponing, not procrastinating. Suppression may also entail avoiding thinking about something at the time because it would distract from engaging in another more pressing activity. Unlike in repression, the individual can call the suppressed material back to conscious attention readily, since it is not forgotten.

Appendix 5

Ego Defense Mechanisms Manual
(Jacobson et al.)*

Overall Success of Defenses

> **Definition:** This scale is a global rating of the effectiveness of the subject's defenses, and an overall measure of the subject's variety and flexibility of responses to internal and external stimuli. Optimal functioning allows for both protection against inappropriate breakthroughs of impulses, thoughts, and actions; and for emotional and cognitive richness through access to a wide range of feelings and fantasies.

1. Minimal: There are many intrusions of autistic ideas, idiosyncratic fantasies, and other manifestations of primary process, and/or there is extreme, disabling rigidity of defenses.

2. Little: The subject demonstrates various breakthroughs of inappropriate ideas and affects, and/or has rigid defenses that impair functioning and decrease richness of response.

3. Moderate: The subject's defenses allow for adequate functioning in structured or comfortable settings, but break down or become rigid in other contexts.

4. Considerable: Defenses are adequate against unwanted intrusions in most situations, but there is some reduction in richness of response and/or breakthrough of anxiety in others.

5. Maximal: The subject has adequate and flexible defenses that both protect against unwanted intrusions and allow for emotional and cognitive richness in almost all situations.

X. Cannot say.

---

*The authors of this manual are Alan M. Jacobson, M.D., William Beardslee, M.D., Stuart T. Hauser, M.D., Ph.D., Gil G. Noam, Ed.D., Sally I. Powers, Ed.D., and Elizabeth Gelfand, Ed.D.

Overall Success of Defenses: Examples

Rating 1: Minimal

The subject shows many inappropriate affective responses and manifestations of primary process. He becomes enraged at the slightest provocation
and lashes out physically at others. He trusts no one and is suspicious and
occasionally paranoid in relationships. This adolescent experiences continu-
ous intrusions of fears and idiosyncratic thoughts and fantasies that severely
impair his ability to function.

This youngster is able to function only within a highly circumscribed
portion of his living quarters, and only by sticking to his extremely rigid
routines. He feels that the most ordinary actions—brushing his teeth, tying
his shoes—have to be performed in an invariant, ritualistic way or something
terrible will happen. If these routines and rituals are disrupted, he becomes
very agitated, and either withdraws into fantasy or immediately resumes the
ritual at its beginning. This rigidity extends to virtually all areas of his behavior and seriously compromises his ability to function.

Rating 2: Little

The subject shows varying breakthroughs of inappropriate affects and ideas.
He describes several impulsive expressions and "temper" episodes during
the interview. At one point he lashes out verbally at the interviewer, belittling her and refusing to answer the anxiety- provoking questions she asks.
After this outburst he almost leaves the interview, but is able to regain his
composure long enough to complete it in a perfunctory way.

Another subject, a young woman, was difficult to interview because she
was so constricted emotionally and intellectually. Her answers to questions
were sparse and conventional, reflecting her inability to express feelings or
to tolerate open-ended questions. She manages to function in school by
keeping to herself and only doing written assignments, since she is unable
to speak spontaneously in class or in social situations.

Rating 3: Moderate

This subject can function adequately within the familiar patterns of his life:
at his structured job and with his family and circle of friends. But he becomes
shy and uncomfortable with new people, or if his routines are disrupted, or
if he has to deal with too many unusual demands.

Rating 4: Considerable

Much of the time this subject is able to talk about significant feelings and
experiences with appropriate affect. But there is at times a flat, colorless

quality to his relating: he occasionally analyzes and interprets, or turns away from rather than feels, aspects of conflictual situations; and sometimes he leaves confrontations in order to deal with them. He is able to postpone most conflicts or impulses that intrude on smooth functioning, but is on occasion unable to relax and get involved with an enjoyable situation.

This adolescent is able to function smoothly in most situations. He is comfortable in school, being able to negotiate the challenges of the academic curriculum and the social setting without undue anxiety or self-doubt. In dating situations with girls, however, he reports that he sometimes becomes shy and a bit tongue-tied—not the funny, easy-going kid that he is with his chums on the basketball team. He says that he feels close to and gets along well with most members of his family, but on occasion "blows up" at his little brother when "he acts too cute in front of the parents."

Rating 5: Maximal

The subject shows adequate and flexible defenses in virtually all situations. She is usually aware of her thoughts, feelings, and impulses, and is free to choose whether to act on them or not; she reports no impulsive behavior. She does not negate or minimize feelings or reactions to situations, and willingly engages in discussing significant persons and events with a full, appropriate range of affects. She describes with richness her feelings, attitudes, and actions in a variety of situations, and can fantasize about wanting to do certain things contrary to her usual behavior without feeling either the need to act on these thoughts or guilt at having them.

Acting Out

Definition: Acting out refers to the behavioral expression of an unconscious wish or impulse in order to avoid the affect that would accompany its conscious recognition. Acting out may occur through the omission of a normally adjustive, appropriate behavior; or it may include the use of physical actions (such as overeating), delinquent, antisocial, or impulsive acts, and "tempers" to avoid awareness of feelings.

1. Minimal: The subject reports no impulsive acts, drug use, self-inflicted injuries, antisocial acts, etc. There may be rare or subtle hints of acting out.

2. Little: The subject gives a few descriptions of minor acting-out episodes, or has apparent interest in acting out.

3. Moderate: The subject reports some impulsive actions. They are a clear aspect of the subject's life.

4. Considerable: The subject describes several episodes of acting out, or a few striking examples that imply a consistent pattern. For example, the subject may report frequent physical fights, or a pattern of sexual promiscuity, or one of substance abuse.

5. Maximal: Almost all experiences of tension, anxiety, or other strong affects are responded to by direct actions or behaviors. Chronic drug use, stealing, binge eating, or self-inflicted injury are examples of behaviors utilized consistently to relieve the experience of affect, and hence constitute acting out.

X. Cannot say.

Acting Out: Examples

Similar examples have been developed for the other defenses in this manual and can be obtained from Alan M. Jacobson, M.D., on request.

Rating 1: Minimal

The subject shows no examples of impulsive or other acting-out behavior during the interview. Indeed, in situations that normally lead to such behavior she neither acts out herself nor indicates any vicarious thrill in others' acting out. For example, when describing how friends of hers use pot and other drugs, she says that she does not use them, and she does not even describe any pleasurable excitement at her friends' behavior.

   In addition, she describes how her mother lets her do a lot of things and trusts her a lot, for example, by letting her borrow money or stay up late, because mother knows that she'll do the right thing. "Like, I can stay up as late as I want because she knows I know what time to go to bed; when I am tired I go to bed, and so she just lets me do a lot of things." As this example demonstrates, the subject does not even hint at a temptation to act out.

   The subject reported no instances during her interview of acting-out behavior or fantasies, although she gave rich descriptions of her feelings, attitudes, and actions in a variety of situations. For example, she discussed at length painful disagreements with a brother who was extremely provocative—teasing and hitting her.

   On no occasion did she describe times where she initiated these fights or where she later made retaliations of an impulsive nature; at most she occasionally hit him back after he had begun hitting her. In describing her friendships she reported that she and some of her friends were involved in sexual activities. These seemed to represent age-appropriate experimentation, rather than acting out.

Rating 2: Little

The subject indicates interest in acting out although he does not generally evidence that interest in his behavior. For example, he fantasizes about getting drunk with friends, but does not engage in drunkenness. During the interview the subject was able to contemplate emotionally laden questions without bringing up past experiences. As a diabetic he sometimes will sneak food he should not have because he cannot stand not to satisfy his sweet tooth. He usually controls his diet well and has had no bouts of diabetic ketoacidosis caused by excessive eating or mis-taking of insulin.

Rating 3: Moderate

This young woman describes a number of impulsive expressions and "temper" episodes during the interview: "I usually . . . . she gets mad at me . . . . she likes to take things away from me, and I'm pretty spoiled, so I stomp and cry, you know." In addition, the subject reports occasional overeating when tense or depressed. These incidents are sprinkled throughout the interview, but do not seem to be a predominant feature in her life; thus, she is rated a 3 and not a 4.

Rating 4: Considerable

Action is a predominant mode of responding for this youngster, who reports antisocial acts, frequent bouts of beer drinking, and temper outbursts at individuals whom he finds irritating. While many of this person's actions are antisocial, it is not this fact that makes them acting out; rather it is the avoidance of affects and the impulsive, unplanned nature of the acts that make them acting out. For example, he planned to attend school one day after skipping excessively: "We'd go sit in the first period class and then say, 'Aw, this ain't for me,' and we'd leave."

On rare occasions this young man can plan. For example, tutoring was being arranged which conflicted with a job. Rather than simply quitting the job, he gave 2 weeks' notice.

But these moments of being able to tolerate feelings are not predictable. When asked what sorts of things really get his temper up, he said, "I dunno. Just something, like once something was said to me that I didn't like, and I just went nuts."

Another subject handles many of her emotional conflicts through acting out. Although she is capable of doing school work when her feelings are in abeyance, this young woman frequently tears up her homework in frustration. Her disagreements with her parents often result in shouting and tears; her reaction to their strict dress rules and curfews is provocative dress and promiscuous sexual behavior away from the home.

Rating 5: Maximal

The subject becomes anxious during the interview and cannot contain his impulses. Asked about school, he gets up and kicks a plant, breaking off a leaf. When the interviewer tries to set a limit verbally, the subject gets angry and pulls the cord of the tape recorder. There is much evidence from snatches of talk that this behavior is consistent with his daily experiences outside the interview.

The subject describes many violent incidents. He recalls pulling a knife on someone when feeling threatened. A short period of work with the Guardian Angels in Boston was followed by participation in street crime. The subject also described physical fights at home during which he threatened the life of his father. From his descriptions, virtually all instances of conflict or arousal end in some form of impulsive action devoid of experienced feeling.

Altruism

Definition: Altruism involves the surrender of direct gratification of needs in favor of vicarious satisfaction gained through service to others. Altruistic activities include philanthropy, well-repaid services, and open giving of oneself and one's time in an interview. Openness or talkativeness in the interview does not by itself constitute evidence of altruism, although it may be suggestive. To rate a subject as altruistic from the interview behavior there should be clear indications that the person intends to be helpful to or considerate of the interviewer and/or the abstract others who may gain benefit from the research.

Altruism differs from projection and acting out in that it provides real, not imaginary, benefits to others; from reaction formation in that it redirects instinctual gratifications rather than opposing them; and from asceticism in that it substitutes indirect gratification for renunciation.

1. Minimal: Few or no altruistic involvements are reported by the subject.

2. Little: The subject does not seek out opportunities for altruistic behavior, but may show some tendency to altruism in close relationships.

3. Moderate: The subject engages in some altruistic activities   through charities, social causes, friendships, or helpfulness in the interview.

4. Considerable: The subject is very interested in helping others, e.g., by becoming a devoted doctor to patients, teacher to students, or a social reformer. Although other relationships exist with people, they are considerably less important to this subject than the helping ones.

5. Maximal: The subject's relationships with others and main activities all center around altruism; he or she is selfless and giving, finding satisfaction in others' happiness.

X. Cannot say.

Altruism: Examples

Rating 1: Minimal

There are no signs of altruistic trends in this subject. He uses others, instead of helping them. If he decides he does not like someone for whatever reason, he will gratify his wish to hurt that person. Money in his pocket feels good to him, and satisfaction comes from spending it on himself, not on others. His interests include fixing motorcycles and cars because "I can make a lot of money on auto body, with everybody's dents, and everybody wants their car to look like a hot rod."

Rating 2: Little

The subject was rated as a 2 because he described only one relationship in which he behaved altruistically. He gave to no charities, he participated in no philanthropic activities, he was not especially generous with his time, nor was he forthcoming with descriptions of himself in the interview. His discussions were spare, and on at least two occasions he looked at the clock in hopes that the interview was over, because he felt it was taking up his time, although he denied that the discussions were particularly painful.

However, in his description of the relationship with his father there was one clear example of altruistic activity. While he and his father apparently had many fights around his problems in school and difficulties with mother, the young man described saving money from a summer job to buy his father a tool set that the father can use in his trade. In addition, he likes to help his father garden in the summertime. When the father offered him money for his work, he turned it down, saying that he just wanted to help out. There are no other examples of altruistic activity or hints at altruistic thinking.

Although another subject displayed some empathic understanding toward a troubled sister, she did not describe any situations where she actually helped others out or where she got pleasure from helping. For example, although she described herself as somewhat concerned about this sister, she only wrote to her twice a year. There were no other examples of altruistic involvement.

Rating 3: Moderate

There are some signs of altruistic trends. The subject is willing to give considerable amounts of information, even about uncomfortable topics. This willingness to talk about such material is based on a self-declared wish to be helpful, rather than a need for relief or self-expression. He describes giving as an important feature of relationships. When asked about wanting to be a dominant figure, he says, "Well, I do in a sense, but no, because when you become the dominant figure you have lost all 'we' relationships; everything is you giving, and I like to receive too, but I don't want to be receiving everything; I like to give, too. I like to be in a definite 'we' relationship." In another statement the subject expresses his desire for aid and assistance to the poor people in foreign countries, and he shows some rather idealistic veneration for certain people who devote their lives to this kind of work.

While another subject reported no specific instances of philanthropy, she was quite willing, in her personal relationship, to surrender direct gratification in order to fulfill the needs of others. For example, during the interview she was open in her discussion of problems and at the end of the interview revealed that this openness stemmed, at least in part, from a wish to help the interviewer in her work. At the end of the interview, the interviewer said that she had asked all the questions she could think of, and asked if there were any important areas that had not been discussed. The subject's response was to say, "No, as long as you know about me as much as you need to know." In describing babysitting work the girl noted that other kids frequently charge more than she did. She mentioned, in explaining how she handles the fees for babysitting, that she really enjoys the work. "People think I get gypped, because usually high school kids ask for $1.50 an hour and if people ask me what I get paid I just say a dollar. But if they don't ask, fine, I'll take what they pay me because that's really the rate. But I don't see why I should charge so much if all I do is put the kids to bed and watch television and have fun. It's an easy job if the kids are quiet, and I like doing it."

The subject was not rated higher than a 3 because there were many instances in which she did not surrender to the needs of others. For example, she reported that when her friends wished to talk about subjects in which she was not interested, for example sex and boys, she was quite willing to tell them that she did not want to talk about these things and to change the subject, or at a slumber party, to roll over and go to sleep. With her brother, who often teased and fought with her, she either avoided his teasing by leaving the room or on occasion fought back verbally and physically.

Rating 4: Considerable

The subject has a strong interest in helping others and in being charitable, thoughtful, and available. This is true in his open and committed behavior with the interviewer and the study, and with friends. He values being supportive to friends when they need him, although this is not the exclusive pattern of his friendships. For example, he has some friends of whom he asks favors, and others whom he feels prompted to protect: "I have a friend who's got to be interviewed, and he's, he's a good kid, but he's got sort of a mixed up family, and I just like to stay with him; I think I can give him support, and he's my friend. I need to study for an exam this afternoon, but I think it's more important to be here for him."

At another point he mentioned passing up an opportunity to look smart in front of a teacher because he knew that the friend he had worked with on the project had not prepared for class and was feeling anxious about being found out.

Rating 5: Maximal

The subject is preoccupied with the welfare of others and puts herself out continuously to help others. She is a volunteer in her town's hospice program, a tutor for non-English speaking students in her high school, and a "candy striper" at a local hospital. These actions make her feel fulfilled and give her a sense of purpose in life. She feels selfish unless others benefit from her actions: personal gain and comfort hold little interest for her.

Asceticism

Definition: Asceticism aims at the elimination or avoidance of pleasurable experience and is directed against all consciously perceived physical enjoyment. Gratification comes from renunciation of needs and pleasures; hence, biological or sensual satisfactions are forbidden, whereas nonsensual joy is countenanced. Asceticism may be part of an ethical, religious, or moral concern, and one may find a moralistic tone present in the judgments of self and others.

1. Minimal: The subject displays no interest in inhibiting pleasure seeking, is not preoccupied with selflessness, is not critical of others for their sensuality, and is almost disinhibited.

2. Little: The subject is not critical of others for excessive pleasures, is not preoccupied with the issue of satisfaction vs. renunciation, and is almost neutral—not controlling but also not wild.

3. Moderate: The subject may eschew certain pleasures, such as drugs or sex, while advocating and enjoying others. He or she holds some "antipleasure" values, but also engages in some sensually gratifying activities such as dancing and contact sports.

4. Considerable: The subject renounces many if not most physical pleasures. He or she has some areas of sensual satisfaction, but they are limited and closely monitored.

5. Maximal: The subject lives an extremely Spartan existence, forswearing physical comfort and material display. S/he is concerned only with spiritual, intellectual, or esthetic satisfactions and finds bodily pleasure irrelevant and distasteful.

X. Cannot say.

Asceticism: Examples

Rating 1: Minimal

The subject gets pleasure from immediate gratification. There is no second-guessing of animal pleasure, or guilt over getting what he wants even if it really does hurt someone else. He likes money in his pocket, and he likes to spend it. "I'd have, like over a hundred dollars on me. And in 2 days, it would be gone. I'd buy pot, I'd buy mescaline—just to get a kick out of the stuff."

Rating 2: Little

The subject is not critical of others for enjoying pleasurable activities. She participates in sports and some mild amounts of drug and alcohol use for pleasure. On the other hand, she is quite capable of controlling these activities and limiting them to social occasions. She works hard in school and at sports, and derives pleasure from her accomplishments in these areas. While she gives no specific examples of renouncing pleasure for herself, or of criticizing others for their pleasures, neither does she give examples of a kind of wild, free pleasure or enjoyment for herself. Thus, by implication, she is not totally without asceticism, and is rated as "little."

Another subject was rated a 2 because there are no descriptions of intense interest in prohibiting pleasure or in seeking pleasure. For example, at no time does he deride others for membership in religious groups that are antipleasure, or criticize people for letting loose at parties. Rather, the transcript is devoid of criticisms in either direction. He does seem to have some fun at making money, although he uses the money for saving for the future rather than for giving himself pleasures now. He would be rated lower if there were examples in which he used the money or described a great deal of interest in occasions of pleasure, e.g., drinking, drug taking, sexual activities. Transcript is, overall, generally neutral regarding asceticism.

Rating 3: Moderate

This adolescent evidences some criticism or renunciation of pleasure for herself and for others, yet also participates in some enjoyable peer activities. She derives satisfaction from "being good," and notes that at times she feels uncomfortable with kids her own age because "I think smoking pot and stuff like that is all right since it's way better than smoking cigarettes, but it's something that I don't want to do." On the other hand, she mentions that she would like to spend more time with certain of her friends, the kids who are "like her": who aren't into partying, but who enjoy going to Harvard Square and tasting different foods, listening to street musicians, and playing touch football.

Rating 4: Considerable

This adolescent strongly criticizes the pleasure-seeking activities of her peers and sets herself apart: "I know 15-year-olds who smoke grass and hang around and start screaming and yelling. It's bad, it looks bad, and I don't want to be in that kind of group." Similarly, sexual activity is perceived as "doing thing together; disgusting, perverted things." She is mistrustful of her peers who enjoy themselves socially at parties: she sees them as "loose and immature" and avoids them. This subject's strong objection to sensual pleasure is a salient feature of the transcript. She is, however, comfortable enjoying folk dancing and nature walks in mixed groups.

Rating 5: Maximal

The subject, a 17-year-old adolescent, has developed an ideology renouncing any form of worldly pleasure. He is highly critical of any form of materialism such as spending money for clothes or other personal comforts. He is also opposed to any sexual intimacies, feeling that they detract from dedication to the spiritual life. He is very intolerant of people who are pleasure-seekers and feels that society should make it impossible to live comfortably. He feels that only the strengthening of body and soul through austerity makes life worth living.

Avoidance

Definition: Avoidance entails an active "turning away" from conflict-laden thoughts, objects, feelings, or experiences. The avoidance can take many forms, including leaving a distressing situation, walking away from a discussion, closing the eyes, or refusing to talk about something. With avoidance there is an evasion of what one feels to be conflictual; with denial there is more likely a lack of awareness of the disturbing stimuli or events.

1. Minimal: The subject rarely turns away from or leaves situations of conflict.

2. Little: The subject occasionally departs from or refuses to face conflictual experiences, thoughts, or objects.

3. Moderate: There are some instances of turning away from and/or physically withdrawing from situations. In the interview, the subject may refuse to talk about certain uncomfortable topics.

4. Considerable: There are many instances of withdrawal or staying away from conflict-arousing situations or topics, both within and without the interview situation. Frequent refusals to speak may occur at this level.

5. Maximal: Turning away from disturbing thoughts, people, and situations is a common occurrence in this subject's life. If difficult situations or occasions arise, the subject almost always withdraws from or evades them.

X. Cannot say.

Avoidance: Examples

Examples of avoidance and the other defenses in this manual can be obtained from Alan M. Jacobson, M.D., on request.

Denial

Definition: Denial involves the automatic refusal to acknowledge painful or disturbing aspects of inner or outer reality. At the low end of the scale denial is evidenced by minor lapses in awareness, and by efforts at minimizing discomfort and looking for the good in difficult situations. At the high end, external reality is denied: "I am not in the hospital; this is my country club." In mid range, the painful or frightening import of events or perceptions is denied, although the evidence itself is acknowledged: "This cough has nothing to do with my cigarette smoking."

Denial contrasts with repression, which allows the affect surrounding a conflict to be experienced without awareness of the content; and with suppression, which entails the conscious or semiconscious decision to postpone, but not to forget or avoid, a painful reality. Denial's effectiveness may be enhanced through exaggeration, negation, and fantasy formation.

1. Minimal: Evidence of denial is rare or negligible.

2. Little: The subject may have occasional lapses in awareness of events or feelings and/or may minimize the importance of certain thoughts or feelings.

3. Moderate: The subject shows some minimizing, unawareness, or negation of, fantasies about, or exaggerations of events, thoughts, or feelings.

4. Considerable: The subject frequently negates thoughts and feelings and/or the implications of events. This pattern may be accompanied by a mild euphoric affect that supports the denial.

5. Maximal: Distortions of thoughts, feelings, and even events through denial are very frequent and may reach psychotic proportions.

X. Cannot say.

Displacement

Definition: Displacement refers to the purposeful (albeit unconscious) redirection of feelings toward a safer or less important object than the person or situation arousing the feelings or impulses. The feelings remain the same, but their object is changed. Displacement involves the discharge of emotions, often angry or erotic, onto things, animals, or people perceived as less dangerous by the individual than those with whom the feelings were originally evoked.

1. Minimal: There is no or only minor evidence of misdirected feelings or thoughts.

2. Little: The subject has occasional episodes of misdirecting thoughts or feelings, e.g. unexplained annoyance with a sibling or pet after a conflict with a friend.

3. Moderate: The subject sometimes defensively redirects thoughts and feelings away from their original targets; at other times, he or she appropriately connects them with the persons or situations that evoked them.

4. Considerable: There are many instances of "taking it out" on others, e.g., punching walls after a frustrating day at school, or studying animal mating behavior to conceal one's own sexual interests.

5. Maximal: Virtually all thoughts and feelings are misdirected to inappropriate people or situations. Only rarely does the subject direct thoughts and feelings toward the persons or situations that evoked them.

X. Cannot say.

Intellectualization

Definition: Intellectualization refers to thinking as a special and limited variety of doing—as a mode of controlling affects and impulses by thinking them instead of experiencing the feelings associated with them. The person employing intellectualization uses the thinking process defensively, as a substitute for and protection against emotion and impulse. As a result, he or she emphasizes reason, devoid of affect, and tends to give blandly abstract, esoteric, or logical explanations of internal and external conditions. Intellectualization differs from rationalization, which is justification of irrational behavior through clichés, stories, and pat explanations.

1. Minimal: Evidence of intellectualization is rare.

2. Little: There is occasional use of abstractions, devoid of feeling, in responding to internal or external stimuli.

3. Moderate: In some situations, the subject interprets or analyzes feelings instead of experiencing them; in other situations, he or she acknowledges the feelings.

4. Considerable: The subject frequently makes bland verbalizations about emotion-laden topics and offers "explanations" of conflicts devoid of feeling. In some situations, however, he or she experiences affect along with ideas.

5. Maximal: Almost all inner experiences and external events are discussed logically or philosophically, as a way of excluding emotion.

X. Cannot say.

Projection

Definition: Projection involves the unconscious rejection of one's own unacceptable thoughts, traits, feelings, or wishes, and the attribution of them to other people. It is the perception and treatment of certain inner impulses, affects, and thoughts as if they were outside the self, as a way of making awareness of them tolerable. The rejected elements may be thoughts or feelings, wishes to do things, or criticisms.

Projection may be expressed through severe prejudice, rejection of intimacy, unwarranted suspicion, hypervigilance to danger, injustice-collecting, or exaggerated attention to others' sexual interests and behavior.

1. Minimal: There is rare evidence of projection. The subject recognizes his or her thoughts and feelings as originating in the self.

2. Little: There are few examples of projection. Only occasionally does the subject misattribute thoughts or feelings to others.

3. Moderate: The subject mistakenly perceives some thoughts or feelings as originating in others, but recognizes other ideas and affects as his or her own.

4. Considerable: The subject often perceives others to be the origins of his or her own disavowed wishes, thoughts, or feelings. This results in marked social anxiety and defensiveness, hyper-alertness, and/or mistrust-fulness.

5. Maximal: The subject perceives virtually all of his or her unacceptable thoughts, feelings, and impulses as originating in others. There are frequent marked distortions of a suspicious or grandiose nature.

X. Cannot say.

Rationalization

Definition: Rationalization refers to common-sense, utilitarian justifications of internal and external conditions. It is an effort to justify attitudes, beliefs, or behaviors that are irrational or otherwise unacceptable by the arbitrary application of a truth—a so-called "logical explanation"—or by the invention of a convincing fallacy.

Rationalization is the unconsciously motivated and involuntary act of giving logical and believable explanations for irrational behaviors that have been prompted by unacceptable, unconscious wishes or by the defenses used to cope with such wishes. It is the use of commonplace expressions or clichés to cover over puzzling, shameful, or embarrassing actions.

Rationalization differs from intellectualization—which also refers to the use of thoughts to handle unacceptable feelings and impulses—in that its aim is self-justification, rather than masking of painful affects.

1. Minimal: Use of false justifications of ideas or behaviors is rare.

2. Little: Infrequent or modest efforts are made at rationalizing views or actions.

3. Moderate: There is some resorting to "logical explanations" or clichés to explain away personal actions or feelings.

4. Considerable: Many attempts are made at justifying irrational behaviors and feelings with "common-sense" explanations. This is a recurrent theme in the interview material.

5. Maximal: The subject attempts to "explain" (away) virtually all irrational behaviors and foibles and is preoccupied with justifying himself or herself.

X. Cannot say.

Repression

Definition: Repression consists of an unconsciously motivated forgetting or unawareness of external events or of internal impulses, feelings, thoughts, or wishes. Although the repressed is not recognized consciously, its effects remain.

Repression may be expressed in a variety of ways that will enable the rater to distinguish it from simple forgetting. When repression is expressed as forgetting, the persistence of the repressed in the unconscious may be sensed directly by the subject—in the feeling that one "ought" to know what has been forgotten, or even that does know it "somehow," that it is "on the tip of the tongue"—or indirectly, when feeling is retained without memory. The forgetting associated with repression is unique in that it may be accompanied by a subjective sense that the repressed is not really forgotten; or by symbolic behavior, such as "accident-proneness," or shaking one's fist while saying that one is not angry. Repression may also be expressed as unawareness, e.g., unawareness that one's behavior is at odds with one's conscious intentions, or unawareness of the impact of one's behavior on others, or of how others will interpret one's actions, or restriction from awareness of certain fantasies or feelings.

Repression differs from suppression [which only postpones awareness] by effecting unconscious inhibition of thoughts, impulses, or memories; and from denial [in which awareness of inner or outer stimuli and of reactions to them is blocked] by restricting conscious awareness of thoughts, impulses, and memories, while leaving the feelings associated with them present. If a man wiped away his tears and said he would wait until later to cry, he would be utilizing suppression; if the weeping man said that he was not crying, he would be using denial; if he said that he didn't know why he was crying, he would be exhibiting repression.

1. Minimal: There are only minor indications of the use of repression.

2. Little: There are only a few examples of repression; the subject does not generally forget significant life experiences.

3. Moderate: There are several instances of forgetting of conflict-laden situations and/or unawareness of how one's actions affect others.

4. Considerable: There are frequent examples of forgetting and restriction of fantasies and impulses from awareness.

5. Maximal: There is marked restriction in awareness of impulses, and inhibition of curiosity. There are very frequent lapses in memory.

X. Cannot say.

Suppression

Definition: Suppression is the conscious or semiconscious decision to postpone (but not to avoid) paying attention to a conscious impulse, feeling, or conflict. It is a mechanism that temporarily removes a disturbing thought, feeling, fantasy, or impulse from awareness so that it can be dealt with at a more convenient or opportune time in the future. Suppression is differentiated from rationalization, where the point is to evade; and from denial and repression, which are attempts at permanent removal from awareness. The person utilizing suppression returns to the subject at a later time.

1. Minimal: Only rarely does the subject elect to postpone concern with a particular thought or anxiety.

2. Little: Occasionally the subject chooses to postpone considering some conflicts and stresses.

3. Moderate: The subject sometimes postpones attending to disturbing feelings, conflicts, or experiences. At other times he or she responds to them as they arise.

4. Considerable: The subject often postpones dealing with disturbing feelings, conflicts, and experiences when it is useful to do so, but will occasionally be unable to postpone attending to a conflict.

5. Maximal: The subject almost always postpones handling conflicts and disturbing thoughts and feelings when it is useful to do so.

X. Cannot say.

Turning Against the Self

Definition: This mechanism entails turning back upon the self an aggressive impulse directed against another person. Turning against the self is displacement onto oneself, the singular displacement of using oneself as the object. This means that the identity of the original object of hostility remains obscure, and sometimes the emotion itself remains outside conscious awareness. When hostility is turned inward on the self, the person may injure himself or herself physically or in other ways—socially, financially, academically, professionally, etc. Certain procrastinations, failures, and provocative behaviors (including passive-aggressive ones) may be reflections of this mechanism. There must be evidence not only of selfdestructive behavior, but also of previous hostility toward another: getting into trouble per se does not indicate turning against the self.

Examples of turning against the self include the following: 1) After being irritated with his mother, the subject refuses to study for the next day's exam, or he punches a brick wall with his bare fist. 2) Angry with his teacher, another subject flagrantly misbehaves in class, thereby provoking public criticism of him by the teacher.

1. Minimal: Instances of turning aggressive impulses against the self are rare or nonexistent in the transcript.

2. Little: Although present, actions directed against the self are not frequent or significant for the subject.

3. Moderate: Some examples are present in which the subject brings down on himself or herself humiliating or otherwise self-destructive consequences following angry arousal toward another.

4. Considerable: Frequent self-induced disturbances appear in the transcript, leading one to consider the subject a self-destructive, masochistic person.

5. Maximal: The subject responds to almost all instances of aggressive stirrings by turning them against the self through self-destructive acts.

X. Cannot say.

Appendix 6

Bond's Defense Style Questionnaire (DSQ)
(1984 Version)

INSTRUCTIONS

This questionnaire consists of 88 statements, each of which is followed by a rating scale:

Strongly Disagree 1 2 3 4 5 6 7 8 9 Strongly Agree

Rate the degree to which you agree or disagree with each statement and write your rating from one to nine on the answer sheet.

Example:

#. **Montreal is a city in Canada.**

Strongly Disagree 1 2 3 4 5 6 7 8 9 Strongly Agree

You would choose 9 and write 9 on the answer sheet beside the statement number.

Asterisk indicates the 67 items used by Vaillant in Chapter 8.

*1. **I get satisfaction from helping others and if this were taken away from me I would get depressed.**

Strongly Disagree 1 2 3 4 5 6 7 8 9 Strongly Agree

*2. **People often call me a sulker.**

Strongly Disagree 1 2 3 4 5 6 7 8 9 Strongly Agree

Questionnaire devised by Michael Bond, M.D.. Scoring manual available from Dr. Bond (see contributors' list for address).

*3. I'm able to keep a problem out of my mind until I have time to deal with it.

Strongly Disagree 1 2 3 4 5 6 7 8 9 Strongly Agree

*4. I'm always treated unfairly.

Strongly Disagree 1 2 3 4 5 6 7 8 9 Strongly Agree

*5. I work out my anxiety through doing something constructive and creative like painting or woodwork.

Strongly Disagree 1 2 3 4 5 6 7 8 9 Strongly Agree

*6. Once in a while I put off until tomorrow what I ought to do today.

Strongly Disagree 1 2 3 4 5 6 7 8 9 Strongly Agree

*7. I keep getting into the same type of frustrating situations and I don't know why.

Strongly Disagree 1 2 3 4 5 6 7 8 9 Strongly Agree

*8. I'm able to laugh at myself pretty easily.

Strongly Disagree 1 2 3 4 5 6 7 8 9 Strongly Agree

*9. I act like a child when I'm frustrated.

Strongly Disagree 1 2 3 4 5 6 7 8 9 Strongly Agree

*10. I'm very shy about standing up for my rights with people.

Strongly Disagree 1 2 3 4 5 6 7 8 9 Strongly Agree

*11. I am superior to most people I know.

Strongly Disagree 1 2 3 4 5 6 7 8 9 Strongly Agree

*12. People tend to mistreat me.

Strongly Disagree 1 2 3 4 5 6 7 8 9 Strongly Agree

*13. If someone mugged me and stole my money, I'd rather he'd be helped than punished.

Strongly Disagree 1 2 3 4 5 6 7 8 9 Strongly Agree

*14. Once in a while I think of things too bad to talk about.

Strongly Disagree 1 2 3 4 5 6 7 8 9 Strongly Agree

*15. **Once in a while I laugh at a dirty joke.**

Strongly Disagree 1 2 3 4 5 6 7 8 9 Strongly Agree

*16. **People say I'm like an ostrich with my head buried in the sand. In other words, I tend to ignore unpleasant facts as if they didn't exit.**

Strongly Disagree 1 2 3 4 5 6 7 8 9 Strongly Agree

*17. **I stop myself from going all out in a competition.**

Strongly Disagree 1 2 3 4 5 6 7 8 9 Strongly Agree

*18. **I often feel superior to people I'm with.**

Strongly Disagree 1 2 3 4 5 6 7 8 9 Strongly Agree

*19. **Someone is robbing me emotionally of all I've got.**

Strongly Disagree 1 2 3 4 5 6 7 8 9 Strongly Agree

*20. **I get angry sometimes.**

Strongly Disagree 1 2 3 4 5 6 7 8 9 Strongly Agree

*21. **I often am driven to act impulsively.**

Strongly Disagree 1 2 3 4 5 6 7 8 9 Strongly Agree

*22. **I'd rather starve than be forced to eat.**

Strongly Disagree 1 2 3 4 5 6 7 8 9 Strongly Agree

*23. **I ignore danger as if I were Superman.**

Strongly Disagree 1 2 3 4 5 6 7 8 9 Strongly Agree

*24. **I pride myself on my ability to cut people down to size.**

Strongly Disagree 1 2 3 4 5 6 7 8 9 Strongly Agree

*25. **People tell me I have a persecution complex.**

Strongly Disagree 1 2 3 4 5 6 7 8 9 Strongly Agree

*26. **Sometimes when I am not feeling well I am cross.**

Strongly Disagree 1 2 3 4 5 6 7 8 9 Strongly Agree

*27. **I often act impulsively when something is bothering me.**

Strongly Disagree 1 2 3 4 5 6 7 8 9 Strongly Agree

*28. **I get physically ill when things aren't going well for me.**

Strongly Disagree 1   2   3   4   5   6   7   8   9   Strongly Agree

*29. **I'm a very inhibited person.**

Strongly Disagree 1   2   3   4   5   6   7   8   9   Strongly Agree

*30. **I'm a real put-down artist.**

Strongly Disagree 1   2   3   4   5   6   7   8   9   Strongly Agree

*31. **I do not always tell the truth.**

Strongly Disagree 1   2   3   4   5   6   7   8   9   Strongly Agree

*32. **I withdraw from people when I feel hurt.**

Strongly Disagree 1   2   3   4   5   6   7   8   9   Strongly Agree

*33. **I often push myself so far that other people have to set limits for me.**

Strongly Disagree 1   2   3   4   5   6   7   8   9   Strongly Agree

*34. **My friends see me as a clown.**

Strongly Disagree 1   2   3   4   5   6   7   8   9   Strongly Agree

*35. **I withdraw when I'm angry.**

Strongly Disagree 1   2   3   4   5   6   7   8   9   Strongly Agree

*36. **I tend to be on my guard with people who turn out to be more friendly than I would have suspected.**

Strongly Disagree 1   2   3   4   5   6   7   8   9   Strongly Agree

*37. **I've got special talents that allow me to go through life with no problems.**

Strongly Disagree 1   2   3   4   5   6   7   8   9   Strongly Agree

*38. **Sometimes at elections I vote for men about whom I know very little.**

Strongly Disagree 1   2   3   4   5   6   7   8   9   Strongly Agree

*39. **I'm often late for appointments.**

Strongly Disagree 1   2   3   4   5   6   7   8   9   Strongly Agree

*40. **I work more things out in my daydreams than in my real life.**
Strongly Disagree 1 2 3 4 5 6 7 8 9 Strongly Agree

*41. **I'm very shy about approaching people.**
Strongly Disagree 1 2 3 4 5 6 7 8 9 Strongly Agree

*42. **I fear nothing.**
Strongly Disagree 1 2 3 4 5 6 7 8 9 Strongly Agree

*43. **Sometimes I think I'm an angel and other times I think I'm a devil.**
Strongly Disagree 1 2 3 4 5 6 7 8 9 Strongly Agree

*44. **I would rather win than lose in a game.**
Strongly Disagree 1 2 3 4 5 6 7 8 9 Strongly Agree

*45. **I get very sarcastic when I'm angry.**
Strongly Disagree 1 2 3 4 5 6 7 8 9 Strongly Agree

*46. **I get openly aggressive when I feel hurt.**
Strongly Disagree 1 2 3 4 5 6 7 8 9 Strongly Agree

*47. **I believe in turning the other cheek when someone hurts me.**
Strongly Disagree 1 2 3 4 5 6 7 8 9 Strongly Agree

*48. **I do not read every editorial in the newspaper every day.**
Strongly Disagree 1 2 3 4 5 6 7 8 9 Strongly Agree

*49. **I withdraw when I'm sad.**
Strongly Disagree 1 2 3 4 5 6 7 8 9 Strongly Agree

*50. **I'm shy about sex.**
Strongly Disagree 1 2 3 4 5 6 7 8 9 Strongly Agree

*51. **I always feel that someone I know is like a guardian angel.**
Strongly Disagree 1 2 3 4 5 6 7 8 9 Strongly Agree

*52. **My philosophy is, "Hear no evil, do no evil, see no evil."**
Strongly Disagree 1 2 3 4 5 6 7 8 9 Strongly Agree

*53. **As far as I'm concerned, people are either good or bad.**

Strongly Disagree 1 2 3 4 5 6 7 8 9 Strongly Agree

*54. **If my boss bugged me, I might make a mistake in my work or work more slowly so as to get back at him.**

Strongly Disagree 1 2 3 4 5 6 7 8 9 Strongly Agree

*55. **Everyone is against me.**

Strongly Disagree 1 2 3 4 5 6 7 8 9 Strongly Agree

*56. **I try to be nice to people I don't like.**

Strongly Disagree 1 2 3 4 5 6 7 8 9 Strongly Agree

*57. **I would be very nervous if an airplane in which I was flying lost an engine.**

Strongly Disagree 1 2 3 4 5 6 7 8 9 Strongly Agree

*58. **There is someone I know who can do anything and who is absolutely fair and just.**

Strongly Disagree 1 2 3 4 5 6 7 8 9 Strongly Agree

*59. **I can keep the lid on my feelings if it would interfere with what I'm doing if I were to let them out.**

Strongly Disagree 1 2 3 4 5 6 7 8 9 Strongly Agree

*60. **Some people are plotting to kill me.**

Strongly Disagree 1 2 3 4 5 6 7 8 9 Strongly Agree

*61. **I'm usually able to see the funny side of an otherwise painful predicament.**

Strongly Disagree 1 2 3 4 5 6 7 8 9 Strongly Agree

*62. **I get a headache when I have to do something I don't like.**

Strongly Disagree 1 2 3 4 5 6 7 8 9 Strongly Agree

*63. **I often find myself being very nice to people who by all rights I should be angry at.**

Strongly Disagree 1 2 3 4 5 6 7 8 9 Strongly Agree

*64. There's no such thing as "finding a little good in everyone." If you're bad, you're all bad.

Strongly Disagree 1 2 3 4 5 6 7 8 9 Strongly Agree

*65. We should never get angry at people we don't like.

Strongly Disagree 1 2 3 4 5 6 7 8 9 Strongly Agree

*66. I am sure I get a raw deal from life.

Strongly Disagree 1 2 3 4 5 6 7 8 9 Strongly Agree

*67. I fall apart under stress.

Strongly Disagree 1 2 3 4 5 6 7 8 9 Strongly Agree

68. When I know that I will have to face a difficult situation, like an exam or a job interview, I try to imagine what it will be like and plan a way to cope with it.

Strongly Disagree 1 2 3 4 5 6 7 8 9 Strongly Agree

69. Doctors never really understand what is wrong with me.

Strongly Disagree 1 2 3 4 5 6 7 8 9 Strongly Agree

70. When someone close to me dies, I don't feel upset.

Strongly Disagree 1 2 3 4 5 6 7 8 9 Strongly Agree

71. After I fight for my rights, I tend to apologize for my assertiveness.

Strongly Disagree 1 2 3 4 5 6 7 8 9 Strongly Agree

72. Most of what happens to me is not my responsibility.

Strongly Disagree 1 2 3 4 5 6 7 8 9 Strongly Agree

73. When I'm depressed or anxious, eating makes me feel better.

Strongly Disagree 1 2 3 4 5 6 7 8 9 Strongly Agree

74. Hard work makes me feel better.

Strongly Disagree 1 2 3 4 5 6 7 8 9 Strongly Agree

75. My doctors are not able to help me really get over my problems.

Strongly Disagree 1 2 3 4 5 6 7 8 9 Strongly Agree

76. **I'm often told that I don't show my feelings.**

   Strongly Disagree   1   2   3   4   5   6   7   8   9   Strongly Agree

77. **I believe that people usually see more meaning in films, plays, or books than is actually there.**

   Strongly Disagree   1   2   3   4   5   6   7   8   9   Strongly Agree

78. **I have habits or rituals that I feel compelled to do or else something terrible will happen.**

   Strongly Disagree   1   2   3   4   5   6   7   8   9   Strongly Agree

79. **I take drugs, medicine, or alcohol when I'm tense.**

   Strongly Disagree   1   2   3   4   5   6   7   8   9   Strongly Agree

80. **When I feel bad, I try to be with someone.**

   Strongly Disagree   1   2   3   4   5   6   7   8   9   Strongly Agree

81. **If I can predict that I'm going to be sad ahead of time, I can cope better.**

   Strongly Disagree   1   2   3   4   5   6   7   8   9   Strongly Agree

82. **No matter how much I complain, I never get a satisfactory response.**

   Strongly Disagree   1   2   3   4   5   6   7   8   9   Strongly Agree

83. **Often I find that I don't feel anything when the situation would seem to warrant strong emotions.**

   Strongly Disagree   1   2   3   4   5   6   7   8   9   Strongly Agree

84. **Sticking to the task at hand keeps me from feeling depressed or anxious.**

   Strongly Disagree   1   2   3   4   5   6   7   8   9   Strongly Agree

85. **I smoke when I'm nervous.**

   Strongly Disagree   1   2   3   4   5   6   7   8   9   Strongly Agree

86. **If I were in a crisis, I would seek out another person who had the same problem.**

   Strongly Disagree   1   2   3   4   5   6   7   8   9   Strongly Agree

87. **I cannot be blamed for what I do wrong.**

Strongly Disagree 1   2   3   4   5   6   7   8   9   Strongly Agree

88. **If I have an aggressive thought, I feel the need to do something to compensate for it.**

Strongly Disagree 1   2   3   4   5   6   7   8   9   Strongly Agree

Appendix 7

Vaillant's Modification of the Haan Q-sort

Q-sort Defense Statements

Legend: M = Mature/adaptive defensive style. N = Neutral/neurotic defensive style. I = Immature/maladaptive defensive style. <u>New</u> = Q-statement not used in Haan. # = Number of five independent raters agreeing on defense label for the Q-statement (Roston, C. Vaillant, G. Vaillant, Haan, McCullough).

Since there are 6, not 3, cards for suppression and isolation, divide totals by 2.

(Front Side of Card) **(Back Side of Card)**

1. Distinguishes between self's own feelings and the facts of situations. Fair in emotional situations.

   M
   1. Suppression
   #3

2. Views self in an objective light. Explicitly acknowledges self's shortcomings.

   N
   2. Isolation
   #3

3. Evaluates both sides of arguments, including those contrary to self's own point of view.

   N
   3. Isolation
   #4

4. Help-rejecting complainer. Angry or belittles others' efforts to help.

   I <u>New</u>
   4. Hypochondriasis
   #4

5. Listener feels assaulted by or
   disbelieving of the intensity of
   subject's suffering.

    I   New
5. Hypochondriasis
    #4

8. Applies abstract, formal ideas in
   solving problems (low if thinks
   concretely). Impartial awareness
   and analysis.

    N
8. Isolation
    #5

10. Produces intellectualizations rather than
    cogent solutions. Talks on a level of
    abstraction not quite appropriate to
    the situation.

    N
10. Isolation
    #5

11. Applies abstract ideas and terms to
    situations to avoid feelings.
    Uses jargon.

    N
11. Isolation
    #5

12. Produces intellectualizations
    that seem self-serving. Does not
    specify how ideas relate to context.

    N
12. Isolation
    #5

16. The subject often shoots self
    in the foot or acts
    the clown.

    I   New
16. Passive aggression
    #4

17. The subject often sacrifices his or her own
    needs for others. Seems incapable of
    assertive behavior.

    I   New
17. Passive aggression
    #4

18. The subject is adept at
    guilt-tripping others.

    I   New
18. Passive aggression
    #3

19. Can defer decisions in complicated
    situations (low if unable to make
    decisions or acts on the spur of
    the moment). Does not need
    to commit self to clear-cut choices
    in complicated situations
    where choice is impossible.

    M
19. Anticipation
    #3

20. "Pays now, flies later," grieves or is modestly anxious before stressful events, relatively calm later.

    M New
20. Anticipation #2

21. Able to wait for other people to make up their minds in complicated situations; tolerates indecision or slowness in others.

    M
21. Anticipation #2

25. Tries to understand others' feelings and perceptions (low if oblivious to others' feelings).

    M
25. Altruism #4

27. Anticipates others' reactions to situations with accuracy, that is, can put himself or herself in other fellow's boots. Interested in feelings of others.

    M
27. Altruism #5

28. Preoccupied with the possibility that others will act badly. Attributes objectionable tendency to another.

    I
28. Projection #5

29. Feels accused and criticized by others. Feels a need to be on guard to avoid being made a "sucker."

    I
29. Projection #5

30. Vigilant in "ferreting" out others' reactions. Attribute objectionable feeling to another.

    I
30. Projection #5

31. Enjoys surprising aspects of situations, for example, situational humor, or sudden insights.

    M
31. Humor #4

32. Plays creatively with ideas and feelings without being constrained by situational demands (low if constrained by situation).

    M
32. Sublimation #3

36. Views self as not being responsible in difficult situations.

    I
36. Dissociation #3

41. Ignores aspects of self's situations that
    are potentially threatening.

    I
41. Dissociation
    #4

42. Focuses attention on the pleasant
    aspects of problems and ignores
    others, for example, "Every cloud
    has a silver lining."

    I
42. Dissociation
    #3

45. Expresses feelings in a variety
    of satisfying, socially tolerated ways.

    I
45. Sublimation
    #2

46. Displaces feelings in form
    (e.g., stomachache instead of
    temper tantrum) or in object
    (kicks dog instead of boss).

    N
46. Displacement
    #5

47. Misdirects positive, warm feelings
    from original aims or object
    (e.g., dogs are better than people).

    N
47. Displacement
    #5

48. Expresses aggressive, even hostile
    feelings in nonrelevant contexts and
    objects (irrelevant irritability).

    N
48. Displacement
    #5

49. Acts fairly even in trying circumstances.
    Genuinely civilized person with
    wide interests.

    M
49. Suppression
    —

51. Regulates expression of feelings
    proportionate to the situation.

    M
51. Suppression
    #2

53. Feels that things that feel good
    may be debilitating. Somehow
    believes pleasure equals sin.

    N   New
53. Reaction formation
    #2

54. Made uncomfortable by praise or
    by being given gifts.

    N   New
54. Reaction formation
    #2

55. Supresses but is aware of feelings
    and thoughts in most circumstances
    (low if expresses or unaware of
    feelings). Holds infeasible and
    inappropriate feelings in abeyance.

    M
    55.   Suppression
          #5

56. Controls expression of affective
    reactions when not appropriate
    to express them, for example,
    older person not hurting children
    even when provoked.

    M
    56.   Suppression
          #5

57. Inhibits self's reactions for
    the time being when appropriate.

    M
    57.   Suppression
          #5

58. Constricts and inhibits self's cognitive
    associations. Constriction in thinking
    not due to low IQ but naive, oblivious,
    unthinking attitude; an unwillingness
    to think broadly.

    N
    58.   Repression
          #5

59. Forgets aspects of trying circumstances.

    N
    59.   Repression
          #5

60. Unable to recall painful experiences.

    N
    60.   Repression
          #5

61. Gets pleasure out of giving to and
    caring for others.

    M   New
    61.   Altruism
          #4

62. Not infrequently expresses emotions
    through art, music, or other
    creative activity.

    M   New
    62.   Sublimation
          #4

63. Not infrequently "regresses in
    the service of ego."

    M   New
    63.   Humor
          #3

64. The subject sometimes deals with
crises with tantrums.

	I	New
64.	Acting out	
	#4	

65. The subject engages in incomprehensible
delinquent activities—or has hurt people
without seeming to care.

	I	New
65.	Acting out	
	#4	

66. The subject escapes conflict through
risk-taking behaviors.

	I	New
66.	Acting out	
	#4	

67. The subject makes interviewer laugh,
and at such times the interviewer
does not feel the subject
is being evasive or clowning.

	M	
67.	Humor	
	#4	

68. The subject often behaves or talks
regarding instinctual issues as if black
were white and white, black.

	N	New
68.	Reaction formation	
	#3	

69. Exaggerates distress often in a way
that makes others feel responsible.

	I	New
69.	Hypochondriasis	
	#4	

70. Some of the subject's best friends
are imaginary.

	I	New
70.	Fantasy	
	#4	

71. The subject can escape the real world
into reverie and imaginary activities,
shared with no one.

	I	New
71.	Fantasy	
	#4	

72. The subject has a vivid inner
emotional life but hardly ever exposes
feelings to others.

	I	New
72.	Fantasy	
	#4	

Index

Page numbers printed in boldface type refer to tables or figures.

Commitment, 92
Compliance, patient, 32, 191
Comprehensive Textbook of Psychiatry
(Kaplan, Freedman, and Sadock),
48, 95
Conscience, 55
Construct validity, 134, 228
Context
clinical treatment of immature
defenses, 82
defenses in developmental
longitudinal, 94
reliability in clinical identification
of defenses, 172
Control
acting out, 78–79
exaggerated belief in personal,
91–92
stress and health, 92
Controlling, 241
Cooper, Steven
competing models of defense
mechanisms, 62–63
Defense Mechanism Rating Scales,
147
empirical assessment of defense
mechanisms, 95, 98, 99
Coping
coding systems, 184
conscious cognitive and ego
defensive styles, 91
as distinct from unconscious
defense mechanisms, 44, 172
need for uniform
nomenclature, 43
transformational, 92
working definition and ego
mechanisms of defense, 44–45
Coping and Defending (Haan), 94
CORE CITY Study
comparison with other study
groups, 110–113
Defense Style Questionnaire and
cross-validation, 159–167
maturity of defenses
gender, education, and class,
118–125
mental health, 113–116
physical health, 116–118
Q-sort approach, 220–221, **229,
230**

sample, 107–108
Counterprojection, 76
Countertransference, 64–70. *See also*
Transference
Cox, N., 134
Cramer, P., 91
Criminal justice system, 66
Criterion validity, 139
Cross-sectional measures, 195–200,
202–206, 208–215

Daydreaming, 13, 256
Defense and Resistance (Blum), 23
Defense Mechanism Rating Scales
(DMRS)
definitions of defenses, 253–259
development, reliability, and
validity, 195–200, 202–206,
208–215
subject responses compared to
Defense Style Questionnaire,
146–156
Defense Mechanisms Inventory
(DMI), 92
Defense mechanisms
adolescent and clinical interviews,
181–192
clinical management of immature
and personality disorders, 59–84
clinical techniques and reliability in
identifying, 171–179
cross-sectional measures and
prediction, 195–200, 202–206,
208–215
Defense Style Questionnaire and
empirical study of styles,
127–156
definitions
DSM-III-R, 237–238
Meissner's glossary, 239–242
need for consensus, 23–24
need for uniform nomenclature,
43–48, 50, 54–56
Perry's Defense Mechanism
Rating Scale, 253–259
Vaillant's glossary, 243–251
diagnostic formulation and
modern clinical practice, 29–41
Ego Defense Mechanisms Manual,
261–278